Extracorporeal Shockwave Therapy:
Technologies, Basics, Clinical results

Ludger Gerdesmeyer
Lowell Scott Weil

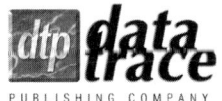

Data Trace Publishing Company

Copyright © 2007 by
Data Trace Publishing Company
Towson, MD 21204
All rights reserved

Printed in the United States of America

ISBN: 978-1-57400-115-0

Authors:

Ludger Gerdesmeyer, MD, PhD, FIPP
Dept. Orthopedic and Traumatology
Technical University Munich
Ismaningerstraße 22
D-81675 Munich, Germany
E-Mail: Gerdesmeyer@aol.com

Lowell Weil, DPM
Fellowship Director
Weil Foot and Ankle Institute
1455 E. Golf Road
Des Plaines, Illinois 60016
U.S.A

Project coordination and Cover design:
Thomas Stierle, Dipl.-Betriebswirt(FH)

Library of Congress Cataloging-in-Publication Data

Extracorporeal shockwave therapy : technologies, basics, clinical results / [edited by] Ludger Gerdesmeyer, Lowell Scott Weil.
    p. ; cm.
Includes bibliographical references and index.
    ISBN-13: 978-1-57400-115-0 (alk. paper)
    ISBN-10: 1-57400-115-9 (alk. paper)
    1. Extracorporeal shockwave therapy. I. Gerdesmeyer, Ludger. II. Weil, Lowell Scott.
    [DNLM: 1. High-Energy Shockwaves—therapeutic use. WB 480 E96 2006]
    RD736.E9E86 2006
    617.4'706—dc22

                                2006036433

Contents

Preface vi

BASICS

1. History of Extracorporeal Shockwave Therapy 1
2. Physical Principles and Generation of Shockwaves 11
3. Physical Principles in Shockwave Generation – Clinical Relevance and Practical Implications. 21
4. Molecular Mechanisms of Shockwaves. 27
5. Biological Mechanism of Musculoskeletal Shockwaves. 37
6. Effects of ESWT on Bone. 55
7. From Nociception to Pain 69
8. rESWT for Pain Therapy in Orthopedics and Sports Medicine 83
9. Effect of Extracorporeal Shockwaves on the Growth of Microorganisms 91
10. Extracorporeal Shockwave Therapy and Avascular Necrosis of the Femoral Head 99
11. Extracorporeal Cardiac Shockwave Therapy as a New Therapeutic Option for Ischemic Cardiomyopathy 111

APPLICATION / THERAPY

12. Clinical Application of the EMS Swiss DolorClast® 199
13. Method Swiss DolorClast® (rESWT) - System Components 129
14. Orthopedic Shockwave Treatment at Urologic Work Stations. 139

INDICATION AND CLINICAL RESULTS

15. Treatment Result of rESWT (Swiss DolorClast®) with the Use of a Focused Handpiece 153
16. Results of rESWT - Treatment of Sports-Induced Diseases 161
17. Efficacy of rESWT for Calcific Tendinitis 177
18. rESWT- in Heel Spur (Fasciitis Plantaris) 193
19. rESWT- A New Method for the Treatment of Epicondylitis Humeri Lateralis 205
20. Efficiency of rESWT for Calcifying Shoulder Tendinitis 217

21. ESWT for the Treatment of Chronic Calcifying Tendonitis of the Rotator Cuff 225
22. Painful Heel - Anatomy, Clinical Study and Therapy. 247
23. Short and Medium-term Results in the Treatment of Epicondylitis Humeri Radialis with rESWT 259
24. rESWT – Benefit in the Treatment of Tendinopathies 267
25. Different Results in Repetitive Low Energy ESWT for Chronic Plantar Fasciitis. 275
26. Morton's Interdigital Neuroma: Indications, ESWT Technique, and Clinical Experience. 281
27. Extracorporeal Shockwave Therapy (ESWT) in Traumatology........ 289
28. Use of ESWT in Adult Osteochondrosis Dissecans and a Case Study of the Treatment of Osteochondral Lesions........................ 303
29. Shockwave Treatment of Femoral Head Necrosis in Adults........... 311
30. ESWT – A Prospective Double Blind Study on Bilateral Plantar Fasciitis. 321
31. Extracorporeal Shockwave Therapy (ESWT) in Skin Lesions Causes of Skin Lesions... 325
32. Radial Shockwaves and Autologous Growth Factors Combined Therapy for Bone Delayed Unions 331

TST - TRIGGER POINT SHOCKWAVE THERAPY
33. Results of Three Prospective Studies 347

SHOCKWAVE ASSOCIATIONS
34. ATRAD - Association for Radial Pain Therapy 355
35. ISMST - International Society for Musculoskeletal Shockwave Therapy 359

Index of Authors

Author	Address Details
Sabine Arentz, MD	Sportmedizinisches Institut Frankfurt am Main e.V., Otto-Fleck-Schneise 10, D-60528 Frankfurt am Main, Germany
Vinzenz Auersperg, MD	Orthopädische Abteilung AKh Linz Krankenhausstr. 9 A, A-4020 Linz, Austria
Wolfgang Bauermeister, MD	Unnützstraße 17a, D-81825 München, Germany
Peter Diehl, MD	Department of Orthopedic, and Traumatology Technical University of Munich, Ismaningerstraße 22, D-81675 München, Germany
Felix Egloff	ATRAD general secretary, Zurich, Switzerland
Ludger Gerdesmeyer, MD, PhD, FIPP	Vice Chairman Department of Orthopedic, and Traumatology Technical University of Munich, Ismaningerstraße 22, D-81675 München, Germany
Hans Gollwitzer, MD	Department of Orthopedic, and Traumatology Technical University of Munich, Ismaningerstraße 22, D-81675 München, Germany
Gerald Gremion, MD	Hôpital Orthopédique de la Suisse Romande, Av. Pierre-Decker 4, CH-1005 Lausanne, Switzerland
Michael Haake, MD, PhD	Department of Orthopedic Surgery, University Regensburg, Kaiser-Karl V.-Allee 3, D-93077 Bad Abbach, Germany
Gerald Haupt, MD, PhD	St. Vincentiuskrankenhaus, Holzstrasse 4a, 67346 Speyer, Germany
Jörg Hausdorf, MD	Department of Orthopedic Surgery, Ludwig-Maximilians-University Munich, Klinikum Großhadern, Marchioninistr. 15, 81377 Munich, Germany
Matthias Hausschild, MD	Department of Orthopedic Surgery University Rostock, Germany
Mark Henne, MD	Department of Orthopedic, and Traumatology technical University of Munich, Ismaningerstraße 22, D-81675 München, Germany
Herve de Labareyre, MD	Clinique des Lilas, 41-49 Avenue du Maréchal Juin, F-93260 Les Lilas, France

INDEX OF AUTHORS

Heinz Lohrer, MD	Sportmedizinisches Institut Frankfurt am Main e.V., Otto-Fleck-Schneise 10, D-60528 Frankfurt am Main, Germany
Carlos Leal, MD	Orthopaedic Research Laboratory – Department of Orthopaedics - Bosque University, Bogotá, Colombia
Petra Magosch, MD	ATOS Praxisklinik Heidelberg, Bismarckstr. 9-15, D-69115 Heidelberg, Germany
Markus Maier, MD, PhD	Ferdinand-Maria Str. 6, 82319 Starnberg, Germany
Jan Dirk Rompe MD, PhD	OrthoTrauma Clinic, Kirchheimer Str. 60, 67269 Grünstadt, Germany
Wolfgang Schaden, MD	Trauma Center Meidling, Landstrasser Hauptstrasse 83, A-1030 Vienna, Austria
Hiroaki Shimokawa, MD, PhD	Department of Cardiovascular Medicine, Kyushu University Graduate School of Medical Sciences, 3-1-1 Maidashi, Higashi-ku, Fukuoka 812-8582, Japan
Jakob Schöll, MD	Sportmedizinisches Institut Frankfurt am Main e.V., Otto-Fleck-Schneise 10, D-60528 Frankfurt am Main, Germany
Thomas Stierle Dipl.- Betriebswirt (FH)	EMS SA, Ch. de la Vuarpillière 31, CH-1260 Nyon, Switzerland
Richard Thiele, MD	Kurfürstendamm 61, 10707 Berlin, Germany
Jürgen Wagner, MD	MD, Assistant Professor, Department of anaesthesiology, technical university Munich, Klinikum rechts der Isar, Ismaninger Strasse 22, 81675 Munich, Germany
Ching-Jen Wang, MD	Department of Orthopedic Surgery, Chang Gung Memorial Hospital at Kaohsiung, 123 Ta-Pei Road, Niao-Sung Hsiang, Kaohsiung, Taiwan 833
Lowell Scott Weil, PDM	Fellowship Director, Weil Foot and Ankle Institute, 1455 E. Golf Road, Des Plaines, Illinois 60016, U.S.A

Preface

"Six pages of equations however all improvable, incomprehensible, ignore quantum mechanics and are incorrect." Science 1929.

This was in response to Einstein's theory of relativity published in Science in 1929. Einstein's theories were controversial and questioned by the scientific community. The same cynicism has been directed toward shockwave therapy. Fifty years ago healing by non-surgical techniques was only realized in science fiction.

This type of non-surgical healing is now a reality. As with the AO teachings of Switzerland and arthroscopy, it has taken approximately ten years for shockwave to cross the Atlantic Ocean and reach North America. Shockwave therapy was first developed twenty-five years ago for use with kidney stones. However, for the last fifteen years it has been used for various musculoskeletal disorders. Drs. Delius, Thiele, Schaden, Rompe, Gerdesmeyer, Wang and others have all helped to advance the understanding and use of shockwave therapy. Through their work, shockwave therapy has gained worldwide recognition as a scientifically proven therapy.

Turkey hosted the first international conference for the International Society for Musculoskeletal Shockwave Therapy in 1998. Each of the subsequent annual conferences has brought forward new ideas and scientific evidence on the uses of shockwave therapy. The most recent conference, held in Vienna in 2005, was attended by physicians from over thirty countries. This enthusiasm keeps growing and I expect many more countries and health care workers will realize the potential of shockwave therapy. In the past two years alone, new types of machines have been developed and accepted for use by the American Food and Drug Administration.

The latest advances in shockwave therapy have generated much excitement and include the treatment of cardiac tissue and non-healing ulcers and trigger point therapy. Ironically as of January 2006, almost ten years after its introduction in North America, there will be CPT billing codes given for shockwave therapy for the treatment of plantar fasciitis and tennis elbow. We are on the brink of general acceptance of shockwave therapy in the North American continent. For shockwave the future is now. The possibilities are limited only by our imaginations.

Dr. Robert Gordon

This treatment in the care of plantar fasciitis as well as calcific tendonitis of the shoulder is now proven as a function of research developed and organized by excellent clinical scientists. The careful (evidence-based) research methodology and controls have allowed the differentiation of placebo from the shockwave treatment. It is now clear that the placebo effect is statistically large and often confusing, especially when statistical filters are not applied. Additionally the placebo controlled shockwave trials have enlightened our understanding of shockwave treatment and placebo effects.

Now that we know that ESWT is better than placebo, it is our task to maximize the clinical efficacy of ESWT treatment.

Refining ESWT treatment with regard to optimizing its effect, clinical outcome and new indications is the task of those reading this excellent book.

Dr. John J. Stienstra, DPM, FACFAS
Past President of
The American College of Foot and Ankle Surgeons
(2005-2006)

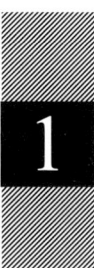

History of Extracorporeal Shockwave Therapy

Michael Haake,[1] Ludger Gerdesmeyer[2]

Clinical Application

As early as 1947 Frank Riber submitted a patent application in the United States for an electrohydraulic shockwave generator for the treatment of brain tumors. However, the first studies on the effect of Extracorporeal Shockwave Therapy (ESWT) did not take place until the mid-fifties. In the early '60s, shockwave research received renewed impetus in connection with non-destructive materials research.

A study commissioned by Germany's Ministry of Defense examined the effect of shockwaves on biological tissue. It was prompted by observations made during World War II in which lung damage was observed due to the detonation of hydrogen bombs without any signs of external injuries. These experiments were the first to systematically determine the disintegrating effect on lung tissue and inner organs. What caught the attention was the fact that shockwaves were able to travel through connecting tissue, fat and muscles without causing major damage to them.

Based on these studies, the first touch-free in vitro fragmentation of kidney stones took place[17]. In 1980 this method was used for the first time to disintegrate kidney stones in a patient[4]. The first Dornier HM1 Lithotrypter was followed in 1983 by the first commercial HM3 model. Developed in Germany, this

---

[1] Dept Orthopedic University Regensburg
[2] Dept Orthopedic and Traumatology, Technical University Munich

method became the treatment of choice for renal and urethral calculi in the past two decades[25].

Once again in Munich, shockwaves were applied in 1985 for the first time for the treatment of a gallbladder stone. Meanwhile the number of indications has increased to include gallstones, pancreatic and salivary duct stones but without gaining such a foothold as it has for the disintegration of kidney stones.

ESWT and the Musculoskeletal System

Karpmann [18] was the first to use ESWT on the musculoskeletal system in 1987. Prior to an endoprosthesis replacement operation on the hip joint, he wanted to proceed with a percutaneous disintegration of the surrounding bone cement in order to reduce the distance between the cement and the prosthesis. However, as successive operations were soon to make clear, the expectations were not met.

The possibility of fragmenting even bone tissue with shockwaves caught the attention of Valchanou, who was the first to use ESWT for the therapy of pseudarthrosis [32], followed by others[27].

The disintegrating effect of shockwaves was also applied to the treatment of tendonitis calcarea of the shoulder in a first series of six patients[5]. Even though very different from kidney stones in terms of composition and structure, the disintegration of calcium deposit may be induced at least in some of the cases in addition to a good clinical effect on pain and function[8].

In another finding, a lasting analgesia of the treated region was observed in the first applications and thus shockwaves were used for pain therapy, first in epicondylitis, then in other chronic insertion enthesiopathies[6].

Despite the absence of any evidence of efficacy based on placebo-controlled prospective studies, the number of applications in orthopedics, estimated at 100,000 to 150,000 patients a year in the mid-nineties, even surpassed the number of lithotripsy applications in urology. In 1996 alone, this trend generated costs of about 30 million Euro not budgeted by Germany's health insurance carriers. Application frequency took another significant jump until 1998.

To date there is no uniform therapy plan or dose recommendations based on studies regarding the different shockwave therapy indications. Gradually, therapy patterns evolved in private practice and in clinics based much more on practicality and insurance coverage than on scientific studies[14].

The example of the treatment of epicondylitis humeri radialis will illustrate this further. In a systematic review of the literature, Haake et al. [12] were able to observe great differences in the original 20 studies in terms of number of therapy sessions and applied impulses. The number of therapy sessions varied considerably in the literature between a single application and more than 20 applications. The number of impulses applied per session also spanned a broad range, varying from 500 to 2500.

In addition, insurance companies as a rule would not refund the costs of the therapy until and unless conventional conservative therapies had been used to a "sufficient" extent but had failed. There were no rules governing the quality or extent of therapy. This state of affairs helps explain why ESWT was used predominantly to treat therapy-resistant chronic cases of insertion enthesiopathies. Once again, this is not documented by scientific studies.

Germany's public [24] as well as private insurance companies [7] demanded that valid studies be conducted on method efficacy, comparisons with conventional therapy methods, identification of side effects and verification of cost-effectiveness.

Since the decision of **7/25/98** by the Federal Physician and Insurance Commission, public insurance carriers are no longer allowed to assume the costs due to the absence of evidence of the method's efficacy on the musculoskeletal system. This limitation is based in essence on an opinion dating back to 1996 and commissioned by the insurance carriers. As a result, ESWT is used today primarily as a so-called individual healthcare service. Exact figures on the frequency of application are not available.

In 1997 the German Orthopedic and Traumatology Society formed the Shockwave Work Group, which initiated clinical studies to bring evidence of ESWT's efficacy in the three most common indications: epicondylitis humeri radialis, tendonitis calcarea and plantar fasciitis. The studies conformed to the current state of clinical research and biometric methodology in accordance with the principles of good clinical practice. These quality studies on ESWT in orthopedics - the world's largest - yielded different results for the individual indications.

For the treatment of tendonitis calcarea of the shoulder, a good clinical effect of "high-energy" ESWT with 0.32 mJ/mm^2 was found after six months compared to a placebo therapy and to a therapy group with 0.08 mJ/mm^2[8]. If this result could be confirmed in further studies, it would bring the first evidence of a clinical use of ESWT on the musculoskeletal system with methods of modern clinical research.

However, in the case of epicondylitis humeri radialis [11] or of plantar fasciitis [10], ESWT was able to demonstrate small effect size without clinically relevant efficacy in terms of application technique or method compared to the control groups. In the therapy of tennis elbow, no clinical difference in success rates was found up to one year in comparing low energetic focused ESWT at ED+ of 0.07 to 0.09 mJ/mm^2 versus placebo therapy combined with local anesthesia.

A similar situation was found for the therapy of plantar fasciitis with three applications of ESWT at ED+ of 0.08 mJ/mm^2 compared to a placebo therapy and local anesthesia, except that the success rates in both groups were higher than for epicondylitis.

Further studies also failed to bring any clear evidence of efficacy even though they demonstrated a slight superiority of ESWT groups compared to control groups[3]. The demonstrated ESWT effect based on 4 studies was sufficient for the method to be approved by the U.S. Federal Drug Administration (FDA) for plantar fasciitis[2, 21]. In the meantime, FDA approval was also obtained for epicondylitis following a study which brought evidence of its efficacy (http://www.sonorex.com/us/physicians/sse.pdf)[23]. In this prospective randomized placebo-controlled study, a clear clinical improvement was found in 60.7% of the ESWT group. In contrast, only 29.3% of the placebo group obtained a comparable result.

In terms of radial extracorporeal shockwave therapy, (rESWT) there are limited data demonstrating clinical relevant effect sizes, but data were not appropriate to prove efficacy. The international multicentered trial to prove the effect of rESWT on chronic plantar fasciitis was recently finished and data submitted to the FDA for approval.

Some scientific groups found excellent outcome after ESWT in new indications like chronic wound healing as well as in infected conditions, aseptic bone necrosis and some enthesiopathies like patella tendon syndrome or chronic Achilles tendonitis. All new indications are described and discussed in several chapters within this book.

Energy Density

In terms of ESWT treatment of insertion enthesiopathies, the literature continues to distinguish between high and low-energy applications. This distinction, however, is relatively voluntary and is not based on physical parameters or their effect on the tendon insertion. According to Rompe [26], energy density is classified as "low energy" up to an energy flux density ED of 0.08 mJ/mm^2, as "medium energy" up to 0.28 mJ/mm^2, and as "high energy" above that level.

A shift in the measuring method in the late '90s [34] as well as the absence in the literature of data on the energy used makes a comparison between different clinical studies and experiments largely impossible.

To date it is not clear which physical parameter or parameters from more than two dozen customary parameters are primarily responsible for ESWT's clinical effects and side effects[13].

Indications and Limitations of Coverage and/or Medical Necessity

Extracorporeal shockwave therapy is a non-invasive treatment option for musculoskeletal conditions that have failed to respond to conservative treatment. ESWT uses technology similar to lithotripsy in an attempt to relieve musculoskeletal symptoms of the specified affected area. The exact mechanism by which ESWT works is not known. There are two theories on the therapeutic effects of the shockwaves. These will be discussed in the later chapters about the ESWT principles. Alleviated pain by increasing blood flow and decreasing inflammation in the affected area as well as local damage of cell membranes, interfering with the transmission of pain signals are the two major principles.

Use of shockwaves in treatment of musculoskeletal conditions has been mainly for chronic calcific tendonitis in the shoulder, chronic tennis elbow and painful heel.

All these conditions have high rates (70-90%) of more-or-less successful treatment with simpler, less expensive and more convenient methods of non-invasive medical or orthotic treatment, although there is no clear consensus on the superiority of one approach over another. Relatively small numbers of such cases are recalcitrant, unresponsive to rest, physical therapy, oral medication, injection of local anesthetics and corticosteroids, splints or plaster casts, heel cushions and heel cups. Surgical methods, whether open or endoscopic, give frequent though inconsistent improvement in responsive cases, but are regarded in the orthopedic community as last-ditch measures.

Although the experience with extracorporeal shockwave therapy in the musculoskeletal field is sparse, the treatment method appears to offer benefit in a significant proportion of cases.

In terms of medical necessity, it is clear that is inappropriate at this time as primary treatment for the musculoskeletal conditions mentioned above. Where available, ESWT may be indicated when simpler, conservative methods have been thoroughly tried but proven ineffective and as an alternative to surgical treatment.

In these limited situations, ESWT will be reimbursed only when used to treat epicondylitis or plantar fasciitis. Claims may be suspended for review of medical records documenting that simpler methods have been employed and failed.

Only services using equipment that is FDA approved for epicondylitis and plantar fasciitis will be considered for payment. The following devices are approved:

Orthospec™ (http://www.fda.gov/cdrh/mda/docs/p040026.html)
OssaTron™ (http://www.fda.gov/cdrh/mda/docs/p990086.html)
Dornier Epos™ Ultra (http://www.fda.gov/cdrh/mda/docs/p000048.html)
Siemens SONOCUR® (http://www.fda.gov/cdrh/mda/docs/p010039.html)
Orbasone (http://www.fda.gov/cdrh/mda/docs/p040039.html)
EMS Swiss DolorClast®, manufactured by EMS, has been submitted to the FDA

The Blue Cross Blue Shield Medical Technology Assessment states some CPT/HCPCS codes, which are listed below (www.bcbsma.com/common/en_US/medical_policies/400.htm). Blue Cross Blue Shield is the largest private medical insurer in the US. This site states that BCBS does cover ESWT for plantar fasciitis as of May 1, 2002, but it did not state the reimbursement amount.

For payment these CPT/HCPCS Codes are used:

0020T	Extracorporeal shockwave therapy, involving plantar fascia
G0279	Extracorporeal shockwave therapy, involving elbow epicondylitis
G0280	Extracorporeal shockwave therapy; involving other than elbow epicondylitis or plantar fasciitis

Literature

1. Böddeker IR, Haake M: Extracorporeal shockwave therapy in treatment of epicondylitis humeri radialis. A current overview. Orthopäde 2000; 5:463-9
2. Buch M, Knorr U, Fleming L, Theodore G, Amendola A, Bachmann C et al. Extracorporeal shockwave therapy in plantar fasciitis: a review. Orthopäde 2002;31:637-44.
3. Buchbinder R, Ptasznik R, Gordon J, Buchanan J, Prabaharan V, Forbes A. Ultrasound-guided extracorporeal shockwave therapy for plantar fasciitis: a randomized controlled trial. JAMA 2002;288:1364-72.
4. Chaussy C, Schmiedt E, Jocham D, Brendl W, Forssmann B, Walther V: First clinical experience with extracorporeally induced destruction of kidney stones by shockwaves. Journal of Urology 1982;127:417-420
5. Dahmen GP, Meiss L, Nam VC, Skruodies B: Extrakorporale Stosswellentherapie (ESWT) im knochennahen Weichteilbereich an der Schulter. Extr Orthopaedica 1992;11:25-27
6. Dahmen GP, Nam VC, Meiss L: Extrakorporale Stosswellentherapie (ESWTA) zur Behandlung von knochennahen Weichteilschmerzen. Indikation, Technik und vorläufige Ergebnisse. Konsensus Workshop der Deutschen Gesellschaft für Stosswellenlithotripsie Attempto-Verlag, Tübingen 1993;143-148
7. Fritze J: Extracorporeal shockwave therapy (ESWT) in orthopaedic indications: a selective review. Versicherungsmedizin 1998;59:180-185
8. Gerdesmeyer L, Wagenpfeil S, Haake M, Maier M, Loew M, Wörtler K, Lampe R, Seil R, Handle G, Gassel S, Rompe JD. Extracorporeal Shockwave Therapy for the Treatment of Chronic Calcifying Tendonitis of the Rotator Cuff: A Randomized Controlled Trial. JAMA 2003;290:2573-2580
9. Gerdesmeyer L, Schraebler S, Mittelmeier W, Rechl H. Gewebeinduzierte Veränderungen der extrakorporalen Stosswellen. Orthopäde 2002;31:618-622
10. Haake M, Buch M, Schoellner C, Goebel F, Vogel M, Mueller I, Hausdorf J, Zamzow K, Schade-Brittinger C, Mueller HH. Extracorporal Shockwave Therapy in the treatment of plantar fasciitis - Randomized multicenter trial. BMJ 2003; 327:75-77
11. Haake M, König IR, Decker T, Riedel C, Buch M, Müller HH for the ESWT Clinical Trial Group. Extracorporal Shockwave Therapy in the treatment of lateral epicondylitis- A randomized multicenter trial. J Bone Joint Surg (Am) 2002;84:1982-1991

12. Haake M, Hünerkopf M, Gerdesmeyer L, König IR. Extrakorporale Stosswellentherapie (ESWT) bei Epicondylitis humeri radialis - Eine Literaturübersicht. Orthopäde 2002; 31:623-632.
13. Haake M, Böddeker IR, Decker T, Buch M,Vogel M, Labek G, Maier M, Loew M, Maier-Boerries OM, Fischer J, Betthäuser A, Rehack HC, Kanovsky W, Müller I, Gerdesmeyer L, Rompe JD. Side Effects of Extracorporeal Shockwave Therapy (ESWT) in the Treatment of Tennis Elbow. Arch Orthop Traum Surg 2002;122:222-228
14. Haake M, Rautmann M, Griss P. Therapieergebnisse und Kostenanalyse der Extrakorporalen Stosswellentherapie bei Tendinitis calcarea und Supraspinatussehnensyndrom. Orthop Praxis 1998;34:110-113
15. Haupt G. Use of extracorporeal shockwaves in the treatment of pseudarthrosis, tendinopathy and other orthopedic diseases. J Urol 1997a; (158): 4-11.
16. Haupt G. [Shockwaves in orthopedics]. Urologe A 1997b; (36): 233-238
17. Häusler E, Kiefer W. Anregung von Stosswellen in Flüssigkeiten durch Hochgeschwindigkeitswassertropfen. Verband Dtsch Physikal Gesellschaft 1971; 6:786
18. Karpmann RR, Magee FP, Gruen TWS, Mobley T: The lithotriptor and its potential use in the revision of total hip arthroplasty. Orth Rev 1987;26:38 – 42. Zitiert nach: Karpman RR, Magee FP, Gruen TW, Mobley T. The lithotriptor and its potential use in the revision of total hip arthroplasty. Clin Orthop. 2001;387:4-7
19. Ludwig J, Lauber S, Lauber HJ, Dreisilker U, Raedel R, Hotzinger H. High-energy shockwave treatment of femoral head necrosis in adults. Clin Orthop. 2001;387:119-26.
20. Magosch P, Lichtenberg S, Habermeyer P. [Radial shockwave therapy in calcifying tendinitis of the rotator cuff—a prospective study]. Z Orthop Ihre Grenzgeb 2003; (141): 629-636.
21. Ogden JA, Alvarez R, Levitt R, Cross GL, Marlow M. Shockwave therapy for chronic proximal plantar fasciitis. Clin Orthop. 2001;387:47-59
22. Perlick L, Schiffmann R, Kraft CN, Wallny T, Diedrich O. Die extrakorporelle Stosswellentherapie bei der chronischen Achillodynie. Experimentelle Untersuchungen und vorläufige klinische Ergebnisse. Z Orthop Ihre Grenzgeb. 2002;140:275-80
23. Pettrone F, CS Lefton, DW Romness, BR McCall, DJ Covall, JR Boatright: Evaluation of extracorporeal shockwave therapy for chronic lateral epicondylitis: AAOS, Paper 271, 2002
24. Polak HJ: Ergebnis der Literaturrecherche der MDK-Gemeinschaft zur ESWT mit orthopädischen Indikatoionen. In: Siebert W, Buch M (Hrsg) Stosswellen-Anwendungen am Knochen - Klinische und experimentelle Erfahrungen.Verlag Dr. Kovac 1997, Hamburg
25. Renner C, Rassweiler J: Treatment of renal stones by extracorporeal shockwave lithotripsy. Nephron 1999;81 Suppl 1:71-81
26. Rompe JD, Krischek O, Eysel P, Hopf C: Chronische Insertionstendopathie am lateralen Epicondylus humeri – Ergebnisse der extrakorporalen Stosswellenapplikation. Schmerz 1998;12:105-111
27. Schleberger R, Senge T: Non-invasive treatment of long-bone pseudarthrosis by shockwaves (ESWL). Arch Orthop Trauma Surg 1992;111:224 – 227
28. Schmitt J, Arendt M, Haake M. Ergebnisse einer prospektiv-randomisierten Studie zur Wirksamkeit hoch- und niedrigenergetischer ESWT beim Supraspinatussehnensyndrom. Z Orthop 2003; 141 Supplement S1: S30 O21-1

29. Schmitt J, Tosch A, Huenerkopf M, Haake M. Die extrakorporale Stosswellentherapie (ESWT) als therapeutische Option beim Supraspinatussehnensyndrom? Ein-Jahres-Ergebnisse einer placebokontrollierten Studie. Orthopaede 2002; 31,652-657.

30. Schmitt J, Haake M, Tosch A, Hildebrand R, Deike B, Griss P: Low energy extracorporeal shockwave therapy (ESWT) of supraspinatus tendinitis - A prospective randomised study. J Bone Joint Surg (Br) 2001; 83: 873-876

31. Speed CA, Richards C, Nichols D, Burnet S, Wies JT, Humphreys H, Hazleman BL. Extracorporeal shockwave therapy for tendonitis of the rotator cuff. A double-blind, randomised, controlled trial. J Bone Joint Surg Br. 2002;84:509-12.

32. Valchanou VD, Michailov P: High energy shockwaves in the treatment of delayed and nonunion of fractures. Int Orthop 1991;15:181-184

33. Wess O, Stojan L, Rachel U: Untersuchungen zur Präzision der Ultraschallortung in vivo am Beispiel der extrakorporal induzierten Lithotripsie. In: Die Stosswelle - Forschung und Klinik. Hrsg. Christian Chaussy et al.: Attempto-Verlag Tübingen, 1995;37-44

34. Wess O, Überle F, Dührssen R N, Hilcken D, Krauss W, Reuner T, Schultheiss R, Staudenraus I, Rattne M, Haaks W, Granz B. Working Group Technical Developments- Consensus Report. In: Chaussy C, Eisenberger F, Jocham D, Wilbert D ed. High Energy Shockwaves in Medicine. Thieme Stuttgart 1997;59-71

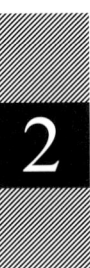

Physical Principles and Generation of Shockwaves

Ludger Gerdesmeyer, Mark Henne, Michael Göbel, Peter Diehl

Introduction

The effect of extracorporeal shockwaves on biological tissue has been known since observations were made during the second World War. At that time, castaways swimming in the water suffered lethal lung damage when water bombs were detonated in a wider radius. The impact of such extracorporeal shockwaves caused lungs to tear without any visible injuries on the outside[12]. The properties of such shockwaves were utilized to develop new test procedures in material research. Another area of application is signaling technology. Indeed, shockwaves propagate (in water, for example) over long distances with only minor energy loss. By measuring acoustic travel time, distances can be deduced as illustrated in laser distance measurement technology[13, 18].

Since they were first used successfully by Chaussy in the treatment of kidney stones in 1980, shockwaves have held their own in medicine and the number of applications has risen considerably[2]. The first gall bladder stones were treated in 1985[15]. Since the study conducted by Valchanov, who described the effect of shockwaves on the healing of bone fractures, the range of indications for ESWT treatment widened significantly in the area of orthopedics[21]. Today, not only kidney and gall bladder stones but also salivary gland stones, pancreatic stones, pseudoarthrosis, lateral epicondylitis humeri radialis, heel spur and calcified shoulder are treated with varying success[5, 6, 9, 11, 15-17]. A precise description of shockwaves was long thought to be unnecessary. What mattered most in the treatment of kidney stones was to be able to fragment the calculi without touching the patient. Side effects such as bleeding or skin lesions were thought to be acceptable. However, the situation in orthopedics is quite different. As a result of the multitude of indications, often very different clinical objectives have been defined. Changing conditions in orthopedic ESWT have brought about a greater need for information on the shockwave itself but also on the equipment to be used and on the possibilities to favor the positive effects of ESWT and to reduce even further any of the rare side effects found to be relevant. To meet such objectives, the information would allow modifying therapy parameters as well as shockwave emission technologies. What is known today about the effects of shockwaves on the treatment of kidney stones does not suffice to determine the reasons for the effect of ESWT on orthopedic treatments, to describe which effects are induced on the cellular level, or to explain the shockwave's analgesic effect[4, 7, 14]. A precise definition of shockwave-relevant parameters is therefore an indispensable requirement to be able to evaluate any observed clinical effects or findings from basic research.

This chapter gives an overview of the physical parameters, the characteristic properties and the generation of extracorporeal shockwaves.

The definition of physical parameters and their characteristic properties is based on the international standard proposal IEC 61846 (International Electrotechnical Commission, Geneva, Switzerland) and on the work of the Shockwave Therapy Consensus Group. They define which parameters are to be described for individual units and therefore provide utmost transparency for the user[23]. However, they do not state which of these parameters has medical relevance or which has specific biological effects. Parameters can be viewed at http://www.ismst.org/. The hope is to define the relation between dose and effect independently of the equipment used, and to look for parameters that may be responsible for the medical efficacy of the shockwave.

Shockwaves are defined as transient pressure oscillations that propagate in three dimensions and typically bring about a clear increase in pressure within a very short time. In most units used in medicine, such maximum pressure is reached within few nanoseconds (ns)[10]. Besides this very rapidly rising positive pressure impulse, shockwaves are also characterized by a tension phase with negative pressure following the pressure phase. Overall, shockwaves are characterized by the following properties (Figure 1)[19, 22, 23]:

PHYSICAL PRINCIPLES AND GENERATION OF SHOCKWAVES 13

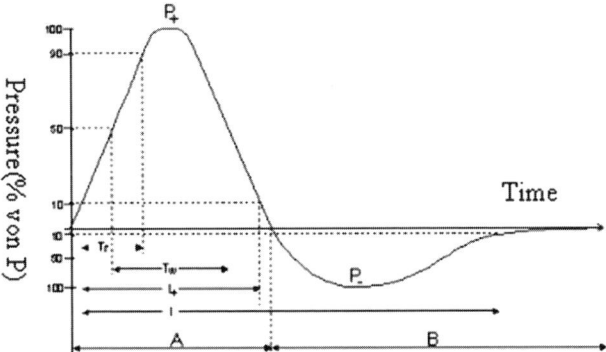

Figure 1a. Illustration of a shockwave. Shockwave pressure is shown as a function of time. A, first portion of the shockwave with positive pressure; B, second portion of the shockwave with negative pressure; P+, positive peak pressure; P-, negative peak pressure; Tr, rise time; Tw, impulse width; I+, standard time interval to calculate the shockwave's so-called "positive energy"; I, standard time interval to calculate the shockwave's so-called overall energy.

- Positive peak pressure (P+): P+ is defined as the difference between maximum positive peak pressure of the shockwave and ambivalent pressure. Depending on equipment type, P+ varies from 5 mega Pascal (MPa) to 120 MPa.

- Negative peak pressure (P-): P- is defined as the maximum negative peak pressure during the second phase of the shockwave. P- reaches values between 10% and 20% of P+.

- Rise time (Tr): Tr is defined as the interval in which pressure rises from 10% of P+ up to 90% of P+. Depending on equipment type, Tr can vary from a few nanoseconds to milliseconds.

- Impulse width (Tw): Tw is defined as the interval between the time when pressure first exceeds 50% of P+ and the time when pressure (during the exponential pressure drop within the first phase of the shockwave) is less than 50% of P+. The duration of Tw is between 200 ns and 500 ns. The term "full-width-half-maximum" (FWHM) is also used as a synonym for Tw. The duration of Tw affects directly the energy flow density of extracorporeal shockwaves.

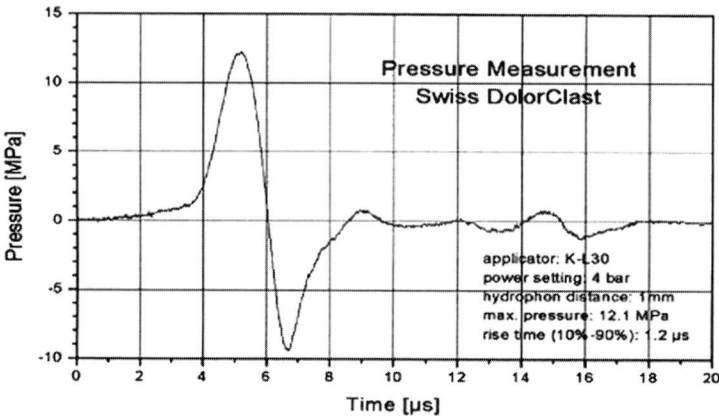

Figure 1b. Pressure measurement of one radial shockwave impulse.

The values of P+, P-, Tr and Tw of a shockwave depend to a large extent on the shockwave source and on the setting used. The tension portion of the shockwave lasts clearly longer than the pressure portion. In contrast, the value of P- is always less than the value of P+. Also, in contrast with P+, P- is limited in its amplitude due to physical principles. In the case of higher tension force, cohesion forces of the surrounding medium may be exceeded whereby gas-filled negative pressure bubbles - so-called cavitation bubbles - appear[11]. A complete shockwave lasts from a few microseconds to milliseconds; the frequency spectrum encompasses a range between 16 Hz and 20 MHz.

Principle of shockwave generation

Different processes have been developed to generate shockwaves. Four techniques in particular are used in clinical applications. All methods so used aim to couple the generated pressure impulse to the tissue while minimizing energy loss. To this effect, several coupling media are used. The units used in medicine to generate pressure impulses rely on some techniques that are basically different[18].

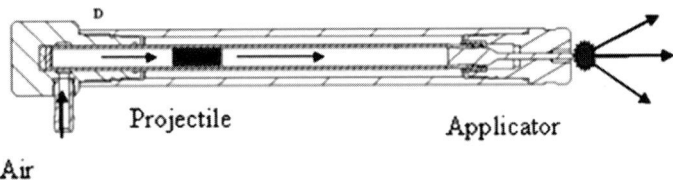

Figure 2a.   Illustration of a ballistic shockwave source

One of the latest but also very common methods is the mechanical generation of shockwaves. Based on ballistics, compressed air significantly accelerates a projectile which hits an applicator placed on the skin at very high kinetic energy. By using a coupling gel such as ultrasound gel or Castor oil, this impact pressure hitting the applicator can be delivered to the tissue in the form of a pressure wave. Then, the shockwave continues to propagate in the body in the form of a spherical or ball-shaped wave. This wave travels in a radial fashion, thus the descriptive term *radial shockwave*.

The main characteristic of this type of unit is that steepening occurs much more slowly compared to focused shockwave devices. Focused technologies are required to treat deep areas. Radial technologies provide no second acoustic focus. In this type of shockwave generation, the applicator surface constitutes the geometric point of highest pressure and highest energy density and so it is called tip-of-the-applicator-focus. Due to radial expansion, the pressure and energy density of the shockwave drop steadily upon leaving the applicator. The same shockwave propagation characteristics could be found in focused technologies behind the acoustic focus. Due to theoretical considerations, they also first appear to be less appropriate for classic indications such as pseudoarthrosis or calcific tendonitis located in deeper tissue layers[23]. In contrast, there is no doubt that indications near the surface are highly appropriate for shockwaves that propagate radially. In the meantime, new and improved techniques have led to a modification in applicator systems used to deliver ballistic shockwaves. Special geometry and changes in applicators allow ballistic shockwaves to focus on areas of higher concentration. Clinical studies will need to demonstrate whether such technical modifications would also be appropriate to treat conditions such as pseudoarthrosis or calcific tendonitis reserved until now for the "classic" shockwave.

Another common method to generate shockwaves is using electromagnetic currents (Figure 3).

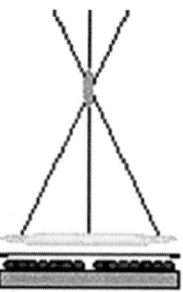

Figure 3. Illustration of an electromagnetic shockwave source

In this process, local electromagnetic currents are induced with a flat coil in a thin copper foil. Due to the Lorentz effect on charges in motion, the foil undergoes an explosion-like deflection. In the process, the associated water column is deflected in proportion to the tension. The pressure impulse so generated is then coupled and transmitted to the next medium. Additional technical features such as acoustic cutoff lenses are able to bundle the pressure waves into a defined focus to be placed in deeper regions of the body. Additional acoustic reflectors can further improve the precision of the focus. Further clinical studies will have to show whether such features would be suitable as part of orthopedic pain therapy. The electro pneumatic principle is an old method by which shockwaves are generated by a spark plug located in the primary focus (Figure 4). The high temperatures reached at the time of spark discharge cause the surrounding liquid to evaporate and a plasma bubble to occur. These radial shockwaves from the primary focus are then bundled into a second focus by using an elliptic acoustic mirror.

By using appropriate coupling media, shockwaves can be transmitted in selected regions. One of the disadvantages of this process is spark plug wear and wear-dependent shockwave energy variations. The rather costly exchange of electrodes must be repeated after a certain number of discharges. In addition, the shockwave generated with this process may fluctuate between shots in terms of energy and geometry [1] but these variations are believed to be clinically irrelevant.

Another method is the piezoelectric principle[20]. A small pressure impulse is emitted in the center of a ball cup by pulse-like local electric impulses of individual piezocrystals. Since the crystals are arranged on a half shell, the individual pressure waves can be bundled in one focus (Figure 5).

PHYSICAL PRINCIPLES AND GENERATION OF SHOCKWAVES 17

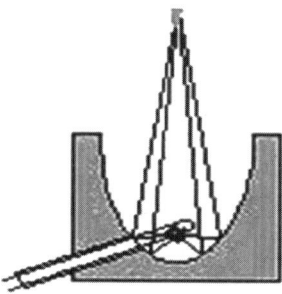

Figure 4. Illustration of an electromagnetic shockwave source

As in the other methods, such focus can then be placed in the body by using appropriate localization systems. The shockwave is coupled based on the same principle as in the other emission methods mentioned earlier.

In terms of shockwave generation methods, a detailed discussion about technical equipment parameters is of little use at this time from a medical point of view. Indeed, today it has not been determined which parameter is significant for possible biological effects or clinical results[8]. However, for the purpose of technical comparisons, it is useful to identify as many shockwave parameters as possible.

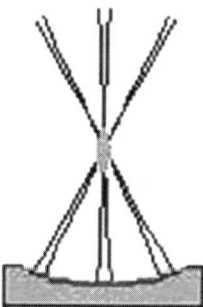

Figure 5. Summary illustration of a piezoelectric shockwave source

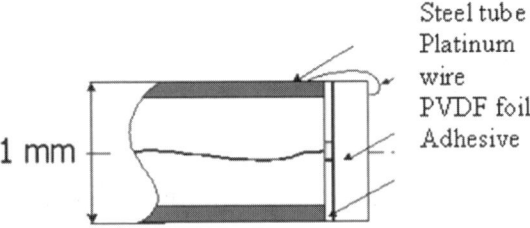

Figure 6. Illustration of a PVDF hydrophone

Measuring Technique

Just like technical progress has led to on-going equipment modifications and new techniques to generate shockwaves, so have technical advances affected the processes involved in measuring technology. In principle, shockwave magnitude can be measured by electrical and non-electrical means. Non-electrical methods include optical methods and the defined fragmentation rate of model stones[7, 18]. However, there is general consensus that only electrical sensors, so-called hydrophones, are suitable for the quantitative measurement of shockwave magnitude.

These are sensors for acoustic pressure in liquids which deliver an electric signal and which are appropriate due to the possibility of calibration for absolute measurements. Among the older hydrophones are PVDF hydrophones. The first dynamic pressure measurements of shockwaves were performed with them. The hydrophone used at the time is based on a concept by Chivers and Lewin dating back to 1981 and originally designed for the low-pressure area. This measuring technique is based on the piezoelectric properties of a polyvinyl fluoride (PVDF) foil applied to a thin steel tube. At the end the generated potential is made transparent via an oscilloscope (Figure 6).

A major disadvantage of this hydrophone is the fact that the tensile part of the shockwave could not be measured precisely due to local cavitation phenomena as well as the limited stability (life) of the hydrophone.

The consensus therefore was to use hydrophones which do not have the PVDF hydrophones related disadvantage. Among them are fiber-optic hydrophones which register acoustic waves as peaks and convert them to proportional output voltage.

Due to the high cost of this technology fiber glass hydrophones have only been used for the past two years. These more recent measurements produce in part significantly higher values for the same parameters. As mentioned before, measurements performed under in vivo conditions raise particular problems[7].

It must be noted once again that until now no link has been established between measurable shockwave parameters and biological or analgesic effect. Today, it is not known whether such equipment-specific parameters are clinically relevant at all or rather serve to animate a technical discussion of lesser clinical relevance.

Literature

1. Bailey MR, Blackstock DT, Cleveland RO, Crum LA (1999): Comparison of electrohydraulic lithotripters with rigid and pressure-release ellipsoidal reflectors. II. Cavitation fields. J Acoust Soc Am 106:1149-1160.
2. Chaussy C, Chaussy C, Brendel W, Schmiedt E (1980): Extracorporeally induced destruction of kidney stones by shockwaves. Lancet. 13:1265-8.
3. Coleman AJ, Draguioti E, Tiptaf R, Shotri N, Saunders JE (1998): Acoustic performance and clinical use of a fiberoptic hydrophone. Ultrasound Med Biol 24:143-151.
4. Delacretaz G, Rink K, Pittomvils G, et al: Importance of the implosion of ESWL-induced cavitation bubbles. Ultrasound Med Biol 21:97-103, 1995.
5. Delius M: Lithotripsy. Ultrasound Med Biol 26 (Suppl 1):55-58, 2000.
6. Gerdesmeyer L, Wagenpfeil S, Haake M, Maier M, Loew M, Wortler K, Lampe R, Seil R, Handle G, Gassel S, Rompe JD.: Extracorporeal shockwave therapy for the treatment of chronic calcifying tendonitis of the rotator cuff: a randomized controlled trial. JAMA. 2003 Nov 19;290(19):2573-80.
7. Gerdesmeyer, L., Maier, M., Haake, M., Schmitz, C.: Physical-technical principles of extracorporeal shockwave therapy (ESWT). Orthopäde 2002, 31: 610-617
8. Haake M, Boddeker IR, Decker T, Buch M, Vogel M, Labek G, Maier M, Loew M, Maier-Boerries O, Fischer J, Betthauser A, Rehack HC, Kanovsky W, Muller I, Gerdesmeyer L, Rompe JD.: Side-effects of extracorporeal shockwave therapy (ESWT) in the treatment of tennis elbow. Arch Orthop Trauma Surg. 2002 May;122(4):222-8
9. Howell DA: Pancreatic stones: treat or ignore? Can J Gastroenterol 13:461-465, 1999.
10. Hundt E. (1974) Die Physik, Bibliographisches Institut Mannheim – Dudenverlag, S.360
11. Iro H, Zenk J, Waldfahrer F, et al: Extracorporeal shockwave lithotripsy of parotid stones. Results of a prospective clinical trial. Ann Otol Rhinol Laryngol 107:860-864, 1998.
12. Krause H: Physik und Technik medizinischer Stosswellensysteme. In Rompe JD (ed). Extrakorporale Stosswellentherapie. Weinheim, Chapman and Hall, 15-34, 1997.

13. Lewin PA, Schafer ME: Shockwave sensors: I. Requirements and design. J Lithotr Stone Dis 3:3-17, 1991.
14. Maier M, Milz S, Wirtz DC, Rompe JD, Schmitz C. Basic research of applying extracorporeal shockwaves on the musculoskeletal system. An assessment of current status. Orthopade. 2002 Jul;31(7):667-77.
15. Mulagha E, Fromm HJ: Extracorporeal shockwave lithotripsy of gallstones revisited: current status and future promises. Gastroenterol Hepatol 15:239-243, 2000
16. Rompe JD, et al: Shockwave application for chronic plantar fasciitis in running athletes – a prospective, randomized, placebo- controlled trial. Am J Sports Med 2003; 31:268-275
17. Rompe JD, Schoellner C, Nafe B.: Evaluation of low energy extracorporeal shockwave application and treatment in chronic plantar fasciitis. J Bone Joint Surg Am. 2002; 84:335-341.
18. Schräbler S (1999): Ein abtastendes Verfahren zur Darstellung und Analyse von Stosswellen in Flüssigkeit, Shaker Verlag.
19. Staudenraus J.(1995) In Vivo Stosswellenmessung. In Chaussy C (Hrsg) Die Stosswelle in Forschung und Klinik. Attempto Verlag, S 21-26
20. Tavakkoli J, Birer A, Arefiev A, Prat F, Chapelon JY, Cathignol D (1997) A piezocomposite shockwave generator with electronic focusing capability: application for producing cavitation-induced lesions in rabbit liver. Ultrasound Med Biol 23:107-115
21. Valchanou VD, Michailov P (1991) High energy shockwaves in the treatment of delayed and nonunion of fractures. Int Orthop 15:181-184
22. Ueberle F (1997) Shockwave technology. In Siebert W, Buch M (Hrsg) Extracorporal shockwaves in orthopaedics. Springer, S.59-87
23. Wess O, Ueberle F, Dührssen RN, et al: Working Group Technical Developements - Consensus Report. In Chaussy C, Eisenberger F, Jocham D, Wilbert D (eds). High Energy Shockwaves in Medicine. Stuttgart, Thieme, 59-71, 1997.

Physical Principles in Shockwave Generation – Clinical Relevance and Practical Implications.

L. Gerdesmeyer, M. Henne, H. Gollwitzer, P. Diehl

In medicine, shockwaves are customarily generated in water in order to facilitate their delivery to tissue with similar acoustic properties. Pressure impulses propagate waves through tissue such as water, gas or inside solid-state bodies.

The typical form of the shockwave has a very steep and short ascent until pressure maximum results from asymmetric attenuation when traveling through tissue. Referred to as steepening, this phenomenon is the result of differences in attenuation of individual frequency parts of the shockwave front and of pressure- and temperature-dependent acoustic conduction velocity. Acoustic velocity is proportional to the density of the medium it travels through. In shockwaves later parts of the acoustic pressure front accelerate in a medium of higher density and therefore catch up with early parts of the shockwave front[14, 21].

This pressure- and temperature-dependent phenomenon and the differences in attenuation of individual shockwave parts finally brings about an asymmetric deformation of the shockwave. This results in pressure impulse steepening and typical shockwave formation[14]. Such typical wave configuration features a very steep ascent slope and a more flat pressure drop flank. These formations were found within the acoustic focus. In its further course, the wave front loses this typical formation. Individual pressure impulse parts, with varying frequency and intensity, spread out and run away from one another (defocusing).

Most shockwave sources generate pulses in a water bath. Older units were connected to a bath tub in which the patient has to lie down. Most of today's units

Medium	Acoustic Speed [m/s]	Impedance [×103 Ns/m³]
Air	343	429
Fat	1,450	1,380
Water	1,483	1,480
Steel	5,790	45,700
Lung	650-1,160	260-460
ZNS	1,560	1,600
Kidney	1,570	1,630
Muscle	1,545-1,630	1,650-1,740
Bone	2,700-4,100	3,200-7,400
Kidney Stone	4,000-6,000	5,600-14,400

Table 1. Velocity and acoustic impedance of different tissue media[?].

deliver the energy via a water-filled medium. Since muscle and fat tissues are essentially not much different in terms of acoustic properties such as impedance, the associated acoustic border areas are most likely clinically negligible[18]. Acoustic impedance is the tissue-typical resistance to acoustic conductivity and decribed as Ns/m³. Table 1 provides a summary of the different acoustic properties.

Because of its outward similarity with Ohm's law in electricity, this impedance is also referred to as Ohm's law for acoustic speed[17].

In the case of wider variations in impedance of the tissue, an altered shockwave in terms of intensity and geometry is to be expected[14]. The reasons are different impedance-dependent velocities of acoustic conductivity in different media. In these areas where tissues interface or join, the shockwave is first affected by refraction. Beyond this point, not the entire part is transmitted via this interface into the subsequent tissue, but is partly reflected[18]. Such impedance differences occur at the interface of tissue media with different physical properties such as calcium deposit/soft tissue or bone/soft tissue interfaces. At these acoustic interfaces, acoustic energy is transformed into mechanical energy. The release of mechanical energy leads to mechanical effects such as calcium deposit disintegration or trabecular fractures[17, 19, 20]. The portion of acoustic energy transformed into mechanical energy varies from the difference of impedance. If, for example, a shockwave travels through water with an average impedance of 1.49 Ns/m3 and reaches a medium of higher impedance such as kidney stones (up to 15 Ns/m3), most of the acoustic energy is transmitted to the stone[21]. But the reverse is true as well: if a shockwave travels from a tissue with high impedance (stone) to a tissue with low impedance (muscle), a large portion of the acoustic energy is reflected in the stone, undergoes a phase return and combines with the subsequent portion of the shockwave. This explains why shockwave-induced effects are to be found on that side which is turned away from the acoustic source. Another synergistic effect is acoustic bending. Shockwaves traveling past a kidney stone or calcium deposit are bent towards the tissue with higher impedance. In the case of stone disintegration a natural focus could be found at the back side of the stone.

The above mentioned phenomena have been measured and identified in lab conditions. However, the tissue induced shockwave modification and alteration has not been analysed. Large experiences in ESWT for nephrolithiasis have shown that the number of shockwaves needed for stone disintegration clearly varies[13]. In actual patients, 5 to 20 times more shockwaves were needed for disintegration, compared to laboratory conditions[14].

The interaction at acoustic interfaces described above causes one part of the shockwave to be transmitted to the next medium while another part is reflected in the tissue. This effect of transmission and reflection is very difficult to predict. Most parts of the shockwave do not reach the acoustic interface perpendicularly, therefore a lateral shift of the pulse waves is to be expected in addition to their attenuation. This has been demonstrated [17] whereby the attenuation effect is significantly more marked.

Earlier measurements have demonstrated that the positive peak pressure is altered more or less significantly in the sense of a reduction[2, 16]. Depending upon the nature of the hydrophone measuring system used, a reduction between 15% and 85% has been found[3, 6].

Our own study demonstrated a reduction in energy by a factor of three by a tissue layer of at least 1.5 cm.

This attenuation effect in terms of energy flux density and clinical impact can easily be used to explain different results in clinical trials. Accordingly, our knowledge of the attenuating effect is clearly much more clinically relevant than any detailed description of parameters concerning technical equipment. From a scientific point of view, the discussion about type of equipment or type of shock wave device is quite inappropriate as is making a conclusion about which specific parameters or equipment parameters correlate with clinical findings. In this context, only clinical studies in accordance with good clinical practice guidelines are able to make a valid contribution to the subject.

Shockwave-induced effects and principles

Pressure pulses act either directly or indirectly independent of the generating source[4, 8, 16]. In addition to proven thermal and chemical effects, shockwaves also result in mechanical action. This effect is sufficiently known from the treatment of kidney stones[2]. But the underlying prerequisite for all these effects is the conversion of acoustic energy into mechanical, thermal or chemical energy if interfaces provide acoustic differences (Table 1). The resulting direct mechanical effect is proportional to the amplitude of the difference in impedance. The clinical effects are known from kidney stone lithotripsy and the treatment of calcific tendonitis[8, 11, 15]. A rather subordinate role seems to be played by thermal effects induced as a result of high pressure amplitudes and the interaction of compression and depression. A strong increase in local pressure produces an increase in temperature which can be measured but without clinical relevance since the time interval of the increase in temperature is extremely short.

An important indirect mechanism is the induction of cavitation[1]. Cavitation is defined as occurrence of gas-filled bubbles if negative pressure gradients exist. Just a few MPa's of negative pressure were observed in shockwaves to exert a negative pressure. Negative pressure cavities occur if cohesion of liquid media, such as water, is below positive pressure forces. The predominant negative pressure causes the liquid to evaporate at the edge of the cavitation bubble, thus causing cavitation bubbles to increase even further. In water, bubbles of several millimeter in diameter, can be generated under laboratory conditions. When the pressure wave has passed the tissue, pressure conditions return to normal isobar conditions and the bubble collapses again. Since such a collapse is rarely absolutely symmetric, local high-speed liquid flows occur during the collapse. These focal effects are called jet stream [16] and may reach local velocity of up to 800 m/s. They also have a mechanically destructive effect. Regarding this effect, shockwave frequency has an important impact if the previous shockwave may not yet have collapsed and is already reached by the next incoming pressure pulse. If the shockwave frequency reaches a certain level, bubbles that have not collapsed get the next shockwave[4, 5]. Under these circumstances the cavitation bubble is forced to an asymmetric collapse in a very short time. The jet streams resulting from such forced asymmetric collapse are clearly more marked and locally destructive effects were also described[7, 9].

Another indirect effect is known as the occurrence of free radicals. Similar to the irrelevant thermal effect, free radicals occur as a result of high temperatures, significant pressure gradients and released mechanical energy. However such free radicals have no clinical or biological effect that can be demonstrated. In principle, these mechanisms have been demonstrated under laboratory conditions. Whether they also apply to clinical applications remains a matter of debate.

The question of a possible biological dose threshold also remains unanswered today. No studies have been done to determine if there is an overdose, or whether there are non-biochemical changes to be induced at the cellular level in order to effect corresponding changes. Therefore it seems to be possible that effector organ systems such as nerve endings or vessel systems must not be destroyed in order to biologically convert the effect induced by shockwaves. More detailed information is found in the next chapter *Molecular Mechanisms of Shock-Waves*.

The use of local anesthesia in ESWT is one of the actual debates in shockwave application. Since the largest portion of prospective placebo-controlled studies showed surprisingly good results after placebo ESWT, current studies seem to indicate that one should conduct low-energy ESWT without local anesthesia[10, 12]. In most of the randomized placebo-controlled trials, local anesthesics were used to blind the patients.

In new smaller applicators designed recently, shockwaves were no longer applied with local anesthesics. Based on the findings of Rompe and Labek, treatments performed with smaller units indicate that better results may be obtained without local anesthesia than when using local anesthesia.

However, further studies have to be conducted to confirm this effect. Also, the smaller shockwave applicators and devices have to demonstrate their effectiveness. Further findings reached in handling ESWT and technical advances will continue to stimulate the debate about optimum ESWT and will bring about an improvement in accordance with evidence-based medicine.

Literature

1. Bailey MR, Blackstock DT, Cleveland RO, Crum LA: Comparison of electrohydraulic lithotripters with rigid and pressure-release ellipsoidal reflectors. II. Cavitation fields. J Acoust Soc Am 106:1149-1160, 1999.
2. Chaussy C, Schmiedt E, Jocham D, Brendl W, Forssmann B, Walther V (1982) First clinical experience with extracorporeally induced destruction of kidney stones by shockwaves. J Urol 127:417-420

3. Cleveland RO, Lifshitz DA, Connors BA, Evan AP, Willis LR, Crum LA (1998) In vivo pressure measurements of lithotripsy shockwaves in pigs. Ultrasound Med Biol 24(2):293-306
4. Delacretaz G, Rink K, Pittomvils G, et al: Importance of the implosion of ESWL-induced cavitation bubbles. Ultrasound Med Biol 21:97-103, 1995.
5. Delius M, Draenert K, Al Diek Y, Draenert Y: Biological effects of shockwaves: in vivo effect of high energy pulses on rabbit bone. Ultrasound Med Biol 21:1219-1225, 1995.
6. Finney R, Halliwell M, Mishriki SF, Baker AC (1991) Measurement of lithotrypsy pulses through biological media. Phys Med Biol 36: 1485-1493
7. Greenstein A, Matzkin H: Does the rate of extracorporeal shockwave delivery affect stone fragmentation? Urology 54:430-432, 1999.
8. Howard D, Sturtevant B: In vitro study of the mechanical effects of shockwave lithotripsy. Ultrasound Med Biol 23:1107-1122, 1997
9. Huber P, Jochle K, Debus J: Influence of shockwave pressure amplitude and pulse repetition frequency on the lifespan, size and number of transient cavities in the field of an electromagnetic lithotripter. Phys Med Biol 43:3113-3128, 1998.
10. Labek G, Auersperg V, Ziernhöld M, Poulios N, Bohler N: Influence of energy and local anesthesia on the outcome of low energy ESWT on plantar heel Spur: ISMST, 5th Congress, p.65, June 2002
11. Loew M, Jurgowski W, Thomsen M: Effect of extracorporeal shockwave therapy on calcific tendinitis of the shoulder. A preliminary report. Urologe 34:49-53, 1995.
12. Rompe JD, Zoellner J, Hofmann A, Nafe B, Auersperg V, Gerdesmeyer L: Low-energy Shockwave Application without Local Anesthesia is more efficient than Low-energy Extracorporeal Shockwave Application with Local Anesthesia for the Treatment of Chronic Plantar Fasciitis. Submitted 2004
13. Schmidt A, Müller M, Wilke J, Eisenberger F (1990) intrakorporale Druckmessungen in Nierenbecken und Harnleiter während der extrakorporalen Stosswellenlithotrypsie. Z. Urologie Poster 4/1990: 264-265
14. Staudenraus J (1995) In vivo Stosswellenmessung. In Chaussy C. (Hrsg) Die Stosswelle in Forschung und Klinik. Attempto Verlag, S 21-26
15. Steinbach P, Hofstaedter F, Nicolai H, Roessler W, Wieland W: Determination of the energy-dependent extent of vascular damage caused by high-energy shockwaves in an umbilical cord model. Urol Res 21:279-282, 1993.
16. Zhong P, Cioanta I, Cocks FH, Preminger GM: Inertial cavitation and associated acoustic emission produced during electrohydraulic shockwave lithotripsy. J Acoust Soc Am 101:2940-2950, 1997
17. Gerdesmeyer L, Maier M, Haake M, Schmitz C. [Physical-technical principles of extracorporeal shockwave therapy (ESWT)]. Orthopade 2002a; (31): 610-617
18. Krause H. Physik und Technik medizinischer Stosswellensysteme. In: Extrakorporale Stosswellentherapie. Grundlagen, Indikation, Anwendung. (Ed.Rompe JD). London: Chapman&Hall, 1997; 1: 15-34
19. Lokhandwalla M, Sturtevant B. Fracture mechanics model of stone comminution in ESWL and implications for tissue damage. Phys Med Biol 2000; (45): 1923-1940
20. Maier M, Milz S, Wirtz D C, Rompe J D, Schmitz C. [Basic research of applying extracorporeal shockwaves on the musculoskeletal system. An assessment of current status]. Orthopade 2002b; (31): 667-677
21. Ueberle F. Acoustic Parameters of Pressure Pulse Sources Used in Lithotripsy and Pain Therapy. In: High Energy Shockwaves in Medicine. (Eds.Chaussy C, Eisenberger F, Jocham D, Wilbert D). Stuttgart: Thieme, 1997; 1: 76-85

4

Molecular Mechanisms of Shockwaves

M. Maier,[1] J. Hausdorf,[2] C. Schmitz[3]

Summary

The biological effect of extracorporeal shockwaves on the musculoskeletal system is still unclear. Distal rabbit femurs were treated in vivo with shockwaves of 0.9 mJ/mm2 (1500 impulses, 1 Hz) in order to verify the hypothesis that changes in the tissue concentrations of substance P and prostaglandin E2 play a role in the biological effect of shockwaves. The concentrations of substance P and prostaglandin E2 were measured in the eluate of the femur periostiumium. Compared to the untreated contralateral side, a clear increase in the release of substance P was found 6 and 24 hours after shockwave treatment; 6 weeks later, concentration in the eluate was lower. Shockwave treatment did not produce any change in the release of prostaglandin E2. There is a close relationship between the evolution of substance P release and the clinically known treatment pain with consecutive pain reduction in the shockwave treatment of tendon insertion diseases. Substance P appears to play an essential role in the molecular mechanisms of extracorporeal shockwaves on the musculoskeletal system.

Introduction

To explain the biological effects of extracorporeal shockwaves on tissue of the musculoskeletal system, the hypothesis of Melzack's concept of hyperstimulation

---

[1] *Orthopedic Department, Ludwig-Maximilians University, Munich*
[2] *Rehabilitationsklinik für Orthopädie und Rheumatologie am Rheumazentrum Oberammergau*
[3] *Department of Psychiatry and Neuropsychology, University of Maastricht*

analgesia continues to be quoted today[25, 29, 39]. In this context it is of great significance that the direct in vivo application of shockwaves on nerves has led to the induction of action potential[33]. When this also applies to unmyelinized nerve fibers, extracorporeal shockwaves could effect the release of substance P. Substance P is a polypeptide made up of 11 amino acids[6]. In the peripheral nerve system a large portion of substance P is found in C-fibers and a subgroup of the slowly conducting A-delta nerve fibers [12, 14] found in the skin, mucous membrane, intestines and vessels of the entire body. Substance P has a pre- and postsynaptic effect on complex synaptic processes in the central nervous system[5]. Following stimulation, substance P is released by nociceptive nerve fibers on central or peripheral endings[24]. Peripheral mechanisms of substance P are the induction of neurogenic inflammation [18], extravasation of plasma [40] and the stimulation of the proliferation of different cell types such as osteoblasts[11].

The study also showed that extracorporeal shockwave therapy on the musculoskeletal system may cause tissue damage as well as inflammatory response[8, 30]. Based on these findings, shockwave application could also lead to a release of inflammation mediators such as prostaglandins. Prostaglandins are a complex group of oxygenated fatty acids found in almost all mammals[17].

For the in vivo study of the molecular principles of extracorporeal shockwaves, we therefore verified whether the application of extracorporeal shockwaves leads to changes in the release of substance P and prostaglandin E2 from the tissue in focus of the shockwaves.

Method

The experiments were conducted on 20 adult female bastard chincilla rabbits (approximately 1 year old). The animals weighed between four and five kilograms. The animals were randomized into three groups according to the respective experiment period. In Group A (n = 4), animals were sacrificed after 6 hours, in Group B (n = 8) after 24 hours, and in Group C (n = 8) after 6 weeks. For each animal, a hind leg was randomly selected for shockwave treatment, the untreated leg served as control. Shockwaves were applied under narcosis using cetamin and xylazinhydrochloride. During narcosis, a breathing mask supplied the oxygen. After shaving both hind legs, the animals were positioned in the shockwave unit[8]. A single shockwave treatment was applied to the selected distal femur using an electrohydraulic shockwave source (XL 1 from Dornier MedTech,

Wessling, Germany). Shockwaves were focused by laser. 1500 shockwave impulses with an energy flux density of 0.9 mJ/mm2 and a frequency of 1 Hz were applied. Duration of the treatment was about 25 minutes per animal.

In each group the animals were sacrificed following the end of the experiment period, the femur bone was immediately exarticulated from hips and knee, and the adjacent soft tissue was carefully removed with a scalpel. During preparation, particular attention was paid to the complete integrity of the periostiumium and the bone. For the measurement of substance P and prostaglandin E2, each femur traveled through a succession of 5 glass cylinders filled with a synthetic interstitial fluid (95% O2, 5% CO2, bicarbonate-containing electrolyte fluid) as eluation medium. Eluation vessels stood in a water bath at 37° C and were continuously shaken. The 6th sample vessel contained a stimulation solution of inflammation mediators bradykinin, serotonin and histamin (each 10-5 molar). Each femur stayed in this solution for five minutes. Since substance P is also found in relevant quantities in bone marrow, a contamination with substances from the bone marrow hole was prevented by individually filling the glass cylinders to the proper height.

Substance P and prostaglandin E2 were measured as established [9, 15, 32] in the eluation fluid of each individual glass cylinder for a total of six times with immunoassays (Substance P Assay Kit from Cayman Chemical Company, Ann Arbor, USA; Prostaglandin E2 Antobodies by Dr. K. Brune, Institute for Pharmacology, University of Erlangen, Germany)[4]. To this effect the content of each glass cylinder was divided into two equal portions and mixed with enzymimmunoassay buffer (Sigma, Steinheim, Germany) to stabilize substance P and prostaglandin E2. One of these two portions was used immediately to measure substance P. The other portion was deepfrozen at - 20° C and the concentration of prostaglandin E2 was determined the following day.

A statistical analysis was performed by calculating average values and standard deviations for the values of concentration of substance P and prostaglandin E2 in each group and in each eluation medium. The effects of extracorporeal shockwave treatment on the concentrations of substance P and prostaglandin E2 in the eluation medium were calculated with the "Two-way Repeated Measures Analysis of Variance" (ANOVA). Taken into consideration was the fact that the findings were to be viewed in dual perspective as linked sample probes. For each animal, several eluation steps were carried out (first matching). Then, for each experiment animal, the treated as well as the

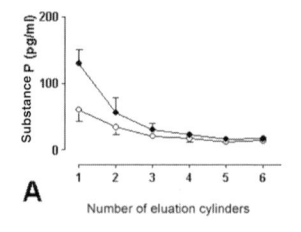

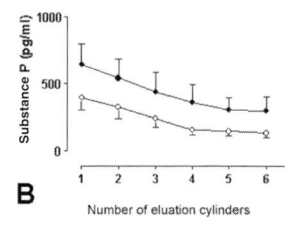

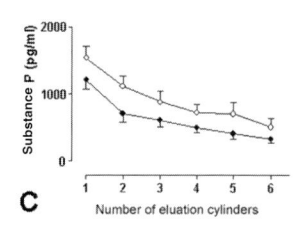

Figure 1.

A: Substance P-concentration in periosteal eluat 6 hours after ESWT (Group A).

B: Substance P-concentration in periosteal eluat 24 hours after ESWT (Group B).

C: Substance P-concentration in periosteal eluat 6 weeks after ESWT (Group C).

In each figure the first eluation step represents the initial eluation (duration: 30 minutes). Eluation steps 2-5 with 5 minutes duration each. The final eluation step was performed after Bradykinin, Serotonin and Histamin were applied.

• = ESWT site

◊ = contol site.

untreated femur was examined (second matching). However, with the two-way repeated measures Analysis of Variance, only one matching can be considered. Accordingly, statistical analysis was conducted twice whereby first the first matching (repeated eluation steps) was considered and then the second matching (treated and untreated femurs). In both cases statistical significance was determined to be $p < 0.05$.

Results

Figure 1 shows concentrations of substance P and Figure 2 concentrations of prostaglandin E2, each time as a function of the eluation step. In summary, the following results were obtained:

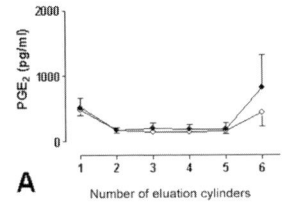

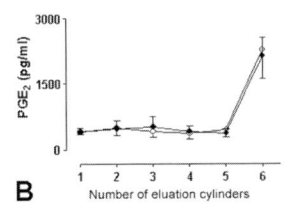

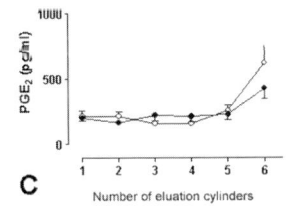

Figure 2.

A: PGE2 concentration in periosteal eluat 6 hours after ESWT (Group A).

B: PGE2 in periosteal eluat 24 hours after ESWT (Group B).

C: PGE2 concentration in periosteal eluat 6 weeks after ESWT (Group C).

In each figure the first eluation step represents the initial eluation (duration: 30 minutes). Eluation steps 2-5 with 5 minutes duration each. The final eluation step was performed after Bradykinin, Serotonin and Histamin were applied.

• = ESWT site
◊ = contol site.

The treatment with extracorporeal shockwaves causes an increase in release of substance P from the treated femur preparations after 6 and 24 hours post EWST compared to the untreated hind legs. In contrast, shockwave treatment brought about a decrease in substance P release from the treated femurs 6 weeks after ESWT.

The more eluation steps were carried out, the lower the substance P concentration in the eluation cylinders.

Extracorporeal shockwave treatment brought about no changes in prostaglandin E2 concentrations, neither after 6 or 24 hours, nor 6 weeks after extracorporeal shockwave treatment.

The successive eluation steps did not affect the concentration of prostaglandin E2 in the corresponding eluation vessels. However, the eluation with synthetic interstitial fluid containing bradykinin, serotonin and histamine produced higher PGE2 concentrations in the eluation medium than eluation with only synthetic interstitial fluid.

Discussion

The sensitivity and specificity of the enzyme immunoassays used in this study is known in the literature[1]. The interindividual variability of the results of this study is comparable to the interindividual variability of similar enzymimmunoassays[1, 9, 15]. We observed a drop in concentration of substance P in the eluation medium with advancing eluation. This could point to eluation of interstitial substance P without resulting in an additional release from nerve endings during the eluation process. In contrast, we found constant PGE2 values in the eluation medium with increasing eluation time and an increase in PGE2 concentration after adding inflammatory mediators.

Basic experiments have shown that the effects of shockwave therapy occur at the junction between tissues of different impedance[8]. The different soft tissues have comparably low impedances whereas the impedance of bone is five times greater[39]. Therefore the greatest effects of extracorporeal shockwave therapy are to be expected at the distal femur in the periostiumium which covers the cortical bone. Substance P-immunoreactive nerve fibers are known to occur in the periostiumium as they do in bone marrow and synovial membranes[2]. However, the special treatment of the samples examined in this study guarantees the release of substance P almost exclusively derived from the periostium.

To date it is not known whether the course in time followed by the release of substance P in those places where clinically the typical pains of tendon and tendon insertion diseases occur is the same as that found in this study on the distal femur of the rabbit. An initial increase and subsequent long decrease in substance P release from the treated region could, however, explain the initial pain during and shortly after shockwave treatment of tendon insertion and subsequent lasting relief from pain. This may be concluded from a recent study examining the possible biological mechanism of capsaicin, a substance whose potent analgesic effect is known[38]. Capsaicin belongs to the vanilloid family and is the substance responsible for the sensory-irritating effect of red hot chilli pepper. Casaicin affects a direct and elective stimulation of polymodal C-fibers (and probably also of A-delta fibers) and brings about the release of substance P through a depolarization of nerve cell membranes followed by a long-lasting depletion of substance P in the initially depolarized nerves. The final result is a long-lasting degeneration of nerve fibers. In humans, capsaicin can be applied directly to the skin. Due to the release of substance P, the surface application of capsaicin initially produces hyperalgesia. When using capsaicin over a longer time period, a depletion of substance P takes place and capsaicin then develops its analgesic effect[26].

However, it must also be noted that substance P may also cause so-called neurogenic inflammations[18]. Inflammatory symptoms in the paratenon of the Achilles tendon of rabbits occurred already one day after high-energy extracorporeal shockwave treatment[30]. Our hypothesis was therefore that following extracorporeal shockwave treatment there is evidence of a modified PGE2 concentration in the treated femurs. However, since no change in PGE2 concentrations occurred, neither 6 or 24 hours, nor 6 weeks after shockwave treatment, this points only to a small inflammatory reaction in the periostium.

In humans the intradermal injection of capsaicin effects a degeneration and a subsequent reingrowth of epidermal nerve fibers[36]. In this regard, the initial increase and subsequent long-lasting decrease in substance P release could be considered as a consequence of damage to the nerves that supply the region. Under these circumstances it is important to note that high-energy shockwave treatment has caused wave-like swelling of axons [27] and other changes in nerve fibers[37]. In addition, it was shown recently that cutting of the nervus mentalis in the rat led to a week-long disappearance of substance P fibers in the skin of the lower lip[31]. This would also bring about an initial pain with subsequent long-lasting relief from pain. However, there is no detailed knowledge about potential nerve damage after application of extracorporeal shockwaves to the musculoskeletal system. This continues to be studied by our work group.

In summary, an initial increase and subsequent decrease in substance P concentration from the periostium of the distal rabbit femur was found following high-energy extracorporeal shockwave treatment. Assuming that the concentration changes in substance P after extracorporeal shockwave treatment also occurs in these places where patients suffer from tendon insertion pain, the findings of this study can be viewed as a first indication of the molecular effect of extracorporeal shockwave treatment.

Literature

1. Averbeck B, Reeh PW (2001) Interactions of inflammatory mediators stimulating release of calcitonin-gene-related-peptide, substance P and prostaglandin E2 from isolated rat skin. Neuropharmacol 40:416-423
2. Bjurholm A, Kreicbergs A, Brodin E, Schultzberg M (1988) Substance P- and CGRP-immunoreactive nerves in bone. Peptides 9:165-171
3. Bretag A (1969) Synthetic interstital fluid for isolated mammalian tissue. Life Sci 8:319-329
4. Brune K, Reinke M, Lanz, R, Peskar BA (1985) Monoclonal antibodies against E- and F- type prostaglandins: High specificity and sensitivity in conventional radioimmunoassays. FEBS Lett 186:46-50
5. Cesaro P (1984) Substance P. Rev Neurol 140:465-478
6. Chang MM, Leeman SE, Niall HD (1971) Amino-acid sequence of substance P. Nat New Biol 232:86-87
7. Delius M, Draenert K, Diek Y, Draenert Y (1995) Biological effects of shockwaves: In vivo effect of high energy pulses on rabbit bone. Ultrasound Med Biol 21:1219-1225
8. Delius M (2000) Lithotripsy. Ultrasound Med Biol 26 (Suppl):55-58
9. Ebersberger A, Averbeck B, Messlinger K, Reeh PW (1999) Release of substance P, calcitonin gene-related peptide and prostaglandin E2 from rat dura mater encephali follwing electrical and chemical stimulation in vitro. Neuroscience 89:901-907
10. Flower RJ (1977) The role of prostaglandins in inflammatory reactions. Naunyn Schmiedebergs Arch Pharmacol 297 (Suppl):77-79
11. Goto T, Yamaza T, Kido MA, Tanaka T (1998) Light- and electron-microscopic study of the distribution of axons containing substance P and the localization of neurokinin-1 receptor in bone. Cell Tissue Res 293:87-93
12. Harper AA, Lawson SN (1985) Conduction velocity is related to morphological cell type in rat dorsal root ganglion neurons. J Physiol Lond 359:31-46
13. Holzer P (1991) Capsaicin: Cellular targets, mechanisms of action, and selectivity for thin sensory neurons. Pharmacol Rev 43:143-201
14. Keen P, Harmar AJ, Spears F, Winter E (1982) Biosynthesis, axonal transport and turnover of neuronal substance P. Ciba Found Symp 91:145-164
15. Kress M, Guthmann C, Averbeck B, Reeh PW (1999) Calcitonin gene-related peptide and prostaglandin E2 but not substance P release induced by antidromic nerve stimulation from rat skin in vitro. Neuroscience 89:303-310
16. Krischek O, Hopf C, Nafe B, Rompe JD (1999) Shockwave therapy for tennis and golfer's elbow - 1 year follow-up. Arch Orthop Trauma Surg 119:62-66
17. Kuehl Jr FA, Egan RW (1980) Prostaglandins, arachidonic acid, and inflammation. Science 210:978-984
18. Levine JD, Clark R, Devor M, Helms C, Moskowitz MA, Basbaum AI (1984) Intraneuronal substance P contributes to the severity of treated arthritis. Science 226:547-549
19. Loew M, Daecke W, Kusnierczak D, Rahmanzadeh M, Ewerbeck V (1999) Shockwave therapy is effective for chronic calcifying tendinitis of the shoulder. J Bone Joint Surg 81B:863-867
20. Maier M, Ueberle F, Rupprecht G (1998) Physical parameters of extracorporeal shockwaves. Biomed Tech 43:269-274

21. Maier M, Staupendahl D, Duerr HR, Refior HJ (1999) Castor-oil decreases pain during extracorporeal shockwave application. Arch Orthop Trauma Surg 119:423-427
22. Maier M, Stäbler A, Lienemann A, Kohler S, Feitenhansl A, Durr HR, Pfahler M, Refior HJ (2000) Shockwave application in calcifying tendinitis of the shoulder: Prediction of outcome by imaging? Arch Orthop Trauma Surg 120:493-498
23. Maier M, Steinborn M, Schmitz C, Stabler A, Kohler S, Pfahler M, Durr HR, Refior HJ (2000) Extracorporeal shockwave application for chronic plantar fasciitis associated with heel spurs: Prediction of outcome by imaging. J Rheumatol 27:2455-2462
24. Malcangio M, Bowery NG (1999) Peptide autoreceptors: Does an autoreceptor for substance P exist? Trends Pharmacol Sci 20:405-407
25. Melzack R (1994) Folk Medicine and the Sensory Modulation of Pain. In: Wall PD, Melzack R (Hrsg) Textbook of Pain. Churchill Livingstone, Edinburgh, S 1209-1217
26. Rains C, Bryson HM (1995) Topical capsaicin. A review of its pharmacological properties and therapeutic potential in post-herpetic neuralgia, diabetic neuropathy and osteoarthritis. Drugs Aging 7:317-328
27. Rompe JD, Bohl J, Riehle HM, Schwitalle M, Krischek O (1998) Evaluating the risk of sciatic nerve damage in the rabbit by administration of low and intermediate energy extracorporeal shockwaves. Z Orthop Ihre Grenzgeb 136:407-411
28. Rompe JD, Hopf C, Kullmer K, Heine J, Burger R (1996) Analgesic effect of extracorporeal shockwave therapy on chronic tennis elbow. J Bone Joint Surg 78B:233-237
29. Rompe JD, Hopf C, Nafe B, Burger R (1996) Low-energy extracorporeal shockwave therapy for painful heel: A prospective controlled single-blind study. Arch Orthop Trauma Surg 115:75-91
30. Rompe JD, Kirkpatrick CJ, Kullmer K, Schwitalle M, Krischek O (1998) Dose-related effects of shockwaves on rabbit tendo Achillis. J Bone Joint Surg 80B:546-552
31. Ruocco I, Cuello AC, Ribeiro-Da-Silva A (2000) Peripheral nerve injury leads to the establishment of a novel pattern of sympathetic fibre innervation in the rat skin. J Comp Neurol 422:287-296
32. Sauer SK, Bove GM, Averbeck B, Reeh PW (1999) Rat peripheral nerve components release calcitonin gene-related peptide and prostaglandin E2 in response to noxious stimuli: Evidence that nervi nervorum are nociceptors. Neuroscience 92:319-325
33. Schelling G, Delius M, Gschwender M, Grafe P, Gambihler S (1994) Extracorporeal shockwaves stimulate frog sciatic nerves indirectly via a cavitation-mediated mechanism. Biophysical J 66:133-140
34. Seil R, Rupp S, Hammer DS, Ensslin S, Gebhardt T, Kohn D (1999) Extracorporeal shockwave therapy in the treatment of chronically painfull calcifying tendinitis: Comparision of two treatment protocolls. Z Orthop Ihre Grenzgeb 137:310-315
35. Simone DA, Nolano M, Johnson T, Wendelschafer-Crabb G, Kennedy WR (1998) Intradermal injection of capsaicin in humans produces degeneration and subsequent reinnervation of epidermal nerve fibers: Correlation with sensory function. J Neurosci 18:8947-8959Shih C, Bernard GW (1997) Neurogenic substance P stimulates osteogenesis in vitro. Peptides 18:323-32
36. Smits GA, Jap PH, Heerschap A, Oosterhof GO, Debruyne FM, Schalken JA (1993) Biological effects of high energy shockwaves in mouse skeletal muscle: Correlation between 31P magnetic resonance spectroscopic and microscopic alterations. Ultrasound Med Biol 19:399-409
37. Snijdelaar DG, Dirksen R, Slappendel R, Crul BJ (2000) Substance P. Eur J Pain 4:121-135

38. Ueberle F (1997) Shockwave Technology. In: Siebert W, Buch M (Hrsg) Extracorporeal Shockwaves in Orthopaedics. Springer, Berlin, 59-87
39. Zochodne DW (1993) Epineurial peptides: A role in neuropathic pain? Can J Neurol Sci 20:69-72

5

Biological Mechanism of Musculoskeletal Shockwaves

Ching-Jen Wang, MD,[1] Feng-Sheng Wang, PhD,[2] Kuender D. Yang, MD, PhD[2]

Abstract

These studies were performed to investigate the biological mechanism of musculoskeletal shockwaves. The investigations were independently performed in tendon, bone and tendon-bone interface in rabbits. The study limbs were treated with shockwaves, whereas the control limbs received sham treatment. The evaluations included histomorphological examination, biomechanical study and immunohistochemical assessments of angiogenic growth indicators including endothelial nitric oxide synthase (eNOS), vessel endothelial growth factor (VEGF), bone morphological protein (BMP-2) and proliferating cell nuclear antigen (PCNA). The results showed that shockwave treatment significantly stimulated the ingrowth of neovascularization associated with increased expressions of angiogenic growth indicators in tendon, bone and tendon-bone interface as compared with the control. The shockwave group also showed higher bone strength and better bonding between tendon and bone at tendon-bone interface. The effects of shockwaves appeared to be time-dependent as well as being dose-dependent. In conclusion, extracorporeal shockwaves produced consistent biological responses in tendon, bone and tendon-bone interface. The biological mechanism of musculoskeletal shockwaves appeared to stimulate the expression of angiogenic growth factors and the ingrowth of neovascularization. Neovascularization may play a role in the improvement of blood supply and healing of tendon and bone.

---

[1] The Department of Orthopedic Surgery, Chang Gung Memorial Hospital at Kaohsiung Taiwan
[2] Medical Research Chang Gung Memorial Hospital at Kaohsiung Taiwan

Introduction

In clinical application, extracorporeal shockwave has been shown to be effective in the treatment of certain orthopedic conditions including non-union of long bone fracture [1, 2, 3, 4], calcifying tendonitis of the shoulder [5, 6, 7, 8, 9], lateral epicondylitis of the elbow [10, 11, 12, 13], proximal plantar fasciitis [14, 15, 16] and Achilles tendonitis[17]. In an animal experiment, shockwave also showed a positive effect in promoting bone healing[18, 19, 20, 21]. However, the exact mechanism of shockwaves in the musculoskeletal system remains unknown. The results of animal experiments showed that shockwave treatment induced neovascularization at the tendon-bone junction[22, 23]. We hypothesized that physical shockwaves might induce biological responses that lead to healing of tendons and bone. The purposes of the study were to investigate the biological responses of shockwaves in musculoskeletal tissues including tendon, bone and tendon-bone interface and to elucidate the biological mechanism of musculoskeletal shockwaves.

Materials and Methods

The Institutional Review Board of our hospital had approved these studies. These studies were performed under the guidelines for the care and use of animals in research. The investigations were independently performed in tendon, bone and tendon-bone interface in rabbits.

1. Experimental study in tendon

Fifty New Zealand white rabbits, 12 months old with body weight ranging from 2.5 to 3.5 Kg, were used in this study. The right limbs (study side) received shockwave treatment to the Achilles tendon near the insertion to the heel bone, while the left limbs (control side) received sham treatment with no shockwaves. The source of shockwave was from an electrohydraulic OssaTron device (High Medical Technology, Kreuzlingen, Switzerland). The shockwave tube was focused on the Achilles tendon near the insertion, and the depth of the treatment was determined with the control guide of the machine and confirmed with C-arm image. Each of the study limbs received a single treatment of shockwave with 500 impulses at 14 kV (equivalent to 0.18 mJ/mm2). The shockwave dosage so selected was based on our previous experiences in animal studies[21, 22, 23]. The sham treatment was performed on the left limbs (control side) using a dummy electrode that did not generate acoustic waves with the impulses.

Histomorphological Examination

Biopsies of the Achilles tendon-bone unit were performed at 0, 1, 4, 8 and 12 weeks with 10 rabbits for each time interval with the first biopsy obtained 24 hours after shockwave application. The decalcified specimens were sectioned and stained with hematoxylin-eosin stain. The histomorphology and the number of new blood vessels including capillary and muscularized vessel were examined microscopically.

Immunohistochemistry Analysis

The angiogenic markers, including vessel endothelial growth factor (VEGF) and endothelial nitric oxide synthase (eNOS), were examined to confirm neovascularization. Proliferating cell nuclear antigen (PCNA) was examined to reflect endothelial cell proliferation with immunohistochemistry stains[24, 25, 26]. The vessels showing positive VEGF expression and cells displaying positive PCNA and eNOS expressions were counted microscopically and the numbers of cells and tissues with positive expression were quantitatively assessed.

Results of Biological Response in Tendon

The results of eNOS, VEGF and PCNA expressions and the number of neo-vessels of the study and the control sides are summarized in Table 1. In the study side, a significant increase of neo-vessels was noted in 4 to 12 weeks, whereas no increase of neo-vessels was noted in the control side, and the difference was statistically significant. It appeared that the ingrowth of neo-vessels after shockwave treatment was time dependent. In the study side, significant increases of eNOS, VEGF and PCNA were noted in as early as one week and lasted for 8 weeks before they declined to normal at 12 weeks, except the PCNA increase which lasted until 12 weeks (Figure 1). In the control side, however, no significant changes in eNOS, VEGF and PCNA expressions were noted, and the differences between the study and control sides were statistically significant. It appeared that shockwaves stimulated the early release of eNOS, VEGF and PCNA expressions, and subsequent ingrowth of neo-vessels and improvement in blood supply.

Time	Growth indicator	Control (N=50) Mean ±SD	Shockwave (N=50) Mean ±SD	P-value
0- week (N=10)	eNOS	112±19	104±21	0.57
	VEGF	14±3	12±4	0.94
	PCNA	145±21	132±24	0.75
	Neo-vessel	22±3	24±4	0.93
1-week (N=10)	eNOS	124±21	293±31	<0.001
	VEGF	17±4	33±5	0.0068
	PCNA	155±37	332±28	0.021
	Neo-vessel	24±4	26±5	0.95
4-week (N=10)	eNOS	131±24	344±32	<0.001
	VEGF	14±5	36±6	0.0018
	PCNA	167±33	320±32	0.011
	Neo-vessel	22±5	42±4	0.024
8-week (N=10)	eNOS	138±26	265±45	0.016
	VEGF	15±4	28±4	0.034
	PCNA	167±33	312±36	0.024
	Neo-vessel	24±5	40±5	0.021
12-week (N=10)	eNOS	136±21	189±42	0.71
	VEGF	17±5	16±4	0.84
	PCNA	154±21	280±28	0.034
	Neo-vessel	25±6	42±4	0.017

Table 1. The results of eNOS, VEGF and PCNA expression and the number of neo-vessels in tendon[23].

2. Experimental study in bone

Twenty-four New Zealand white rabbits,12 months old with body weight ranging from 2.7 kg to 3.6 kg, were used in this study. A 1.5 mm Kirschner pin was inserted retrograde into the canal of the femur through a mini-arthrotomy of the knee. A closed fracture of the right femur was created with a three-point bend method and confirmed with radiographs. The rabbits were randomly divided into three groups with eight rabbits in each group. The first group (the control) received sham treatment with no shockwave. The second group received low-energy shockwave with 2000 impulses at 14 kV (equivalent to 0.18 mJ/mm2 energy flux density). The third group received high-energy shockwave with 4000

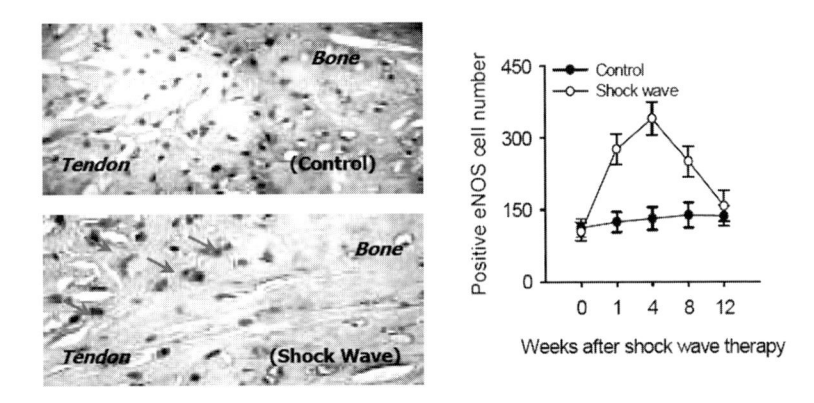

Figure 1a. Number of eNOS released after ESWT.

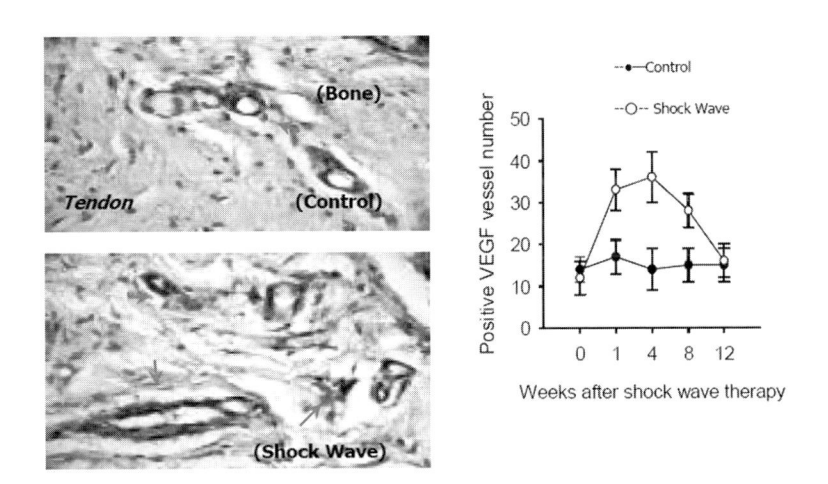

Figure 1b. Number of VEGF released after ESWT.
In the study group, significant increases of eNOS, VEGF and PCNA noted in as early as one week and lasted for 8 weeks before they declined to normal at 12 weeks, except PCNA increase lasted until 12 weeks on immunohistochemical stains. In the control side, however, no significant changes in eNOS, VEGF and PCNA expressions were noted, and the differences between the study and control sides were statistically significant[23].

impulses at 14 KV. How is there a difference in energy if it is the same energy flux density with different numbers of impulses? Shockwaves were applied one week after the operation when the surgical wounds had healed. The location of the fracture site and the depth of the treatment were confirmed with the control guide of the machine and C-arm imaging. The sham treatment was performed with a dummy electrode that did not generate acoustic waves with the impulses.

Radiographs of the right femur in AP and lateral views were performed at 1, 4, 8 and 12 weeks. The fracture healing was evaluated with clinical assessment and confirmed with radiographic examination.

Biomechanical Examination

The animals were sacrificed at 12 weeks, and a 5-cm long femur bone including the callus was harvested. The specimens were subject to biomechanical testing on Material Testing System (MTS, Minneapolis, MN) including peak load, peak stress and modulus of elasticity. The biomechanical testing was similarly performed in the high-energy, low-energy and control groups.

Histomorphological Examination

After biomechanical testing, the specimens were decalcified and sectioned and subjected to hematoxylin-eosin, alcian blue or alizarin red stains (Sigma Chemicals Inc, St. Louis, MO) for the purpose of distinguishing fibrous tissue, cartilaginous and bony tissues within the region of interest.

Immunohistochemical Examination

The angiogenic activities including eNOS, VEGF, BMP-2 and PCNA were examined with immunohistochemistry stains for verification of neo-vessels. The specimens were immunostained for eNOS, VEGF, BMP-2 and PCNA (Santa Cruz Biotechnolog Inc, Santa Cruz, CA). An antibody against von Willebrand factor (vWF) was used to identify the immunolocalization of neo-vessels in the fracture sites. The number of positive immuno-labeled cells and total cells in each area were counted and the percentage of positive labeled cells were calculated.

Tendon   **(Shockwave)**

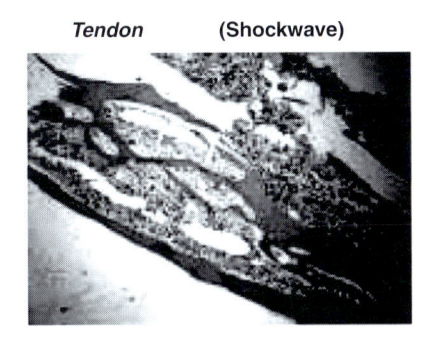

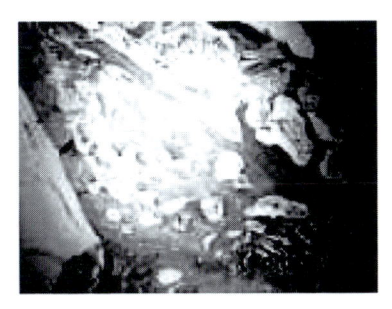

Figure 2. The histomorphological features. Histomorphology showed that high-energy shockwaves produced significantly more cortical bone, less fibrous tissue and comparable woven bone than the control and low-energy shockwaves[39].

Results of Biological Response in Bone

The histomorphological features showed that high-energy shockwaves produced significantly more cortical bone, less fibrous tissue and comparable woven bone than the control and low-energy shockwaves (Figure 2). The results of low-energy shockwave did not differ significantly from the control group.

The results of the biomechanical study showed that high-energy shockwaves demonstrated better bone strength including peak load, peak stress and modulus of elasticity than low-energy shockwave and the control (Figure 3). The low-energy shockwaves showed comparable results to the control.

The results of positive eNOS, BMP-2, VEGF and PCNA immunostained cells and the numbers of neo-vessels in the fracture sites of the control, low- and high-energy groups are summarized in Table 2. The numbers of neo-vessels and cells with positive eNOS, BMP-2, VEGF and PCNA expressions are significantly higher in the high-energy shockwave group than in the control and low-energy groups (Figure 4). The data of the low-energy group did not differ significantly from the control group. The biological effects of shockwaves appear to be dose-dependent.

3. Experimental study in tendon-bone interface

Thirty-six New Zealand white rabbits, 12 months old with body weight ranging from 2.79 Kg to 3.65 Kg, were used in this study. Arthrotomy of the knee was

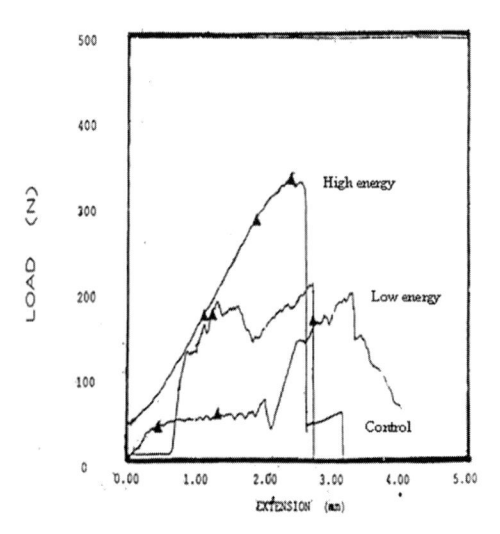

Figure 3. Results of the biomechanical study. Biomechanical testing showed that high-energy shockwaves demonstrated better bone strength including peak load, peak stress and modulus of elasticity than low-energy shockwaves and the control. The low-energy shockwaves showed comparable results to the control[39].

carried out and the anterior cruciate ligament (ACL) was excised. The long digital extensor tendon was dissected off distally at the musculotendinous junction while the proximal end was left intact. A tibia tunnel was created with a graft size-matched drill bit. The distal end of the graft was pulled through the tibia tunnel to complete ACL reconstruction.

Shockwave Application

The left knees received sham treatment with no shockwave, and were used as the control group. The right knees received shockwave treatment immediately after surgery, and were regarded as the study group. The shockwave tube was focused on the mid-portion of the tibia tunnel with the control guide of the device, and the depth was estimated clinically and determined with an ultrasound guide. Each knee was treated with 500 impulses of shockwaves at 14KV (equivalent to 0.18 mJ/mm^2) to the right knee. In sham treatment, a dummy electrode was used that generated no acoustic waves with the impulses.

Shockwaves	Control	Low-energy	High-energy
Neo-vessel and growth indicator	N = 8 Mean ±SD	N = 8 Mean ±SD	N = 8 Mean±SD
BMP-2	211±21	207±28	348±19
P-value 1		0.74	0.015
P-value 2			0.026
eNOS	179±16	192±18	272±21
P-value 1		0.89	0.026
P-value 2			0.014
VEGF	168±20	186±20	257±21
P-value 1		0.62	0.036
P-value 2			0.024
PCNA	196±26	213±18	306±21
P-value 1		0.87	< 0.01
P-value 2			0.017
Neo-vessels	37±10	43±12	78 ±17
P-value 1		0.72	0.012
P-value 2			0.006

Table 2. The results of positive eNOS, VEGF, BMP and PCNA immunostained cells and the number of neo-vessels in bone. The data were analyzed using a general linear model followed by a Duncan's multiple range test to determine the significance between treatments. (40x magnification)
P-values: Comparison of the control with the shockwave side was based on Mann-Whitney test. (40x magnification)
P-value 1: comparison of the control with low- and high-energy groups.
P-value 2: comparison of low-energy with high-energy groups.

Histomorphological Studies

Twenty-four rabbits were sacrificed at different time intervals with 4 rabbits each at 1, 2, 4, 8, 12 and 24 weeks. The central portion of the proximal tibia including the tendon graft was harvested. The specimens were decalcified, sectioned and stained with hematoxylin-eosin stain. The distribution of the tissues surrounding the tendon graft and the bonding of trabecular bone to tendon were examined microscopically.

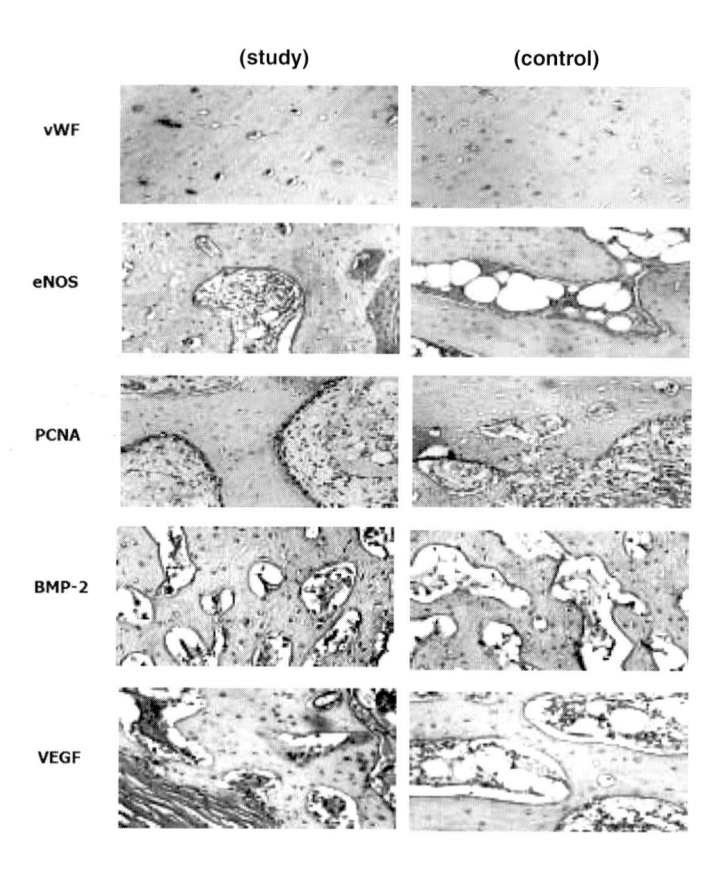

Figure 4. The results of positive eNOs, VEGF, BMP and PCNA immunostained cells and number of neo-vessels. The numbers of neo-vessels and cells with positive eNOS, BMP-2, VEGF and PCNA expressions are significantly higher in the high-energy shockwave group than the control group.

Biomechanical Examination

The remaining twelve rabbits were sacrificed at 12 and 24 weeks with 6 rabbits at each time interval. The ligament structures of the knee were removed and only the ACL graft was retained. The tensile strength of the graft was measured with a load distraction curve on Material Testing Machine (MTS, Minneapolis, MN). The pullout strength, the failure load and the modes of failure were analyzed.

Immunohistochemical Examination

The decalcified specimens were cut into sections in longitudinal and axial directions. Sections were immunostained for eNOS, VEGF, BMP-2 and PCNA (Santa Cruz Biotechnolog Inc., Santa Cruz, CA) for the purpose of identifying angiogenic growth indicators. An antibody against von Willebrand factor (vWF) was used to identify the immunolocalization of neo-vessels. The numbers with positive expression were quantitatively assessed.

Results of Biological Response in Tendon-Bone Interface

The trabecular bone in the surrounding tissues of the tendon graft increased significantly with time in the study group ($P < 0.05$), whereas, the changes in the control group were statistically not significant ($P > 0.05$). The difference in the amount of trabecular bone around the tendon graft between the study and control groups was statistically significant after 4 weeks. The bonding between tendon and bone was much more intimate in the study group than the control group, and the difference in the percentage of bonding between tendon and bone was statistically significant between the study and control groups ($P < 0.05$) (Figure 5).

The biomechanical testing showed that higher tensile strength and better pullout failure were noted in the shockwave group than the control group (Figure 6).

The results of eNOS, VEGF-A, PCNA and BMP-2 expressions and the number of neo-vessels in the tendon-bone interface at different time intervals are summarized in Table 3. The numbers of neo-vessels and the cells with positive immunostaining are significantly higher in the shockwave group than the control group, and the difference was statistically significant at different time intervals (Figure 7).

Discussion

Some authors speculated that shockwaves relieve pain in insertional tendinopathy by hyper-stimulation analgesia [28], while others hypothesized the theoretical mechanism of shockwaves in bone healing including micro-disruption of

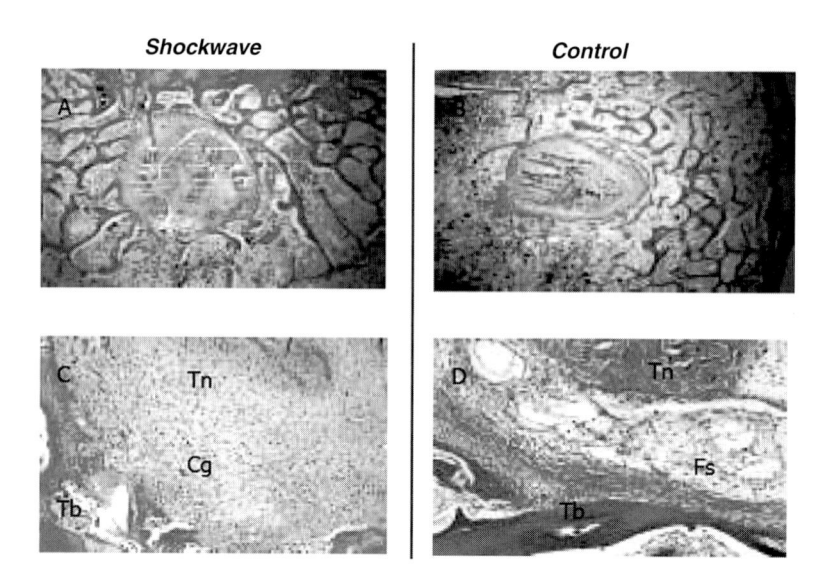

Figure 5. Bonding between tendon and bone. The trabecular bone surrounding the tendon graft increased significantly in the shockwave group as compared with the control group. The bonding between tendon and bone was much more intimate in the study group than the control [37].

avascular or minimally vascular tissue to encourage revascularization and the recruitment of appropriate stem cells conductive to bone healing. [27, 28] However, there are insufficient data to scientifically substantiate either theory concerning the mechanism of shockwaves in the musculoskeletal system. Many recent studies in animals demonstrated the modulations of shockwave treatment including neovascularization, osteogenic differentiation of mesenchymal stem cell and local release of osteogenic and angiogenic growth factors. [22, 23, 29-37] Therefore, extracorporeal shockwaves produced a regenerative or tissue-repairing effect in musculoskeletal tissues, not merely a mechanical disintegrative effect as generally assumed.

Many studies demonstrated that over-expression of eNOS and VEGF induced angiogenesis. [24, 25] The results of the current studies demonstrated for the first time that mechanical shockwaves stimulated the ingrowth of neovascularization associated with early expression of angiogenic markers including eNOS, VEGF and PCNA in tendon, bone and tendon-bone interface.

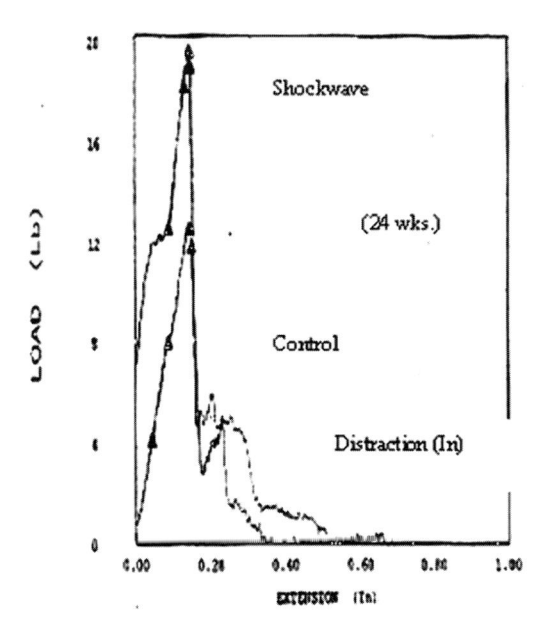

Figure 6. Biomechanical testing. Biomechanical testing showed higher tensile strength and better pull-out failure load in the shockwave group than in the control group [37].

Rompe et al. [38] reported a dose related effect of shockwave on rabbit Achilles tendon. Wang et al. [39] demonstrated that shockwave treatment showed dose-dependent enhancement of bone mass and bone strength after fracture of the femur. The results of these studies showed that the effect of shockwave treatment in musculoskeletal tissues appeared to be time-dependent as well as being dose-dependant. Neovascularization may play a role to improve blood supply and healing of tendon and bone. Therefore, it seemed likely that physical shockwaves raise the mechanotransduction and convert into biological signals that lead to a cascade of biological responses in tendon, bone and tendon-bone interface (Figure 8).

Conclusion

The biological mechanism of musculoskeletal shockwaves appeared to stimulate the release of angiogenic growth factors, and the ingrowth of neovascularization

Time	Growth indicator	Shockwave Mean±SD	Control Mean±SD	P-value
1-week (N=3)	eNOS	256±21	112±18	<0.001
	VEGF-A	246±36	228±25	0.82
	PCNA	122±15	123±17	0.63
	BMP-2	89±11	94±13	0.58
	Neo-vessels	47±9	41±2	0.534
2-weeks (N=3)	eNOS	224±24	106±18	0.006
	VEGF-A	389±42	254±27	0.014
	PCNA	234±21±	138±19	0.023
	BMP-2	143±22	98±17	0.014
	Neo-vessels	53±12	46±13	0.619
4-weeks (N=3)	eNOS	202±20	108±21	0.016
	VEGF-A	432±41	268±32	0.002
	PCNA	278±26	143±21	0.016
	BMP-2	184±24	104±16	0.007
	Neo-vessels	82±14	52±11	0.017
8-weeks (N=3)	eNOS	142±18	122±25	0.14
	VEGF-A	452±37	276±28	0.004
	PCNA	316±23	149±19	0.022
	BMP-2	212±21	98±15	<0.001
	Neo-vessels	93±15	47±9	<0.01
12-weeks (N=6)	eNOS	123±19	108±23	0.57
	VEGF	463±26	284±26	0.013
	PCNA	308±21	158±25	0.017
	BMP-2	168±24	106±18	0.023
	Neo-vessels	87±14	44±12	0.0085
24-weeks (N=6)	eNOS	132±23	98±19	0.68
	VEGF	476±31	271±25	<0.001
	PCNA	312±28	154±17	<0.001
	BMP-2	152±27	115±16	0.026
	Neo-vessels	86±12	47±12	0.0046

P-values were based on Mann-Whitney test. (40x magnification)
Table 3. The results of eNOS, VEGF-A, PCNA and BMP-2 expressions and the number of neo-vessels in tendon-bone interface.

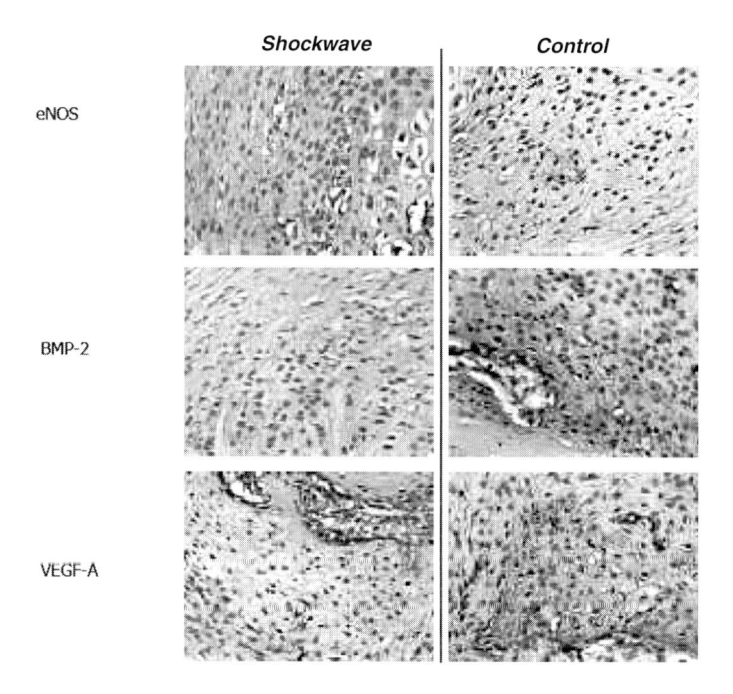

Figure 7. The results of positive eNOS, VEGF-A, PCNA and BMP-2 immunostained cells and number of neo-vessels. The numbers of cells with positive immunostain for eNOS, BMP-2 and VEGF-A at the tendon-bone interface are significantly higher in the shockwave group than the control group [37].

and improvement in blood supply leading to repair of tendon and bone. Musculoskeletal shockwaves produced consistent biological responses in tendon, bone and tendon-bone interface. In contrast to lithotripsy where shockwaves are used to disintegrate urolithiasis, shockwaves are not being used to disintegrate tissues in orthotripsy, but rather to microscopically cause interstitial and extracellular biological responses and tissue regeneration.

Acknowledgement

These studies were partially or totally supported by grants. The sources of grants are from Chang Gung Research Fund (CMRP 83001) and National Science Council (NSC91-2314-B-182A-068). No fund was received or will be received from a commercial party directly or indirectly related to the subjects of this article.

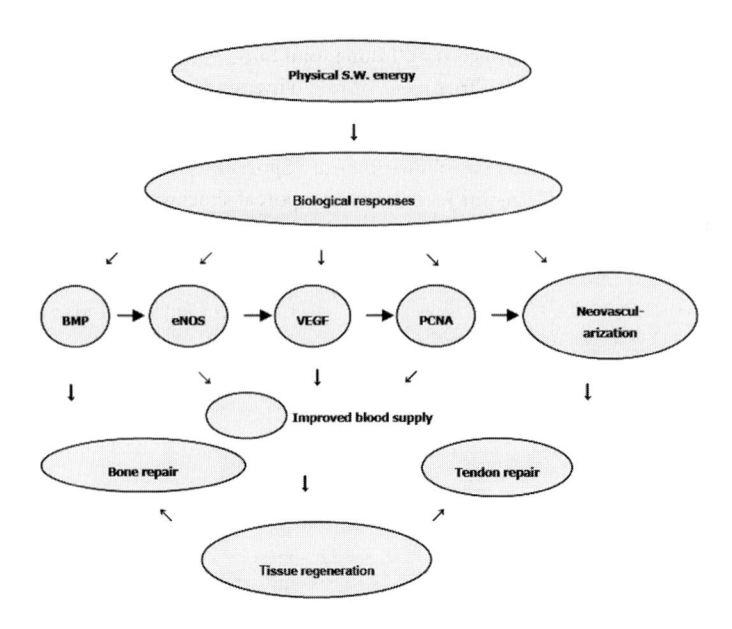

Figure 8. Biological responses to shockwaves. A proposed cascade of biological mechanism of extracorporeal shockwaves in musculoskeletal tissues.

The authors would like to thank Ya-Zu Yang, Yi-Chi Sun and Ya-Hsieh Chuang for their technical assistances and collection of data in the studies.

Literature

1. Haupt G. Use of extracorporeal shockwave therapy in the treatment of pseudoarthrodesis, tendinopathy and orthopaedic disease. J Urology 1997; 158:4-11.
2. Rompe JD, Rosendahl T, Schöllner C, et al. High-energy extracorporeal shockwave treatment of nonunions. Clin Orthop 2001; 387: 102-111.
3. Schaden W, Fischer A and Sailler A. Extracorporeal shockwave therapy of nonunion or delayed osseous union. Clin Orthop 2001; 387: 90-94.
4. Wang CJ, Chen HS, Chen CE, et al. Treatment of nonunions of long bone fractures with shockwaves. Clin Orthop 2001; 387: 95-101.
5. Loew M, Daecke W, Kuznierczak D, et al. Shockwave therapy is effective for chronic calcifying tendonitis of the shoulder. J Bone Joint Surg 1999; 81B: 863-867.
6. Rompe JD, Rumler F, Hopf C, et al. Extracorporeal shockwave therapy for calcifying tendinitis of the shoulder. Clin Orthop 1995; 321:196-201.

7. Speed CA, Richards C, Nichols D, Burnet S, Wiles JT, Humphrey H, Hazlemann BL. Extracorporeal shockwave therapy for tendonitis of the rotator cuff. A double-blind, randomized, controlled trial. J Bone Joint Surg. (Br) 2002; 84: 509-12
8. Wang CJ, Ko JY, Chen HS. Treatment of calcifying tendonitis of the shoulder with shockwave therapy. Clin Orthop 2001;387: 83-89.
9. Wang CJ, Yang KD, Wang FS. Shockwave therapy for calcifying tendinitis of the shoulder. A two- to four-year follow-up. Am J Sports Med 2003; 31(3):425-30.
10. Hammer DS, Rupp S, Ensslin S, et al. Extracorporeal shockwave therapy in patients with tennis elbow and painful heel. Arch Orthop Trauma Surg 2000; 120:304-307.
11. Ko JY, Chen HS, Chen LM. Treatment of lateral epicondylitis of the elbow with shockwaves. Clin Orthop 2001; 387: 60-67.
12. Rompe JD, Hopf C, Kullmer K, et al. Analgesic effect of extracorporeal shockwave therapy on chronic tennis elbow, J Bone Joint Surg 1996; 78B: 233-237.
13. Speed CA, Nichols D, Richards C, Humphrey SH, Wiles JT, Burnet S, Hazlemann BL. Extracorporeal shockwave therapy for lateral epicondylitis – a double-blind, randomized, controlled trial. J Orthop Res. 2002; 20: 895-8.
14. Chen HS, Chen LM, Huang TW. Treatment of painful heel syndrome with shockwaves. Clin Orthop 2001; 387: 41-46.
15. Ogden JA, Alvarez R, Levitt R, et al. Shockwave therapy for chronic proximal plantar fasciitis. Clin Orthop 2001; 387:47-59.
16. Rompe JD, Hopf C, Nafe B, et al. Low-energy extracorporeal shockwave therapy for painful heel. A prospective controlled single-blind study. Arch Orthop Trauma Surg 1996; 115:75-79.
17. Perlick L, Schifmann R, Kraft CN, Wallny T, Diedrich O. Extracorporeal shockwave treatment of the Achilles tendonitis: Experimental and preliminary clinical results. Z Orthop Ihre Grenzgeb 2002; 140(3): 275-80.
18. Delius M, Draenert K, Al Diek Y, et al. Biological effect of shockwave: In vivo effect of high-energy pulses on rabbit bone. Ultrasound Med Biol 1995; 21:1219-1225.
19. Johannes EJ, Kaulesar-Sukul DM, Metura E, et al. High-energy shockwaves for the treatment of nonunions: An experiment on dogs. J Surg Res 1994; 57:246-254.
20. Kaulesar Sukul DM. Johannes EJ. Pierik EG. van Eijck GJ. Kristelijn MJ. The effect of high-energy shockwaves focused on cortical bone: An in vitro study. J Surg Res 1993; 54: 46-51.
21. Wang CJ, Huang HY, Chen HH, et al. Effect of shockwave therapy on acute fractures of the tibia. A study in a dog model. Clin Orthop 2001;387: 112-118.
22. Wang CJ, Huang HY, Pai CH: Shockwave therapy enhanced neovascularization at the tendon-bond junction: an experiment in dogs. J Foot Ankle Surg 2002; 41: 16-22.
23. Wang CJ, Yang KD, Wang FS, Huang CC, Yang LJ. Shockwave induces neovascularization at the tendon-bone junction. A study in rabbits. J Orthop Res 2003; 21:984-989.
24. Babaei S, Stewart DJ. Overexpression of endothelial NO synthase induces angiogenesis in a co-culture model. Cardiovascular Res. 2002; 55: 190-200.
25. Spyridopoulos I, Luedeman C, Chen D, Kearney M, Murohara T, Principe N, Isner M, Losordo DW. Divergence of angiogenesis and vascular permeability signaling by VEGF: inhibition of protein kinase C suppresses VEGF-induced angiogenesis, but promotes VEGF-induced NO-dependent vascular permeability. Arteriosclero, Thrombo and Vas Biol 2002; 22: 901-6.
26. Nagashima M, Tanaka H, Takahashi A, Tanaka K, Ishiwata T, Asano G, Yoshino S. Study of the mechanism involved in angiogenesis and synovial cell proliferation in

human synovial tissues of patients with rheumatoid arthritis using SCID mice. Lab Invest 2002; 82(8): 981-8.
27. Ogden JA, Toth-Kischkat A, Schultheiss R. Principles of shockwave therapy. Clin Orthop 2001; 387: 8-17.
28. Thiel M: Application of shockwaves in medicine. Clin Orthop 2001; 387: 18-21.
29. McCormack D, Lane H, McElwain J. The osteogenic potential of extracorporeal shockwave therapy: An in-vivo study. Ir J Med Sci 1996; 165:20-22.
30. Maier M, Milz S, Wirtz DC, Rompe JD, Schmitz C. Basic research of applying extracorporeal shockwaves on the musculoskeletal system. An assessment of current status. Orthop 2002; 31: 667-77.
31. McCormack D, Lane H, McElwain J. The osteogenic potential of extracorporeal shockwave therapy: An in vivo study. Irish J Med Sci 1996; 165: 20-22.
32. Wang FS, Wang CJ, Sheen-Chen SM et al. Superoxide mediates shockwave induction of RRK-dependent osteogenic transcription factor (CBFA 1) and mesenchymal cells differentiation toward osteoprogenitors. J Biol Chem 2002; 277: 10931-7
33. Wang FS, Yang KD, Wang CJ, et al. Extracorporeal shockwave promotes bone marrow stromal cell growth and differentiation toward osteoprogenitors associated with TGF-b 1 induction. J Bone Joint Surg 2002; 84B: 457-61.
34. Wang FS, Wang CJ, Huang HC, et al. Physical shockwave mediates membrane hyperpolarization and Ras activation for osteogenesis in human bone marrow stromal cells. Biochemical Biophysical Research Communications 2001; 287: 648-655.
35. Wang FS, Yang KD, Kuo YR, Wang CJ, Huang HJ, Chen YJ. Temporal and spatial expression of bone morphogenetic proteins in extracorporeal shockwave-promoted healing of fracture defect. Bone 2003; 32:387-396.
36. Yang C, Heston WDW, Gulati S, Fair WR. The effect of high-energy shockwaves (HESW) on human bone marrow. Urol Res 1988; 16:427-42.
37. Wang CJ, Wang FS, Yang KD, Weng LS, Sun YC, Yang YL. The effect of shockwave treatment at the tendon-bone interface – A histomorphological and biomechanical study in rabbits. J Orthop Res 2004 (In press).
38. Rompe JD, Kirkpatrick CJ, Küllmer K, et al. Dose related effects of shockwaves on rabbit tendon Achilles. A sonographic and histological study. J Bone Joint Surg 1998; 80B: 546-552.
39. Wang CJ, Yang KD, Wang FS, Hsu CC, Chen HS. Shockwave treatment shows dose-dependent enhancement of bone mass and bone strength after fracture of the femur. Bone 2004; 34:225-230.

6

Effects of ESWT on Bone Histological and Radiological Findings

Gerald Haupt

Introduction

Extracorporeal shockwaves have been successful in inducing osteoneogenesis in animal as well as human experiments[1]. The equipment necessary to generate such an effect is substantial. Underlying such medical shockwave research were pneumatically generated shockwaves. Initially, such shockwaves were produced by shooting a high-speed projectile to a metal plate[2]. The same principle was used in the Swiss DolorClast® System and is called radial shockwave therapy (rESWT). This study is to examine the effect of rESWT on the bone.

Material and Method

White New Zealand rabbits were chosen for the study with the Lithoclast (modified prototype) as a source of radial shockwaves. They were used already during earlier experiments as a model for bone regeneration. Shockwave therapies with extracorporeal shockwave units (HM3 and XL1) were conducted on this model, for example, at the Urological Clinic of Ruhr University Bochum [3], thus allowing for a direct comparison.

A total of 40 white New Zealand rabbits were used. The animals were maintained under standard laboratory conditions and fed with a standard diet (Altromin international, Lage, Germany). Water was available ad libitum. An accommodation period of at least one week was observed.

Group	Number	Survival Period (days)	Treatment Pressure (bar)	Impulses per Treatment Point
1	4	2	2,0	1000
2	4	14	1,8	1000
3	4	14	1,8	2000
4	4	2	3,0	2000
5	4	13	3,0	2000
6	4	19	4,0	2000
7	4	60	4,0	2000
8	4	2	4,0	3×2000
9	3*	14	4,0	3×2000
10	4	60	4,0	3×2000

* 1 animal died before the treatment 4 months following ovarectomy (see below)
Table 1. Treatment parameters and survival times

Two treatment areas were chosen: the left iliac crest and the left lower jaw at the mandibular angle. Treatments were mostly performed under general anesthesia with Ketanest 50 mg/kg bodyweight (Ketavet®, Parke-Davis, Berlin) and Xylazin 5 mg/kg bodyweight (Rompun®, Bayer, Leverkusen). Treatment parameters and survival times are summarized in Table 1. At the end of the experiment, the animals were sacrificed with T61 (embutramide and mebezoniumjodid, Hoechst, Bad Soden).

A macroscopic inspection followed. Skin, skeleton muscles and bones of both treatment areas were prepared histologically. The contralateral sides served as a control. A Formaline fixed evaluation was conducted (4%) and bones were decalcified with an Ossa-fix solution (formaldehyde 3%, zinc chloride 2%, Trichloracetic acid 10%, Distilled water Wilhelms-University, Münster). Coloration was fixed with hematoxylin-eosin (HE), Trichrom (Goldner) and according to Ladewig.

In Groups 8 to 10, an ovarectomy was conducted on both sides to induce osteoporosis. After 6 months, 3 treatment areas, located very close together on the lower jaw, received rESWT.

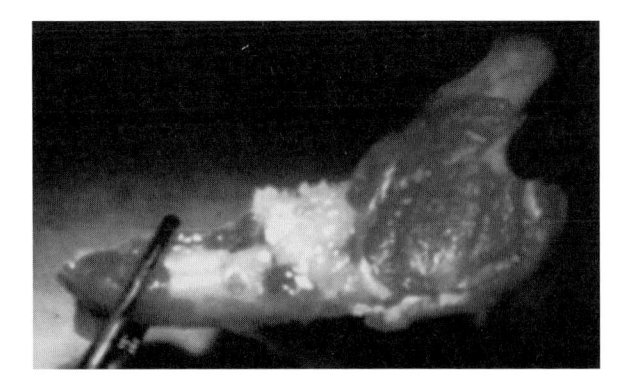

Figure 1. Lower jaw, 60 days after treatment with 2000 impulses at 4.0 bar, shows minor thickening of the compacta with light subperiostal bleeding.

Results

Postoperative findings

The treatment areas were inspected immediately at the end of the treatment, during the treatment and during biopsies of the animals.

At the end of rESWT treatment, we regularly found minor skin lesions caused by the applicator. Petechial bleeding or punch lesions of the skin were observed in 7 animals regardless of the chosen treatment parameters.

The postoperative clinical outcome was ordinary for all animals. Food absorption was not reduced for any animal.

Biopsy findings

Skin, skeletal muscles and bones were subjected to macroscopic inspection at autopsy. At this point in time (2 to 60 days after treatment), there was no evidence of change on the skin of any animal. In 3 animals, local hematomata were found in the muscles 2 days after the treatment. These were classified as minor. Later on, no muscular pathologies were found. No animal showed any macroscopic irregularities at the iliac crest. However, subperiostal bleeding occurred at the lower jaw in 6 animals from treatment groups receiving higher energies (Figure 1).

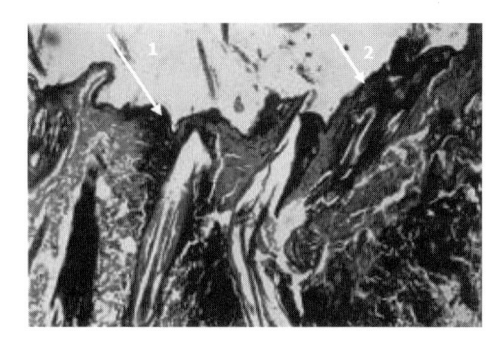

Figure 2. Skin, 2 days after treatment with 1000 impulses at 1.8 bar (Goldner, magnification 60x), shows moderate epithel degeneration (1) in addition to subcutaneous inflammatory infiltrates (2).

Histological results

After 2 days, focal degeneration of the epithel and immigration of inflammation cells are found (Figure 2).

An aseptic muscular inflammation was found as well. In addition, a few preparations showed hyaline degeneration with focal necrosis of muscle fibers (Figure 3). At later times, very few pathological changes in skin or muscles were found. These involve fibrotic processes such as scar formation.

Apart from mild hyperemia found 2 days after rESWT on the ilium in only 2 animals, no other histological changes were observed at any time.

In contrast, a wide spectrum of reactions was found on the lower jaw. They vary from normal histology to marked osteoneogenesis. The nature of the tissue reactions was dependent upon the time of the autopsy after treatment and the dose used. Contrary to expectations, no osteoporosis was found in animals with ovarectomy. Accordingly, all untreated lower jaws showed a normal appearance of compacta and spongiosa.

In 3 out of 12 animals, histological preparation of the treated lower jaw produced a normal microarchitecture 2 days after treatment. In all other animals, a hyperemia was found in the treatment area 2 days following treatment. In this

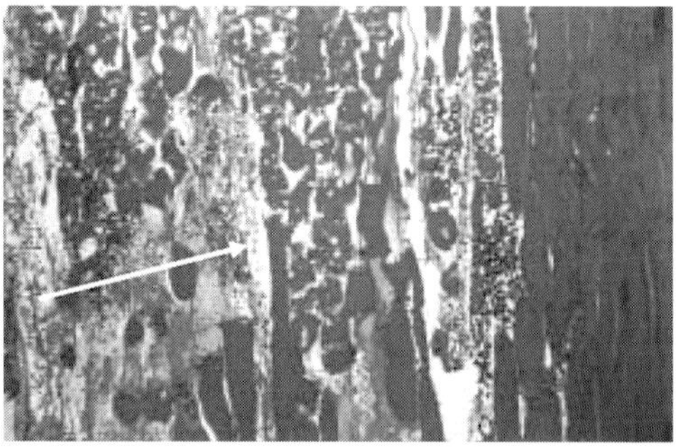

Figure 3. Skeletal muscles, 2 days after treatment with 1000 impulses at 1.8 bar (HE, magnification 60x), shows hyaline-cartilage degeneration (↗) of muscle fibers with initial reactive inflammatory infiltration.

regard, hyperemia occurred more frequently in animals treated with higher energies (Table 2). No other changes were found; trabeculae and osteocytes were intact (Figure 4).

The results are summarized in Table 2.

Group	Survival Period (days)	Treatment Pressure	Impulses	Hyperemia (n)	Osteoneo-genesis (n)
1	2	2,0	1000	2	-
2	14	1,8	1000	-	-
3	14	1,8	2000	-	-
4	2	3,0	2000	4	-
5	13	3,0	2000	3	3
6	19	4,0	2000	4	4
7	60	4,0	2000	2	2
8	2	4,0	3*2000	3	-
9	14	4,0	3*2000	2	2
10	60	4,0	3*2000	3	3

Tabel 2. Hyperemia and Osteoneogenesis.

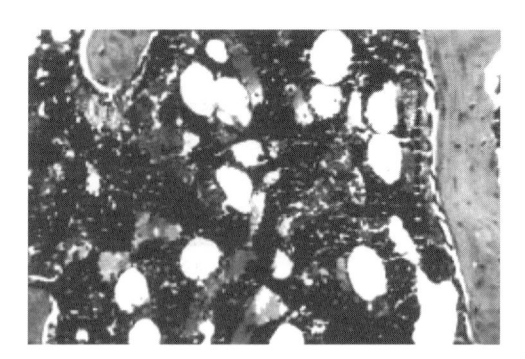

Figure. 4. Lower jaw, 2 days after treatment with 1000 impulses at 1.8 bar (Goldner, magnification 150x), shows intact osteocytes in the trabeculae and hyperemic sinus in bone marrow.

In other words, in the absence of any clear dependency on treatment pressure, hyperemia is the leading pathological-anatomic correlate after 2 days (Figure 5).

After 2 weeks, no difference was found at the lower jaws between those treated with 1000 impulses at 2.0 bar and control. However, all animals from Group 5 (3.0 bar) and 3 of 4 animals from Group 11 (4.0 bar) histologically showed endostal oestoneogeneration. Osteoide was formed appositionally on mature trabeculae and even completely new trabeculae (Figure 6). Apart from medular osteoneogenesis, additional osteoneogenesis was observed at the marrow side of the compacta. The transition of newly formed fiber to lamella bones may be smooth in this area (Figure 7).

With the chosen experimental setup, osteoneogenesis was induced only if treatment pressure was applied between 2 and 3 bar (Figure 8).

The animals surviving 60 days were treated with 4.0 bar. Four of them received treatments with 2000 impulses, the other 4 received three times 2000 impulses on adjacent treatment areas on the same side of the lower jaw. A normal microarchitecture of the lower jaw was found on the control side even among these animals with ovarectomies.

After 60 days, a massive generation of new bone was the major finding on the treatment side. The spongious vascular system was dilated and hyperemic. Osteoblast activity was increased with extended osteoid formation and restructuring of

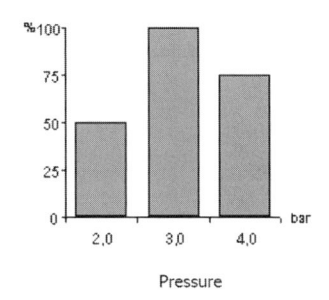

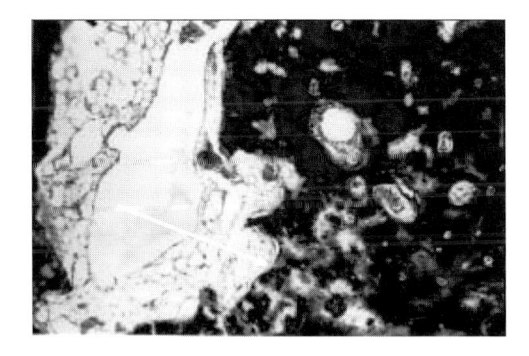

Figure 5. Hyperemia 2 days after treatment.

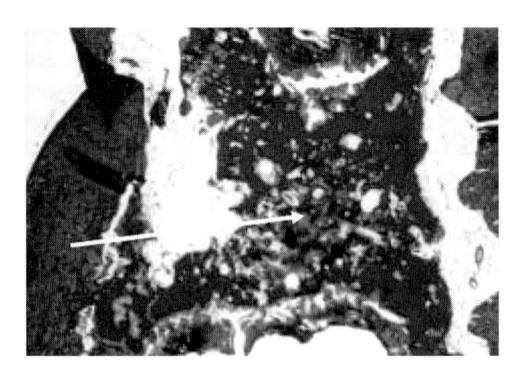

Figure 6. Lower jaw, 13 days after treatment with 2000 impulses at 3.0 bar (Ladewig, magnification 60x), shows medular neogenesis of bone tissue in treatment area as a result of higher dose with greater magnification and newly formed osteoid (↗)

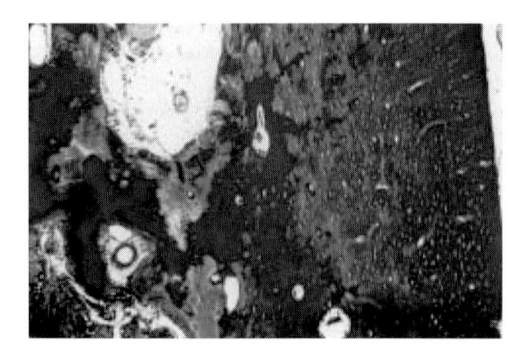

Figure 7. Lower jaw, 13 days after treatment with 2000 impulses at 3.0 bar (Ladewig, magnification 24x), shows greater degree of osteoneogenesis with smooth transition between the lamella bone of the compacta and the bone marrow on the treatment side.

of the microarchitecture (Figure 9). In part, osteoneogenesis was completed but there remain many active osteoblasts on the edge of newly formed bones that continued growing and elsewhere (Figure 10).

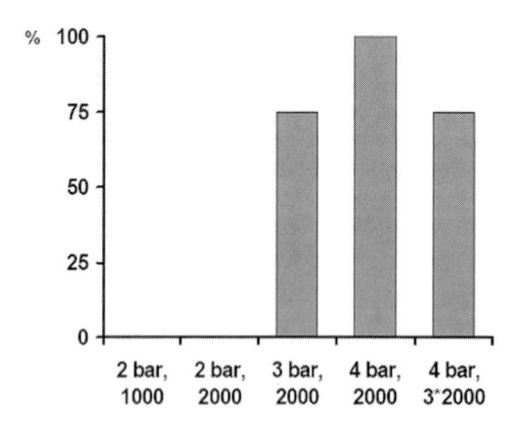

Figure 8. Percentage of animals with osteoneogenesis after 2 weeks depending on dose.

EFFECTS OF ESWT ON BONE   63

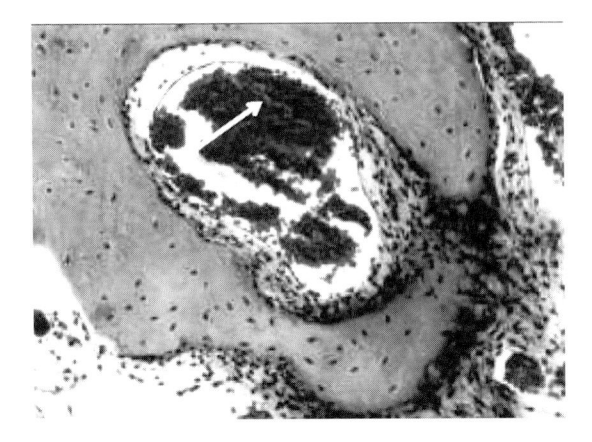

Figure 9. Lower jaw, 60 days after treatment with 2000 impulses at 4.0 bar (Goldner, magnification 150x), shows osseous consolidation of free trabecular endings with high osteoblast activity (↗) and hyperemic, dilated sinus (↗).

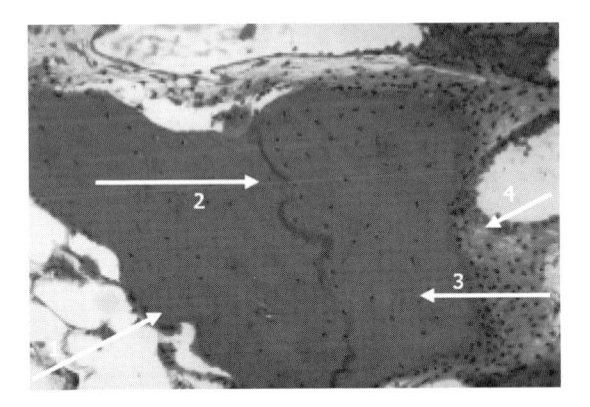

Figure 10. Lower jaw, 60 days after treatment with 2000 impulses at 4.0 bar (HE, magnification 150x), shows trabecular structure with inactive osteocytes (↗) through a clear conjunction line (↗) of newly formed trabecular bone with functional cellular core swelling of the osteocytes (↗) osteoblast activity as a sign of advancing osteoneogenesis (↗).

Discussion

Extracorporeal shockwaves were used in 1986 for stimulating healing processes rather than disintegrating calculi. At that time, various shockwave doses were applied to superficial skin wounds in pigs. In the process, a correlation with administered dose was found: low energies showed a stimulating effect but at high energy levels an inhibiting effect was found. In the model with delayed wound healing through preradiated skin, shockwaves increased the reepithelialization rate[4-6]. The osteogenetic potential of shockwaves was discovered with the experimental Dornier XL 1 lithotripter in the fracture model of rats. Radiological, histological and biochemical results showed a stimulation of fracture healing by shockwaves[7-9].

In terms of a wide availability of extracorporeal shockwaves, the need for substantial equipment - regardless of shockwave source - and the high costs are a disavantage. It is therefore desirable to develop an economical but equally effective process.

A radial shockwave system was used for this study. It is characterized by the absence of any parts subject to wear. The shockwave characteristic of the rESWT unit is different from that of various other extracorporeal shockwaves: the radial shockwave is delivered directly at the end of the applicator and loses intensity as it passes through tissue. In contrast, extracorporeal shockwaves develop their maximum energy density in one focus point and therefore gain intensity as the distance from the shockwave source increases. The effect of radial shockwaves on bone tissue was to be tested.

The rabbit was selected as the experimental animal for bone processes; this allowed us to make comparisons with studies conducted in our clinic with extracorporeal shockwaves[3]. Graff studied the effects of shockwaves traveling through tissue for the treatment of kidney and gall stones. He described only minor effects on skin and muscles. Even with the pneumatic system, macroscopic and histological results on skin and muscles showed minor side effects of the treatment only. After just 14 days a complete restitution had occurred. Local inflammation and bleeding correspond to the reactions to mild trauma [3] but without clinical relevance.

Even with intact bones, Graff found macroscopically small hematomata and petechial bleeding such as those following moderate trauma. Macroscopic fractures were not found. While hyperemia, bleedings and necrosis were found more frequently after 48 hours, aseptic necrosis of the bone marrow and osteocyte damage with hyperosteoneogenesis occurred 2 and 3 weeks after rESWT especially in animals treated with high energy. From an osteologic perspective, this involved a fracture healing process with multidirectional formation of new trabeculae without previous fracture[3, 10-12]. Graff's results were confirmed by Johannes[13]. The Municn Grosshadern study group found an energy-dependent osteoneogenetic effect as well, even outside the direct focus zone[24, 25].

A comparable course was found in lower jaw bones treated with radial shockwaves. After 2 days, hyperemia of different magnitude appeared. These were present in three quarters of the animals. All animals that had been treated at 3.0 or 4.0 bar, showed this reactive hyperemia. A mere one-fourth of the animals showed hyperemia at the ilium. Bone marrow necrosis, as described following extracorporeal shockwave therapy, was not observed. Instead, a beginning osteoneogenesis appeared of different magnitude depending on the applied energy.

Osteoneogenetic changes were also found in animals from the longer-surviving groups when high energies were used. In addition, up to 60 days after the treatment a large number of osteoblasts and osteoclasts were found in these animals. The osteoblasts still showed a high osteogenetic activity. Osteoclasts resorbed simultaneously overshooting newly formed trabecular bone. This morphologically points to overshooting osteoneogenesis, adapted to the physiological load. Therefore the effect of radial shockwaves on bony tissue (at least in rabbits) seems to be comparable to bony effects found after application of high energetic focused shockwaves, as described in the study on rabbit femur and tibia as a function of dose[14].

Another complication of extracorporeal shockwaves is the alteration of the epiphyseal plate. In 3 of 8 rats the application of 1500 shockwaves at 20 kV with the experimental Dornier XL1 lithotripter on the epiphyseal region showed an inhibition of longitudinal growth. In 8 animals the epiphysis was partly replaced by bone spikes[15]. A statement on the effect of radial shockwaves on the epiphysis cannot be made based on this study. However, similar effects are to be expected so that a therapy in this area is not advised.

No osteoneogenesis was found on the ilium and hyperemia in isolated cases. This was also found in a few studies about extracorporeal shockwave therapy.

With 1000 shockwaves at 18 kV (Dornier HM-3), no effect was found on the femur of rabbits[16]. No improved healing following shockwave therapy was found on standardized fibula osteotomies or tibia defects[17]. Both studies used lower energies. A lesser effect of radial shockwaves on the ilium compared to osteoneogenesis induced at the jaw may also result from lower energy application. The pelvis bone is largely covered by soft tissue. This buffer consisting of skin, muscle, nerves, vessels and collagen tissue attenuates the applied energy. Unlike the extracorporeal shockwave, the depth of penetration of the non-focused radial shockwave is limited to a short distance.

With shockwave induced extrusion of bone marrow the authors derived the risk of fat emboli[18]. This complication was never observed in clinical applications. None of the bones treated with radial shockwaves showed such an extrusion. When evaluating the shockwave effects on bone [14, 18, 19] the ex vivo model leads to results contradicting in vivo studies and has limited relevance. Wang observed a neovascularization following shockwave therapy on dogs and confirmed his finding with a higher number of new vessels as well as increased angiogenesis-associated markers such as eNOS, VEGF and PCNA in a study on rabbits.

The osteologic results on live rabbits cannot always be transferred to the situation in other mammals or humans. With extracorporeal shockwaves, however, experiments on larger animals showed similar results. In a pseudarthrosis model of dogs, 4 out of 5 animals were found with bony consolidation within 12 weeks but only one was found in the control group[20]. In a standardized fracture model on sheep, we observed increased end- and periostate osteogenesis as well as a significant transformation in laminar stable bones 4 and 7 weeks after extracorporeal shockwave therapy administered with a modified Dornier HM3[21-24].

A similar transferability could apply to osteologic results achieved with a radial shockwave unit in rabbits. This results in several potential applications for radial shockwaves[25]:

a) Induction of osteoneogenesis in diseases of bone degeneration (e.g. parodontitis)
b) Therapy for pseudarthrosis
c) Therapy for soft-tissue disorders

Conclusion

The local treatment with radial shockwaves leads to histological changes in treated areas. These are in part dose dependent. The effects are as follows:

A focal degeneration of the epithel and a focal infiltration of inflammation cells occur on the skin; furthermore, almost complete restitution occurs. Focal necrosis of muscle fibers and associated inflammatory reaction were also found but showed complete disappearance in course of time. While almost no effects are substantiated on the ilium, a medullary osteoneogenesis is induced on the lower jaw.

The verifiable morphological changes correspond to the effects of shockwave treatments on tissue. Osteoneogenesis is induced at the lower jaw bone. Such osteoneogenesis depends upon dose when high energy is used; in contrast, lower energy remains without effect. The absence of any effect at the ilium is explained by the shockwave attenuation due to the thick muscle layer.

Literature

1. Haupt, G., Extracorporeal shockwaves in the treatment of pseudarthrosis, tendinopathy and other orthopedic diseases. J. Urol., 1997. in press.
2. Chaussy, C., et al., The use of shockwaves for the destruction of renal calculi without direct contact. Urol. Res., 1976. 4: p. 175.
3. Graff, J., Die Wirkung hochenergetischer Stosswellen auf Knochen und Weichteilgewebe. 1989b, Bochum: Habilitationsschrift, Ruhr-Universität Bochum.
4. Haupt, G. and M. Chvapil, Effect of shockwaves on the healing of partial-thickness wounds in piglets. J. Surg. Res., 1990. 49: p. 45-48.
5. Haupt, G., et al., Wound and fracture healing: New indication for extracorporeal shockwaves? J. Endourol., 1990. 4: p. S54.
6. Haupt, G., et al., Extrakorporale Stosswellen in der Therapie von Wund- und Frakturheilung? Urologe A, 1990. 29: p. A72.
7. Haupt, G., et al., Enhancement of fracture healing with extracorporeal shockwaves. J. Urol., 1990. 143: p. 230A.
8. Haupt, G., et al., Der Einfluß extrakorporaler Stosswellen auf die Knochenbruchheilung. Hefte zur Unfallheilkunde, 1991. 220: p. 524.
9. Haupt, G., et al., Influence of shockwaves on fracture healing. Urology, 1992. 39: p. 529-532.
10. Graff, J., K.-D. Richter, and J. Pastor, Wirkung von hochenergetischen Stosswellen auf Knochengewebe. Verh. Ber. Dt. Ges. Urol., 1987. 39: p. 76.
11. Graff, J., K.-D. Richter, and J. Pastor, Effect of high energy shockwaves on bony tissue. Urol. Res., 1988a. 16: p. 252.

12. Graff, J., C. Berding, and M. Beck, Transmission of shockwaves through bone: Is it possible to treat iliac ureteral stones with patient in supine position?, in Shockwave lithotripsy, J.E. Lingeman and D. Newman, Editors. 1989a, Plenum Press: New York. p. 115-120.
13. Johannes, E.J., et al., Non-operative treatment of non-unions in bone with extracorporeal shockwaves. Eur. Surg. Res., 1992. 24(Suppl. 2): p. 24.
14. Sukul, K., et al., The effect of high energy shockwaves focused on cortical bone: an in vitro study. J. Surg. Res., 1993. 54: p. 46-51.
15. Yeaman, L.D., P.J. Christopher, and D.L. McCullough, Effects of shockwaves on the structure and growth of the immature rat epiphysis. J. Urol., 1989. 141: p. 670-674.
16. van Arsdalen, K.N., et al., Effects of lithotripsy on immature bone and kidney development. J. Urol., 1991. 146: p. 213-216.
17. Seemann, O., et al., Effect of low-dose shockwave energy on fracture healing: an experimental study. J. Endourol., 1992. 6: p. 219-223.
18. Braun, W., et al., Untersuchungen zur Wirksamkeit von Stosswellen auf die Festigkeit des Verbundes von Knochen und Polymethyl-Methacrylat. Z Orthop., 1992. 130: p. 236-243.
19. Ekkernkamp, A., Die Wirkung extrakorporaler Stosswellen auf die Frakturheilung. 1991, Bochum: Habilitationsschrift, Ruhr-Universität Bochum.
20. Ekkernkamp, A., et al., Effects of extracorporeal shockwaves on standardized fractures in sheep. J. Urol., 1991. 145: p. 257A.
21. Ekkernkamp, A., et al., Der Einfluß der extrakorporalen Stosswellen auf die standardisierte Tibiafraktur am Schaf, in Aktuelle Aspekte der Osteologie, T. Ittel, G. Sieberth, and H. Matthiass, Editors. 1992, Springer: Berlin Heidelberg New York. p. 307-310.
22. Haupt, G., et al., Einfluß extrakorporal erzeugter Stosswellen auf standardisierte Haupt, G., A. Menne, and M. Schulz, Medizinisches Instrument zum Erzeugen und Tibiafrakturen im Schafmodell. Urologe A, 1992. 31: p. A43.
23. Weiterleiten von extrakorporalen nicht fokussierten Druckwellen auf biologisches Gewebe. Patent.
24. Maier M, Milz S, Tischer T, Munzing W, Manthey N, Stabler A, Holzknecht N, Weiler C, Nerlich A, Refior H J, Schmitz C. Influence of extracorporeal shockwave application on normal bone in an animal model in vivo. Scintigraphy, MRI and histopathology. J Bone Joint Surg Br 2002; (84): 592-599.
25. Tischer T, Milz S, Anetzberger H, Muller P E, Wirtz D C, Schmitz C, Ueberle F, Maier M. [Extracorporeal shockwaves induce ventral-periosteal new bone formation out of the focus zone-results of an in-vivo animal trial]. Z Orthop Ihre Grenzgeb 2002; (140): 281-285.

From Nociception to Pain

Wagner, Sprenger, Gerdesmeyer

Introduction

Pain is defined by the International Association for the Study of Pain (IASP) as "an unpleasant sensory and emotional experience associated with actual or potential tissue damage, or described in terms of such damage"[1]. Peripheral nerves represent the initial pathway by which noxious somatic and visceral stimuli gain access to the central nervous system (CNS). When these noxious thermal or mechanical stimuli get in touch with the human body, a chain of events is set in motion that results as a final step in the perception of the complex and multidimensional sensation of pain.

There are two types of pain: nociceptive and neuropathic pain. Nociceptive pain implies activation of nociceptors in the periphery which transduce noxious stimuli into electrochemical impulses. These impulses are then transmitted to the spinal cord and higher centers in the CNS. Somatic and visceral pain are the two subtypes of nociceptive pain. The neural pathways of the latter are less well defined than those of somatic pain. While both subtypes of pain can occur intermittently or constantly, somatic pain is usually characterized as being well localized and described as "aching, gnawing, throbbing or cramping." Visceral pain is felt as diffuse and less topographically distinct. It is described to be "colicky or squeezing."

Neuropathic pain results from injury to neural structures within the peripheral or central nervous system and is often described as "sharp or burning." However, although the clinical descriptions of the pain characteristics by adjectives may help to differentiate pain syndromes in daily practice, they possess low specificity for systematic evaluation.

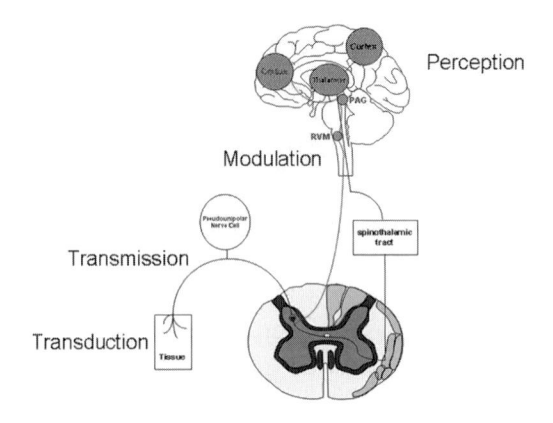

Figure 1. Transduction, transmission, modulation and perception of pain

The mechanisms of how acute pain converts to chronic pain are under intensive investigations. An insight into this complex network of interactions is given at the end of the text.

Between the delivery of a noxious stimulus and the subjective experience of pain a series of complex electrical and chemical events takes place. Thereby, four physiological processes can be identified and are described in detail in the following sections: transduction, transmission, modulation and perception (Figure 1).

Pain transduction

The human somato-sensory system processes four distinct modalities: tactile, proprioceptive, thermal sensations and pain. Each sensory modality is mediated by separate receptors and a distinctive neuroanatomical pathway. Transduction or receptor activation is the process by which external noxious energy is converted into electrophysiological energy in nociceptive primary afferents. The primary sensory afferent fiber dealing with nociception is termed the "nociceptor." Nociceptors in the skin and other somatic tissues are morphologically free nerve endings or very simple receptor structures. A variety of nociceptors have been found to innervate the skin, muscles, viscera, periosteum and joint surfaces. Nociceptive input is mediated via A-delta and C-fibers. The A-delta mechanoreceptors respond to intense mechanical and thermal stimulation. Their receptive fields consist of multiple discrete spots that cover less than 1 mm^2. As many as 20 spots may be grouped over an area from 1 mm^2 to 8 cm^2 to create a receptive field of a single neuron. However, most of the nociceptive input (95% of fibers) from cutaneous tissue is from polymodal nociceptor C-fibers. They respond to intense mechanical, thermal and chemical stimuli. Polymodal nociceptors respond differently to different stimuli, e.g. repeated mechanical stimuli produce fatigue, repeated thermal stimuli produce sensitization (this means the threshold is lowered to a subsequent stimulus). Deep tissues also have nociceptive afferents that are A-delta and C-fibers. Muscle C-fibers produce deep, aching and poorly localized pain. Pain fibers are responsive to various degrees of pressure, violent contraction or stretch, ischemia and inflammation. In cutaneous tissue, there are subtypes of receptors, including mechanoreceptors, polymodal nociceptors and several types of thermoreceptors. Cancellous bone is well supplied with nociceptors and periosteum has the lowest pain threshold for all deep tissue. It is supplied by a dense plexus of A-delta and C-multimodal nociceptors. They are the most numerous of somatic nociceptors and respond to a full range of mechanical, thermal and chemical noxious stimuli as well as to various molecules associated with tissue injury and inflammation, e.g. substance P and prostaglandins. Tissue damage results in inflammation, which affects the response of the nociceptor to further stimuli. Part of the inflammatory process is the release of intracellular contents from damaged cells and inflammatory cells such as macrophages, lymphocytes and mast cells. Nociceptive stimulation also causes a neurogenic inflammatory response with the release of substance P, neurokinin A and calcitonin gene-related peptide (CGRP) from the peripheral terminals of nociceptive afferent fibers[2]. Release of these peptides results in changed excitability of sensory and sympathetic nerve fibers, vasodilation and extravasation of plasma proteins as well as release of chemical mediators by inflammatory cells. As a result, a mixture of inflammatory mediators such as potassium, serotonin, bradykinin, substance P, histamine, cytokines, nitric oxide and products of the cyclooxygenase and lipoxygenase pathways of the arachidonic acid metabolism are released[3]. These chemicals sensitize high-threshold nociceptors which results in the phenomenon of peripheral sensitization. After sensitization, low intensity mechanical stimuli which would not normally cause pain are now perceived as painful ("hyperalgesia"). There is also an increased responsiveness to thermal stimuli at the site of injury. This hyperalgesic zone surrounding the site of injury is commonly observed following surgery and other forms of trauma.

It is noteworthy that the physical and biochemical steps by which the diverse stimuli specifically activate receptors are not known yet. In contrast, the following process, pain transmission, is well investigated and consists of the transmission of the action potential toward the spinal cord via finely myelinated fast conducting (A-delta) and unmyelinated slow conducting (C-fibers) afferent nerve fibers.

Pain transmission

Transmission refers to the process by which the coded information in primary afferent neurons is relayed to those structures of the CNS concerned with pain. The dorsal horn of the spinal cord, representing the major interface between the peripheral and central nervous systems, has been investigated in detail in the past.

The majority of somatic sensory afferents reach the spinal cord through the dorsal root with the cell body of this primary afferent neuron located in the dorsal root ganglion of a spinal nerve. Each of these dorsal root ganglia neurons possesses two branches, the longer branch extending to the periphery and the shorter branch to the CNS, where it couples with dorsal horn neurons. A-delta fibers primarily transmit sharp initial pain and C-fibers transmit so-called "second pain", which is qualitatively dull, aching or burning and persists longer than the noxious stimulus. Nociceptive afferents have the smallest diameter of all somatic, muscular, or visceral sensory fibers. The nociceptive fibers conduct action potentials at average velocities of about 1 m/s (unmyelinated C-fibers) or 15 m/s (finely myelinated A-delta fibers), which is quite slow compared to the conduction velocity of afferent fibers innervating tactile or muscle stretch receptors (75-100 m/s).

Several peptides released by primary afferent neurons play a role in nociception. While certain amino acids and neuropeptides play a relatively predominant role such as glutamate, there is no evidence for the existence of a single "pain neurotransmitter." Moreover, there is evidence for a coexistence of up to four different peptides within a single dorsal root ganglion.

There are a number of other receptor systems that are involved in nociceptive transmission and modulation. Most extensive research was done on the opioid, alpha adrenergic, GABA, serotonin and adenosine receptor systems. Knowledge about this complex system of inhibitory and excitatory effects is the basis for pharmacological analgesic interventions and is currently under intensive investigation. Pharmacologically induced alterations in gene expression and selective modification of the expression of specific receptors that are involved in the transmission of nociceptive information is only one project of research in this field[4].

Pharmacological studies have helped to identify a variety of neurotransmitters and neuromodulators involved in pain processes in the dorsal horn. Non-peptides like monoamines (norepinephrine, serotonin), inhibitory amino acids like GABA and glycine, excitatory amino acids (glutamate, aspartate), nitric oxide, acetylcholine, peptides (opioids), and nonopioids (substance P, CGRP, bradykinin) and others (e.g. adenosine) have been identified. Among these, the excitatory amino acids glutamate and aspartate play a major role[5]. The excitatory amino acids act among others at NMDA-receptors. These receptors seem to play a major role in processes such as "wind-up" and central sensitization and can be blocked by NMDA-antagonists like ketamine which is a promising approach in the prevention of chronic pain.

The dorsal horn is not just merely an interstation for the transmission of sensory signals. It acts as an integration system where incoming tactile and nociceptive sensory input is filtered, attenuated by axons descending from the brain or amplified before being relayed to other segments or the cortex. In 1952, Rexed subdivided the gray matter of the spinal cord according to its cytoarchitecture into 10 laminae (Rexed laminae I-X). The dorsal horn consists of laminae I-VI and differentiates morphologically and functionally[6]. Nociceptive fibers terminate primarily in the superficial dorsal horn or "marginal layer" (lamina I) and in lamina II ("substantia gelatinosa"). Some A-delta fibers also project more deeply and terminate in lamina V. In the dorsal horn, nociceptive afferents form connections with projection neurons or local excitatory or inhibitory interneurons to regulate the flow of nociceptive information to higher centers. These neurons are also located in laminae V and VI. Lamina VI is most prevalent at lumbosacral and cervical cord segments. These cells receive convergent input from limb, muscular and cutaneous afferents. Laminae VII-IX are in the ventral horn and project to spinothalamic and spinoreticular tracts. Input is from interneuronal connections from other laminae. Lamina X consists of a group of cells surrounding the spinal canal. Input is received bilaterally and is nociceptive and high-intensity specific. Projections are to other laminae throughout the length of the spinal cord. Both nociceptive and tactile afferent neurons also have a convergent input into lamina V neurons, either directly or via interneurons. This feature is of clinical importance since these two laminae represent central convergence between somatic and visceral inputs, representing one possible explanation for the clinical phenomenon of "referred pain" described with visceral injury[7].

Functionally, a neuron in the dorsal horn is either a projection neuron, an inhibitory or an excitatory interneuron. Projection neurons are responsible for the transmission of afferent information to higher centers and can be distinguished into three different types: nociception specific cells, low threshold neurons and so called "wide dynamic range neurons." Specific nociceptive cells have only small receptive fields and respond exclusively to noxious stimuli, whereas low threshold neurons respond solely to innocuous stimuli. Wide dynamic range neurons respond to a range of sensory stimuli and receive converging inputs from various primary afferent neurons of disparate sensory modalities and therefore process large receptive fields.

The initial step of pain transmission from the primary afferent neuron to the dorsal horn neuron is followed by a projection through dorsal horn neurons to the higher brain centers like the brain stem and thalamus via relay neurons using ascending pathways such as the spinothalamic tract (classically considered as the major pain pathway), the spinoreticular and the spinomesencephalic pathways. The axons of these second-order neurons cross close to their level of origin to the contralateral side at the spinal cord level.

The third step of pain transmission consists of the projection of impulses from the brain stem and thalamus to various regions of the human cortex via thalamocortical projections.

Pain modulation

Pain modulation is the process whereby nociceptive signal transmission is modified through various influences leading to pain inhibition or facilitation.

Segmental modulation at the level of the dorsal horn and a second system of descending projections from supraspinal sites are responsible for the phenomenon that nociceptive stimuli do not always result in pain perception and, on the other hand, pain may be even perceived in the absence of nociception.

Segmental / spinal control

Spinal modulation of nociceptive activity involves the endogenous opioid system, a variety of other neurotransmitters and segmental inhibition. Dorsal horn neuron activity is further the result of the balance in activity between nociceptive input and other non-nociceptive afferent neuronal input[8].

A number of endogenous opioid peptides play a predominant key role in the production of analgesia. They are derived from three precursor proteins (proopiomelanocortin, proenkephalin, prodynorphin), all located in the CNS at sites associated with the processing or modulation of nociception, and in particular in laminae I and II of the dorsal horn. Opioids have two well-established actions: first, they inhibit voltage-sensitive calcium channels on presynaptic nerve terminals. This action inhibits the release of neurotransmitters, including substance P and glutamate, that are active in spinal nociceptive transmission. Second, opioids can hyperpolarize and thus inhibit postsynaptic neurons by opening potassium channels. Opioid receptors are found in ascending pain pathways and in pain-modulating descending pathways and are nearly ubiquitous in the human cortex. In ascending pathways, opioids act in the peripheral nerve terminals and in the dorsal horn of the spinal cord. All three classical opioid receptor subtypes (μ, δ, κ) are present in high concentrations in the dorsal horn of the spinal cord. They are found presynaptically on terminals of primary afferent neurons and postsynaptically on second-order pain transmission neurons. Opioid agonists therefore inhibit release of excitatory neurotransmitters (e.g. glutamate, substance P) from the primary afferent neurons and directly inhibit second-order pain transmission neurons. These actions (together with supraspinal action) form the basis for the analgesic activity of perispinal (epidural, intrathecal) administered opioids to generate profound analgesia e.g in the perioperative setting and in severe cancer pain treatment.

Other important neurotransmitters supposed to be involved in segmental control of pain modulation are GABA, glycin, cholecystokinin, galanin and endocannabinoids.

GABA is well known to modulate the afferent transmission of nociceptive information by presynaptic and postsynaptic mechanisms. GABA and glycine are colocalized in many neurons in the dorsal horn, and in fact, nearly every glycine-immunoreactive neuron in laminae I-III also contains GABA. The concentration of GABA is the highest in the dorsal horn of the spinal cord, where it is a major inhibitory transmitter. Glycine modulates afferent transmission in the dorsal horn by postsynaptic inhibition.

Cholecystokinin (CCK) appears to have an important but complex involvement in nociceptive transmission and modulation. The most investigated and apparently physiological role of CCK is that it is a functional antagonist of opioid-induced analgesia. CCK antagonists are potentially interesting targets to enhance opiate analgesia.

Galanin is a neuropeptide which is widely distributed in the nervous system and occurs in a small population of primary sensory neurons and also in spinal interneurons. Overwhelming evidence supporting an antinociceptive role for galanin has been obtained from electrophysiological studies in which galanin hyperpolarizes the majority of dorsal horn neurons. Under physiological conditions, galanin is released upon C-fiber stimulation and plays an inhibitory role in spinal cord excitability. Studies on the interaction between galanin and morphine support an antinociceptive role for galanin: it is suggested that the spinal effect of morphine is mediated in part by the inhibitory action of galanin.

The potential antinociceptive action of endocannabinoids has been well demonstrated. The mechanisms of action of endocannabinoid antinociception includes both a spinal and a supraspinal action as well as a more recently recognized peripheral mechanism. Cannabinoid receptors have been identified in the spinal cord and on primary afferent neurons, where they are located to modulate dorsal horn neuron activity. Evidence suggests that cannabinoids and endocannabinoids may act on spinal interneurons to modulate the release of neurotransmitters and thus pain transmission. Finally cannabinoid receptors have been found on mast cells which may participate in the anti-inflammatory effects of cannabinoids.

Local circuits in the dorsal horn of the spinal cord play a critical role in processing nociceptive afferent input and in mediating the actions of descending pain-modulating systems (e.g. noradrenergic neurons via alpha2-adrenergic receptors) on primary afferent neurons in the dorsal horn of the spinal cord. Sensory, spinal and descending neurons that all converge in the dorsal horn of the spinal cord also contain a variety of other neurotransmitters that are undoubtedly involved in transmission and modulation of nociceptive information. However, little is known about these neurotransmitter systems underlying endogenous pain control circuits.

In summary, segmental modulation of nociception has been studied extensively and many neurotransmitters and receptors located in the dorsal horn of the spinal cord have been identified, but the role of some of these substances in pain processing remains obscure whereas the involvement of others has been relatively well established. Finally, additional complexity is provided by the fact that some of the implemented peptides are localized not only in primary afferent neuron terminals but also in intrinsic neurons and descending fibers and by the coexistence of several peptides and classic neurotransmitters in the same neuron.

Descending modulating system

One descending control system that originates in the somatosensory cortex with corticospinal fibers courses along the dorsal lateral funiculus and terminates in dorsal horn laminae I and II. These fibers exert direct control on dorsal horn neurons and probably enhance the inhibitory functions of other descending systems[9]. Among other descending pain control systems that originate in the midbrain (periaqueductal gray, locus coeruleus) and medulla (nucleus raphe magnus, nucleus reticularis gigantocellularis) the most important system appears to be the periaqueductal gray (PAG) / rostral ventromedial medulla (RVM) system. The PAG receives input from (cingulo-)frontal and insular cortex, limbic system, hypothalamus and the reticular system[10]. In this circuit, multiple neurotransmitters are involved: neurons can receive input via several transmitters and each neuron itself may release multiple neurotransmitters. The serotoninergic (5-HT) and noradrenergic (noradrenaline) neurons descend through the dorsolateral funiculus from the brainstem to the spinal cord and terminate in the dorsal horn. They significantly contribute to the modulation of pain together with local circuits, mediating the modulatory actions of the descending pathways and constituing a gating mechanism that controls impulse transmission in the dorsal horn. Electrical stimulation of the midbrain PAG or the nucleus raphe magnus in various species induces powerful analgesia and inhibition of pain responses[11]. This inhibition compares in potency to that achieved by high doses of systemically administered morphine. In the clinical setting, several neurosurgical groups have successfully applied this technique to the alleviation of chronic pain states in man. Evidence exists that activation of the descending pain pathway is mediated by opioids inhibiting inhibitory interneurons[12]. Further support derives from the fact that even minute quantities of opiates injected into the periaqueductal gray induce analgesia as complete and powerful as vast and larger systemic injections.

Interestingly, under certain circumstances, pain perception is not necessarily a consequence of tissue injury and nociception. To explain this finding the hypothesis that the "pain pathway" has a more complex role than just relaying sensory information from the nociceptor to the brain, but can also regulate the passage of nociceptive activity information, was created. Growing information about the process of "pain perception" is available and described in the following paragraph.

Pain perception

Pain perception is the final process whereby transduction, transmission and modulation interact with the unique psychology of the individual to create the final, subjective, emotional experience we perceive as pain. Without perception and a concomitant emotional experience, we do not have pain but only a series of complex physiologic and biochemical mechanisms. In the early days of pain research anatomic and physiologic investigations focused on the identification of the projection pathways originating in the nociceptive areas of the spinal cord dorsal horn, to shed light on possible brain regions associated with nociceptive function. Anatomic and electrophysiologic data show that these cortical regions receive direct nociceptive input through lateral and medial thalamic nuclei.

However, the final processing step towards the experience of "pain" is "perception" in which the pain message is relayed to the brain, producing an unpleasant multidimensional sensory experience, e.g. with affective, defense and perspective components. This multidimensional experience furthermore includes sensory-discriminative and affective-motivational components. Today, the view that pain is perceived only as a result of thalamic processing is overturned and has been replaced by the question of what functions can be assigned to individual cortical areas or networks. Major progress in the understanding of central mechanisms of pain processing was gained by application of functional brain imaging techniques like positron emission tomography (PET) and functional magnetic resonance imaging (fMRI). These techniques have been used in neurophysiological / pharmacological studies as well as in a variety of clinical pain settings. [13] By correlating the obtained results to psychological assessments it has been possible to attribute the processing of specific pain dimensions to distinct anatomical substrates. This extensive central network associated with pain perception consistently includes the thalamus, the primary (SI) and secondary (SII) somatosensory cortices, the insula and the anterior cingulate cortex (ACC). From the results of human studies there is growing evidence that these different cortical structures encode different dimensions of pain: the SI cortex appears to be mainly involved in sensory-discriminative aspects of pain whereas the SII cortex seems to have an important role in recognition, learning, and memory of painful events. The insula has been proposed to be involved in autonomic reactions to noxious stimuli and in affective aspects of pain-related learning and memory. [14] The experience that we call pain always comprises a distinct unpleasantness and desire to escape. Evidence exists that the ACC is closely related to the experience of unpleasantness and may subserve the integration of general affect, cognition, and response selection.

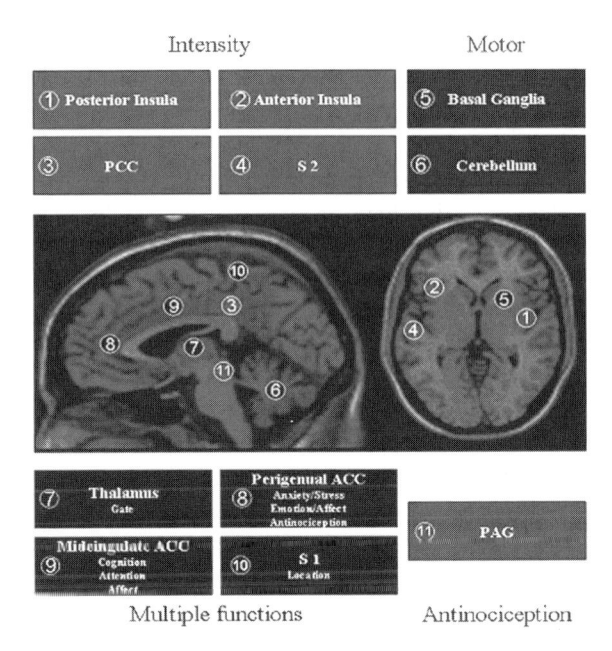

Figure 2. The supraspinal network of pain

Pain intensity seems to be encoded in cerebral structures like SI and the posterior cingulate cortex, whereas the pain threshold is a function which is shared by the anterior cingulate cortex, the frontal inferior cortex and the thalamus (Figure 2). [15]

Chronic pain

Besides the classification of pain into nociceptive and neuropathic pain, for practical purposes, it is useful to distinguish further between acute and chronic pain.

Acute pain results from disease, inflammation or injury to tissue. This type of pain generally begins suddenly, for example, after trauma or surgery, and may be accompanied by anxiety or emotional distress. The cause of acute pain can usually be diagnosed and treated, and the pain is self-limiting, that is, it is confined to a given period of time and severity. In some rare instances, it can become chronic.

According to the definition of the IASP, "pain should be considered chronic when it has persisted nearly continuously for 3 months or longer." [16] It is commonly accepted that chronic pain represents a disease by itself which can be worsened by environmental and psychological factors. Chronic pain persists over a longer period of time than acute pain and is often resistant to most medical treatments. Chronic pain is defined by four basic criteria: 1.) pain lasts longer than the usual expected time for healing, 2.) pain interferes with daily life and/or prohibits the ability to work, 3.) pain has not subsided after multiple interventions, such as medications, physical therapy or surgery, and 4.) pain has lost its physiological "warning" function for a disease or injury and represents in contrast a disease state on its own. Specialist knowledge is required for chronic pain treatment which can not be provided by a single medical discipline. Therefore, multidisciplinary pain clinics have been established where different medical disciplines provide an interdisciplinary approach to guarantee an expert patient treatment.

Focus of basic and clinical research is being shifted presently towards the mechanisms of how acute pain becomes chronic and how this process can be influenced by therapeutic regimes.

How acute pain becomes chronic

Usually the nociceptors, of our joints for example, respond only to overload and lesions and thus serve protective functions. In case of surgery or trauma, local inflammatory mediators including cytokines are released and result in a dramatic enhancement of peripheral nervous system sensitivity. If the corresponding dorsal horn neuron mediating nociception is repetitively affected by stimuli of sufficient intensity to activate C-fibers, the frequency of discharge of this neuron will dramatically increase over time. [17] In case of a long-lasting pain condition, mechanisms emerge in the nervous system that result in an increased sensitivity of the neuronal pain system. Such ongoing noxious input to the spinal cord can expand the receptive fields of dorsal horn neurons as well as induce processes like "central sensitization" or "wind-up." "Wind-up" will occur also in the absence of sensitization of nociceptors and is thought to represent a mechanism for long-term enhancement of nociception by an increase in the frequency of dorsal horn neuron firing. N-methyl D-aspartate (NMDA) receptors seem to play a key role in this process.

However the nociceptor can also be sensitized to repeated noxious stimuli, resulting in "peripheral sensitization." These processes underline that the human nervous system is not a rigid structure. In fact its most striking characteristic may be its plasticity, the ability to learn and to modify output or reactions as a result of experience or circumstances. The processes described above are followed by plastic changes in the central neurotransmitter systems. Possible consequences are long term potentiation of synaptic transmission, induction of immediate-early genes, long-term changes in the expression of target genes and adaptations in neuronal gene transcription, ultimately leading to structural plasticity instead of functional plasticity only. Interactions between the nervous and immune system as well as learning processes may further increase pain sensitivity-the initial step toward the state of chronic pain.

Efforts to reduce chronic pain within the setting of surgical injury (such as perioperative) have concentrated on pain preventive regimes directed at decreasing sensitization in pain pathways. Clinical and experimental data suggest that there is a crucial time interval during the first minutes to hours after injury and a second phase of inflammatory sensitization which depends on the first period. The characteristics of "wind-up" are similar to responses induced by excitatory amino acids that act at the NMDA-receptor. Because nociceptive transmission and synaptic plasticity are closely related to the activation of this receptor type, research and possible therapeutic regimes that aim to reduce changes in the NMDA-receptor system have been initiated. In fact, NMDA-receptor antagonists, such as ketamine, can abolish central sensitization without altering the usual response of dorsal horn neurons to noxious stimulation and may therefore provide a promising tool to prevent chronic pain in the future. [18,19]

In conclusion, a combination of sensitization processes in the peripheral nervous system, spinal cord and brain often constitutes the pathophysiological basis leading to chronic pain. Therefore, the primary aim is to reduce nociceptive activation of the peripheral and central nervous system through multimodal analgesia, in the future possibly in combination with NMDA antagonistic drugs.

In cases of persisting pain, treatment should be started as early as possible to prevent long-term changes and the initiation of chronic pain.

Literature

1. Pain terms: a list with definitions and notes on usage. Recommended by the IASP Subcommittee on Taxonomy. Pain 1979; 6: 249

2. Levine JD, Fields HL, Basbaum AI: Peptides and the primary afferent nociceptor. J.Neurosci. 1993; 13: 2273-86
3. Dray A, Urban L, Dickenson A: Pharmacology of chronic pain. Trends Pharmacol.Sci. 1994; 15: 190-7
4. Akopian AN, Abson NC, Wood JN: Molecular genetic approaches to nociceptor development and function. Trends Neurosci. 1996; 19: 240-6
5. Coderre TJ: The role of excitatory amino acid receptors and intracellular messengers in persistent nociception after tissue injury in rats. Mol.Neurobiol. 1993; 7: 229-46
6. REXED B: A cytoarchitectonic atlas of the spinal cord in the cat. J.Comp Neurol. 1954; 100: 297-379
7. Wall PD, Melzack R: Textbook of Pain. Edinburgh, Churchill Livingstone, 1994, pp 129-51
8. Melzack R, Wall PD: Pain mechanisms: a new theory. Science 1965; 150: 971-9
9. Ruda MA, Bennett GJ, Dubner R: Neurochemistry and neural circuitry in the dorsal horn. Prog.Brain Res. 1986; 66: 219-68
10. Sprenger, T, Berthele, A, Platzer, S, and Boecker, H Toölle T R. What do we learn from in vivo opioidergic brain imaging? Eur J Pain . 2004.Ref Type: In Press
11. Reynolds DV: Surgery in the rat during electrical analgesia induced by focal brain stimulation. Science 1969; 164: 444-5
12. Basbaum AI, Fields HL: Endogenous pain control systems: brainstem spinal pathways and endorphin circuitry. Annu.Rev.Neurosci. 1984; 7: 309-38
13. Wagner KJ, Willoch F, Kochs EF, Siessmeier T, Tolle TR, Schwaiger M, Bartenstein P: Dose-dependent regional cerebral blood flow changes during remifentanil infusion in humans: a positron emission tomography study. Anesthesiology 2001; 94: 732-9
14. Kenneth L.Casey: Pain Imaging, First Edition Edition. Seattle, IASP Press, 2000,
15. Treede RD, Kenshalo DR, Gracely RH, Jones AK: The cortical representation of pain. Pain 1999; 79: 105-11
16. Classification of Chronic Pain: Descriptions of Chronic Pain Syndromes and Definitions of Pain Terms. Seattle, IASP Press, 1994,
17. Woolf CJ: Evidence for a central component of post-injury pain hypersensitivity. Nature 1983; 306: 686-8
18. Dickenson AH: A cure for wind up: NMDA receptor antagonists as potential analgesics. Trends Pharmacol.Sci. 1990; 11: 307-9
19. Stubhaug A, Breivik H, Eide PK, Kreunen M, Foss A: Mapping of punctuate hyperalgesia around a surgical incision demonstrates that ketamine is a powerful suppressor of central sensitization to pain following surgery. Acta Anaesthesiol.Scand. 1997; 41: 1124-32

rESWT for Pain Therapy in Orthopedics and Sports Medicine Development and Application

H. Lohrer,[1] J. Schöll,[1] S. Arentz[1]

Introduction

Extracorporeal shockwave therapy was developed some 50 years ago in urology for the non-invasive treatment of kidney stones. In the past 10 years, this method has also been described for the effective treatment of different orthopedic disorders. In addition to "standard" indications (fasciitis plantaris, EHR, calcific tendonitis and tendopathies of the rotator cuff), specific degenerative sports injuries have now also become an indication for radial extracorporeal shockwave therapy thanks to new technological developments. To date, evaluated data in terms of treatment energy, treatment frequency and post-treatment show inhomogeneity. Experimental bases for rESWT's mechanism are largely inexistent. Currently the reflex-therapeutic use of radial extracorporeal shockwave therapy for trigger point-induced pain is discussed. Just a few papers reported a good outcome after rESWT.

Urologic technology for the treatment of pseudarthrosis

With growing popularity of low-risk extracorporeal shockwave therapy in urology, it was to be expected that other medical disciplines would also become interested in this innovative technology.

---

1 Department of Orthopedics, Institute for Sports Medicine, Frankfurt/Main e.V.

Basic experimental urologic research was conducted especially to study the tissue effects of high-energy extracorporeal shockwaves adjacent to the focus during extracorporeal lithotripsy. Special attention was paid to bone because of the significant impedance differences to soft tissue, just like the treated stone. When examining the side effects, it was shown in vitro and in the animal model that high-energy extracorporeal shockwaves induce osteoneogenesis [7] in addition to energy related aseptic bone marrow necrosis and lesions of osteocytes.

The similarity between shockwave-induced osteoneogenesis on the intact bone and the physiology of fracture healing prompted further experiments. Hereby a stimulation of fracture healing [11] or pseudarthrosis healing was described [14] in a standardized model following high-energy extracorporeal shockwave application.

The first clinical trials for the therapy of pseudarthrosis with high-energy extracorporeal shockwave therapy were reported by Valchanov[26]. Urologic lithotripters were used that necessitated general anesthesia for the patient. Another disadvantage was the necessity to immerse the patient in a bath.

Calcified shoulder - pain relief by fragmentation?

The possibility to disintegrate stones in urolithiasis by extracorporeal shockwaves offers the transfer to pathological neocalcifications in musculoskeletal disorders. Loew & Jurgowski first described calcific tendonitis of the rotator cuff in 1993[15]. Since then many studies have been published showing the therapeutic benefit[12]. Mostly high energies were applied for calcific tendonitis. The dissolution of calcium deposits documented by X-rays appears to increase therapeutic safety. However, it is not a condition that guarantees a good treatment result, but a soft positive correlation was found[6].

Insertion tendinosis - Therapeutic effects of shockwaves at the tendon-bone junction

At an early stage already, enthesiopathic neocalcifications of the tendon insertion area of fascia plantaris were reasonable enough to prompt exploration of the effects of ESWT in chronic plantar heel pain. The initial mechanical idea was to desintegrate the heel spur by ESWT, but no study exists reporting spur disappearance. However, initial observations [3] and controlled studies published later [18] already showed a high effectiveness of extracorporeal shockwave therapy for plantar heel spur. It is well known that only 10% of heel spurs identified by X-rays correlate with clinical findings[19]. Apparently extracorporeal shockwaves also act at the tendon-bone junction where high jumps in impedance exist and pathologically and symptomatically relevant damage resides in fasciitis plantaris.

With the destruction of tissue as observed with high-energy shockwaves, the applied energies were increasingly lowered. Today low energies are routinely used in chronic heel pain. In the meantime, the treatment of chronic fasciitis plantaris has turned out to be the best scientifically documented indication for extracorporeal shockwave therapy[12]. With an average success rate of 81% [17], it is superior to conservative [9] or operative treatment options. It is therefore not surprising that FDA approval has been granted for this indication for several devices.

Similar to fasciitis plantaris, lateral epicondylitis (tennis elbow) involves a degenerative lesion of the tendon insertions of wrist and/or finger extensors. Once again this lesion is extremely common in orthopedic practice and often resists conservative therapies as well as surgery. Not surprisingly, tennis elbow became part of treatment experiments with extracorporeal shockwave therapies[2]. Further studies were conducted in sufficient numbers in controlled randomized clinical experiments mostly with low energy shockwaves[12]. Compared to fasciitis plantaris, epicondylopathy humeri radialis shows a lower success rate of about 60%. Even the less common epicondylopathy humeri ulnaris was regularly treated with extracorporeal shockwaves. Recently, clinical trials performed in accordance to good clinical guidelines are still missing and a proven efficacy has not been shown yet.

Evolution of the equipment

The first findings from the use of extracorporeal shockwave therapy in orthopedics (pseudarthrosis) were gathered with conventional large urologic equipment. These treatments were arduous. The in-patient procedure required the patient in water placement, x-ray controlled application and general anethesia. In the mid-90s the introduction of the first generation of special orthopedic equipment for extracorporeal shockwave therapy appeared. Most of these devices used high-energetic technologies. Like before, radiologic systems (floroscopy) were used for localization purposes. The shockwave was now applied directly through a fixed water-distance secured to the unit, retained by a Silikondrape and delivered via a commercially available ultrasound gel to the patient's skin. Regional or local anesthesia normally was required.

Until now the focusing systems were modified. Ultrasound sonographic units were more often used than x-ray controlled shockwave device. In addition, these units featured a variable energy spectrum (low, medium or high energy). This leads to a significant simplification. Outpatient shockwave procedures now became possible even at a physician's private practice.

A new technological variation in energy generation brought about another significant simplification of the shockwave application. A completely new concept was introduced by the radial shockwave technology. Once again, the principle came from urology[10]. Due to the spheric expansion of the shockwave, comparably larger volumes are treated in a low-energy range. Additional imaging localization procedures are no longer required. The application is biofeedback-controlled. As a rule, anesthesia is no longer required. See Table 1 for a direct comparison of the properties of ESWT devices.

Side effects of extracorporeal shockwave therapy

Extracorporeal shockwave therapy is an extremely uncomplicated therapeutic method. Siebert reported that among "all shockwave treatments performed worldwide in urology and orthopedics no significant side effects could be found[24]."

device	costs ( )	weight (kg)	mobiliy	localizing	energy	analgesia
Urological devices (focused)	0,5 - 1 Mio	250 - 1500	fixed	x-ray or ultrasound	high	general anesthesia
Orthopedic devices First Generation (focused)	55 - 150 T	80 – 200	mobile	ultrasound	high-low energy	local
Orthopedic devices Second Generation (focused/radial)	22 T	30	mobile	Biofeedback	low energy	non

Table 1. Properties of different ESWT devices

Absolute contraindications	Relative contraindications
Lung tissue in direction of sound fields	Degenerative disease
Disturbance of coagulation	Allergy of local anesthetics
tumor	Cervical syndromes
Nerval or vascular structures in direction of shockwaves	Full Rotator cuff defects
pregnancy	Pace maker
infection	
Application to growth joints	

Table 2. Contraindications of ESWT

Specifically, Sistermann & Katthagen conducted a prospective study on the side effects of medium and high-energy extacorporeal shockwaves[25]. In 542 treatments they found smaller and superficial hematomata in 39.8%. Hyperventilation tetanies and blood pressure in excess of 200 mm Hg occurred in 0.7% and 0.6% respectively of treated patients.

Nevertheless the international society of musculoskeletal shockwave therapy (ISMST) listed a series of absolute and relative contraindications for high and medium-energy extracorporeal shockwave therapy (Table 2).

Expected side effects and complications are even less for low-energy extracorporeal shockwave therapy and radial extracorporeal shockwave therapy.

When evaluating the side effects in our own cases treated with radial extracorporeal shockwave therapy, the frequency is 70%. They involve almost exclusively minor side effects such as reddening of the skin. With (local) anesthesia in principle not required with radial extracorporeal shockwave therapy, allergic side effects are not expected with this method and no severe side effect was observed.

Use in highly competitive sports - Use in Olympic Games

Since 1996 international top athletes have been treated with extracorporeal shockwave therapy by the Institute for Sports Medicine in Frankfurt am Main. Since 1998 focussed shockwaves have been almost completely replaced by radial extracorporeal shockwave therapy. In 1996, 2000 and 2004 the German Olympic team used extracorporeal shockwaves in musculoskeletal disorders. Since the side effects of infiltration therapy could possibly interfere with sports performance and international doping requirements, extracorporeal shockwave therapy could be used without limitations regarding these restrictions. It must be noted that competitive performance is not advised immediately following the treatment with extracorporeal shockwaves. During a period of several hours following treatment, pain has been shown to be lower, but the treatment could increase the risk of injury in the event of competitive practice.

Radial extracorporeal shockwave therapy - Quo vadis ?

Today focused extracorporeal shockwaves are used only in few indications like bone pathologies or calcific tendonitis of the shoulder. The radial extracorporeal shockwave technology is now indicated in most soft tissue disorders.

In the future further indications will expand the treatment spectrum. Most recently rESWT is now used in some generalized orthopedic diseases like myofascial pain syndromes, trigger point-associated disorders and in chronic wound care.

Literature

1. Arentz S, Schöll J, Lohrer H. (2004): Kongressband 3. Dreiländertreffen der Österreichischen, Schweizer und Deutschen Fachgesellschaften, Maier, Gillesberger, ISBN 3-8330-0423-1
2. Dahmen G, Haupt G, Rompe J, Loew M, Haist J, Schleberger R (1995): Standortbestimmung der Arbeitsgruppe „Orthopädische Stosswellenbehandlungen". In: Chaussy C, Eisenberger F, Jochum D, Wilbert D (Hrsg.): Die Stosswelle – Forschung und Klinik. Attempo. Tübingen: 137-142
3. Dahmen GP, Franke R, Gonchars V, Poppe K, Lentrodt S, Lichtenberger S, Jost S, Montigel J, Nann VC, Dahmen G (1995): Die Behandlung knochennaher Weichteilschmerzen mit Extracorporaler Stosswellentherapie (ESWT). Indikation. Technik und bisherige Therapie. In: Chaussy C, Eisenberger F, Jochum D, Wilbert D (Hrsg.): Die Stosswelle – Forschung und Klinik. Attempo. Tübingen 175-186
4. Diesch R, Haupt G (1997): Anwendung der hochenergetischen extracorporalen Stosswellentherapie bei Pseudarthrosen. Orth Praxis 33: 470-471
5. Dreisilker (2004): Kongressband 3. Dreiländertreffen der Österreichischen, Schweizer und Deutschen Fachgesellschaften, Maier, Gillesberger, ISBN 3-8330-0423-1
6. Gerdesmeyer L, Wagenpfeil S, Haake M, Maier M, Loew M, Wortler K, Lampe R, Seil R, Handle G, Gassel S, Rompe J D. Extracorporeal shockwave therapy for the treatment of chronic calcifying tendonitis of the rotator cuff: a randomized controlled trial. JAMA 2003; (290): 2573-2580.

7. Graff J, Richter K-D, Pastor J (1988) : Effect of high energy shockwaves on bony tissue. Urol Res 16: 252- 258
8. Gremion G, Augros R, Gobelet Ch, Leyvraz PF (2000): Wirksamkeit der extrakorporalen Stosswellentherapie bei der Calcific tendinitis der Schulter. Schweizerische Zeitschrift für Sportmedizin und Sporttraumatologie. 48: 8-
9. Hammer DS, Rupp S, Kreutz A, Pape D, Kohn D, Seil R (2002): Extracorporeal shockwave Therapy (ESWT) in patients with chronic proximal plantar fasciitis. Foot & Ankle Int. 23: 309-313
10. Haupt G (1997) Use of extracorporeal shockwaves in the treatment of pseudarthrosis, tendinopathy and other orthopedic diseases. J Urol 158: 4-11
11. Haupt G, Haupt A, Gerety B, Chvapil M.(1990): Enhancement of fradure healing with extracorporeal shockwaves. J Urol 143: 230A
12. Heller K-D, Niethard FU (1998): Der Einsatz der extrakorporalen Stosswellentherapie in der Orthopädie – eine Metaanalyse. Z Orthop 136: 390-401
13. Iro H, Schneider TH, Födra C, Waitz G, Nitsche N, Heinritz HH, Benninger J, Ell CH (1992): Shockwave lithotripsy of salivary duct stones. Lancet 339: 1333-1336
14. Johannes EJ, Kaulesar Sukul DM, Pierik EG, Kristelijn M.J, Van Eijck GJ, Bras J (1992) : Non-operative treatment of nonunions in bone with extracorporeal shockwaves. Eur Surg Res 24 (Suppl. 2): 24
15. Loew M, Jurgowski W (1993): Erste Erfahrungen mit der extrakorporalen Stosswellen-Lithotripsie (ESWT) in der Behandlung der Calcific tendinitis der Schulter. Z Orthop 131; 470-473
16. Moll, F, Fischer N, Deutz F-J (1990); Entwicklung von Lithotripsie und Litholayaxie. Urologe 30: 95-100
17. Ogden JA, Alvarez RG, Marlow M (2002): Schockwave therapy for chronic proximal plantar fasciitis: A meta-analysis. Foot & Ankle Int. 23: 301-308
18. Rompe JD, Schöllner C, Nafe B. (2002): Evaluation of low-energy extracorporeal shockwave application for treatment of chronic plantar fasciitis. J Bone Joint Surg 84-A: 335-341
19. Rubin, G., M. Witton (1963): Plantar calcaneal spurs. Am J Orthop 5: 38
20. Sauerbruch T, Delius M, Paumgartner G, Holl J, Wess O, Weber W, Hepp W, Brendel W (1986): Fragmentation of Gallstones by Extracorporeal shockwaves. New Engl J Med 314: 818-822
21. Sauerbruch T, Holl J, Sackmann M, Werner R, Wotzka R Paumgartner G (1987): Disintegration of a pancreatic duct stone with extracorporeal shockwaves in a patient with chronic pancreatitis. Endoscopy 19: 207-208
22. Schöll J, Lohrer H (2000): Radiale Stosswellentherapie des Fersensporns. Orthopädie Mitteilungen 2: A 14
23. Schöll J, Lohrer H, Arentz S (2004): Behandlungsergebnisse der sportindizierten Krankheitsbilder (Achillodynie, Patellaspitzensyndrom und Tibiakantensyndrom) mit radialen Stosswellen. Radiale Extrakorporale Stosswellentherapie): in Gerdesmeyer: Extrakorporale Stosswellentherapie, 2004
24. Siebert W (1996): 1. Kasseler Symposium über die Stosswelllen Therapie in der Orthopädie. Orthopädie-Informationen BVO. Mitteilungen DGOT: 234
25. Sistermann R, Katthagen B-D (1998): Komplikationen, Nebenwirkungen und Kontraindikationen der Anwendung mittel- und hochenergetischer extrakorporaler Stosswellen im orthopädischen Bereich. Z Orthop 136: 175-181
26. Valchanov VD, Michailov P (1991): High energy shockwaves in the treatment of delayed and nonunion of fractures. Int Orthop 15: 181-184

27. Vogel J, Hopf C, Eysel P, Rompe JD (1997): Application of extracorporeal shockwaves in the treatment of pseudarthrosis of the lower extremity – Preliminary results. Arch Orthop Trauma Surg 116: 480-483

Effect of Extracorporeal Shockwaves on the Growth of Microorganisms and Consequences for the Daily Clinical Practice in Orthopedics

Hans Gollwitzer, Carsten Horn, Mark Henne, Ludger Gerdesmeyer

While Extracorporeal Shockwave Therapy (ESWT) already addresses a wide spectrum of indications in modern orthopedics, infections such as the infected pseudoarthrosis are considered contraindications. This study examines the effect of ESWT on infectious foci, and specifically on growth of microorganisms.

The available literature only refers to isolated studies on the interaction of microorganisms and shockwaves. The results of in vitro experiments described in these studies largely depend on the test setup and an inappropriate test setup may conceal antibacterial and other effects of extracorporeal shockwaves. Nevertheless, in some examinations, extracorporeal shockwaves showed a clear bactericidal effect on clinically relevant infectious agents. Consequently, bone infections must be reconsidered as contraindications for ESWT and further studies must be conducted to verify any possible clinical relevance.

Since the introduction of Extracorporeal Shockwave Therapy (ESWT) in the year 1980 for the treatment of nephrolithiasis, the spectrum of indications for ESWT has expanded continuously. Apart from the classic indication of nephrolithiasis, extracorporeal shockwaves today are also applied to treat gallstones, pancreatic calculi and urethral stones[1-3]. For more than 10 years, enthesopathies such as epicondylitis, calcific tendonitis and plantar fasciitis have been classic indications in orthopedics[4-7]. Similarly, pathologies such as pseudoarthroses are being treated with ESWT ever since the positive stimulating effect on bone metabolism was discovered[8, 9]. One exclusion criteria for shockwave therapy is local infected conditions because of the risk of spreading bacteria with subsequent systemic propagation through microdamage to epithelia and vessel walls. The release of microorganisms from deposits in kidneys and gall bladder during ESWT is also viewed as a risk factor for secondary infection. Especially in orthopedics, infections close to the bone or infected pseudoarthroses are generally viewed today as contraindications for ESWT[10,11].

Do microorganisms spread due to ESWT?

Some clinical urologic and gastroenterologic studies reported the appearance of bacteremia following ESWT[12,13]. In 22% of the cases, the Kullman study group observed bacteria circulating in the blood following the ESWT of gallstones. This phenomenon was also documented after the treatment of kidney stones[12-14]. In a prospective study, Westh et al. did not observe any increase in the presence of bacteremia following ESWT for nephrolithiasis[15]. Another controversy surrounds the need for antibiotic prophylaxis during shockwave application[16-18]. Reports of secondary infections such as the development of abscesses, endophthalmitis, spondylodiscitis and even endocarditis following lithotrypsy continue to be limited to individual case descriptions [19-22] and might be due to secondary bacterial spreading after epithelial injury due to sharp stone fragments. Until now, no relevant effect of bacterial spread or secondary infection has been documented with certainty in any clinically controlled studies. In addition, no systemic bacterial complication has occurred to date due to the ESWT treatment of infected pseudoarthroses[23].

Direct bactericidal effect of shockwaves

Several publications have examined the effects of shockwaves on human cells. While complex interactions are already known for human cells - such as an increased transfer of molecular markers to the cells [24] and a more intensive gene transfer in tumor cells [25] - few studies are available on the interaction with microorganisms. Stoller and Workman first reported the effect of extracorporeal shockwaves on the microbiological flora of urinary calculi[26]. In vitro fragmentation of clinically isolated deposits occurred either purely mechanically or with ESWT (up to 1000 impulses), followed by an analysis of the bacterial flora. The authors were unable to identify any antibacterial effect as a result of the shockwaves. The same result was obtained by Kerfoot et al. with a variety of bacterial strains in suspension treated with up to 4000 impulses[27]. In contrast, the Reid work group published studies which pointed to a significant bactericidal effect of extracorporeal shockwaves on suspended bacteria in urine[28]. The antibacterial effect of ESWT was neutralized by embedding bacteria in agar and calcium carbonate crystals for the simulation of struvite stones. Finally, Von Eiff et al. were able to demonstrate that a certain amount of impulses was necessary to induce an antibacterial effect[29]. In suspension, Staphylococcus aureus growth was reduced by more than 3log10 with 350 impulses or more. However, no antibacterial effect was observed with fewer impulses. Complete disinfection was even achieved in the majority of sufficiently treated samples.

In vitro results depend upon test setup

The author's own findings corroborate the data published in the literature. Our experiments pointed to a threshold value for the impulse count as well as for the applied energy flux density. The varying findings referred to in the literature demonstrate that the test setup has a decisive effect on the rate of reduction in bacterial growth due to ESWT. In addition to impulse count and energy flux density, exogenous factors such as test setup, sample positioning in the focus, probe vessel with vessel wall and volume are also important when it comes to determining the antibacterial effect. Table 1 presents an overview of the published in vitro experiments.

The physical parameter "energy" shown in the table does not allow us to conclude the amplitude of the applied energy flux density in the focus of the shockwave. Therefore, a comparison of the studies is not possible. Moreover, the studies involved different test setups with varying media, bacterial strains and vessels.

Physical effects of shockwaves on microorganisms

Apart from ESWT, an antibacterial effect was also described with other physical processes. The inactivation of bacteria through high hydrostatic pressure (200 to 600 MPa) is an established process in the food industry[31,32]. At high hydrostatic pressure, gram positive bacteria have a significantly higher resistance to continuous pressure buildup than gram negative bacteria[33,31]. Our studies did not allow us to extrapolate this phenomenon to shockwaves.

Author	Bacterial strain	Medium	Max. Impulse	Energy [kV]	Bacterial Growth after ESWT
Stoller [26]	miscellaneous	Urinary calculi	1000	18	no sign. difference
Reid [28]	P. mirabilis	Urine, Agar, CaCO3	1000 2000 2000	19	55%
Von Eiff [29]	S. aureus	PBS	1000	20	no sign. difference
Kerfoot [27]	E. coli, S. aureus,	Suspens.	4000	20	no sign. difference
Gollwitzer [30]	S. aureus, S. faecalis, S. epidermidis, P. aerusinosa	NaCl	4000	20	1,1-29,7%

Table 1. In vitro experiments on the antibacterial effect of extracorporeal shockwaves

Beyond the positive pressure buildup during the application of impulses, shockwaves also have additional physical properties already described in previous chapters. Ultrasound is a process widely used in microbiology laboratories to disintegrate bacteria and to clean laboratory equipment[34-36]. However, the level of energy used in these laboratory methods clearly exceeds those applicable in humans. On the contrary, the antibacterial effect of ESWT can already be achieved with clinically applicable energy flux densities.

Beside the thermal and chemical effects of ESWT, sound waves also create a mechanical effect. The prerequisite for all effects is the conversion of acoustic energy into mechanical, thermal or chemical energy. Another possible important indirect mechanism is the induction of cavitation[37,38]. In terms of higherapplication rates, an increased occurrence of cavitation is to be expected at high frequencies. The resulting jet streams are clearly more marked and have a greater mechanical effect than the primary shockwave[39]. This may further strengthen the antibacterial effect as well. In order to minimize the possibility of cavitation effects in our own studies, bacteria were treated with a low frequency of 2Hz[30].

Biological effects are of decisive importance for antibacterial action. In addition to the direct bactericidal effects of high-energy shockwaves, growth of microorganisms may also be inhibited by affecting metabolism and through other molecular effects. Such mechanisms were already described for human cells[25,24]. With basic studies lacking for bacteria, such mechanisms can only be discussed hypothetically.

Respecting the pathology of infection as an entity, biological effects also play an essential role in vivo[40]. Several work groups already demonstrated an improved perfusion in the treated area during and after ESWT. Recent animal experiments demonstrated that ESWT also generates increased vascularization in addition to local hematoma[41,42]. These reactions are of decisive importance for the antibacterial and antiinfectious action of ESWT.

Schaden et al. studied the clinical effect of ESWT under infected and non-infected conditions on pseudoarthrosis. The authors observed healing of infected pseudoarthroses in more than 77% of the cases and were unable to find any differences with the success rate in aseptic pseudoarthroses[23]. Also, this same study did not reveal any systemic spread of infection, secondary infection or septic complication. The published in vitro studies with evidence of direct antibacterial action of shockwaves, the findings of the Schaden work group and the findings regarding the biological effect of ESWT raise the question of whether a local infection is to be considered at all as a contraindication for ESWT. In addition, controlled clinical studies are needed to show whether systemic antibiotic prophylaxis is necessary when treating potentially infected tissue with shockwave therapy and whether healing of bone infections can be induced with ESWT.

Literature

1. Delhaye M, Vandermeeren A, Baize M, Cremer M. Extracorporeal shockwave lithotripsy of pancreatic calculi. Gastroenterology 1992; 102: 610-620.
2. Iro H, Schneider HT, Fodra C, Waitz G, Nitsche N, Heinritz HH, Benninger J, Ell C. Shockwave lithotripsy of salivary duct stones. Lancet 1992; 339: 1333-1336.
3. Sauerbruch T, Delius M, Paumgartner G, Holl J, Wess O, Weber W, Hepp W, Brendel W. Fragmentation of gallstones by extracorporeal shockwaves. N Engl J Med 1986; 314: 818-822.
4. Dahmen GP, Nam VC, Meiss L. Extrakorporale Stosswellentherapie (ESWA) zur Behandlung von knochennahen Weichteilschmerzen, Indikation, Technik und vorläufige Ergebnisse. In: Deutsche Gesellschaft für Stosswellenlithotripsie (ed.): Konsensus Workshop der Deutschen Gesellschaft für Stosswellenlithotripsie. Tübingen: Attempto-Verlag, 1993: 143-148.
5. Loew M, Jurgowski W. [Initial experiences with extracorporeal shockwave lithotripsy (ESWL) in treatment of calcific tendinitis of the shoulder]. Z Orthop Ihre Grenzgeb 1993; 131: 470-473.

6. Rompe JD, Hopf C, Kullmer K, witzsch U, Nafe B. [Extracorporeal shockwave therapy of radiohumeral epicondylopathy-- an alternative treatment concept]. Z Orthop Ihre Grenzgeb 1996; 134: 63-66.
7. Rompe JD, Hope C, Kullmer K, Heine J, Burger R. Analgesic effect of extracorporeal shockwave therapy on chronic tennis elbow. J Bone Joint Surg Br 1996; 78: 233-237.
8. Kaulesar Sukul DM, Johannes EJ, Pierik EG, van Eijck GJ, Kristelijn MJ. The effect of high energy shockwaves focused on cortical bone: an in vitro study. J Surg Res 1993; 54: 46-51.
9. Schleberger R, Senge T. Non-invasive treatment of long-bone pseudarthrosis by shockwaves (ESWL). Arch Orthop Trauma Surg 1992; 111: 224-227.
10. Rompe JD, Buch M, Gerdesmeyer L, Haake M, Loew M, Maier M, Heine J. [Musculoskeletal shockwave therapy--current database of clinical research]. Z Orthop Ihre Grenzgeb 2002; 140: 267-274.
11. Sistermann R, Katthagen BD. [Complications, side-effects and contraindications in the use of medium and high-energy extracorporeal shockwaves in orthopedics]. Z Orthop Ihre Grenzgeb 1998; 136: 175-181.
12. Kullman E, Jonsson KA, Lindstrom E, Dahlin LG, Ansehn S, Borch K. Bacteremia associated with extracorporeal shockwave lithotripsy of gallbladder stones. Hepatogastroenterology 1995; 42: 816-820.
13. Muller-Mattheis VG, Schmale D, Seewald M, Rosin H, Ackermann R. Bacteremia during extracorporeal shockwave lithotripsy of renal calculi. J Urol 1991; 146: 733-736.
14. Cochran JS, Robinson SN, Crane VS, Jones DG. Extracorporeal shockwave lithotripsy. Use of antibiotics to avoid postprocedural infection. Postgrad Med 1988; 83: 199-204.
15. Westh H, Knudsen F, Hedengran AM, Weischer M, Mogensen P, Andersen JT. Extracorporeal shockwave lithotripsy of kidney stones does not induce transient bacteremia. A prospective study. The Copenhagen Extracorporeal Shockwave Lithotripsy Study Group. J Urol 1990; 144: 15-16.
16. Deliveliotis C, Giftopoulos A, Koutsokalis G, Raptidis G, Kostakopoulos A. The necessity of prophylactic antibiotics during extracorporeal shockwave lithotripsy. Int Urol Nephrol 1997; 29: 517-521.
17. Pearle MS, Roehrborn CG. Antimicrobial prophylaxis prior to shockwave lithotripsy in patients with sterile urine before treatment: a meta-analysis and cost-effectiveness analysis. Urology 1997; 49: 679-686.
18. Pettersson B, Tiselius HG. Are prophylactic antibiotics necessary during extracorporeal shockwave lithotripsy? Br J Urol 1989; 63: 449-452.
19. Greenwald BD, Tunkel AR, Morgan KM, Campochiaro PA, Donowitz GR. Candidal endophthalmitis after lithotripsy of renal calculi. South Med J 1992; 85: 773-774.
20. Kamanli A, Sahin S, Kavuncu V, Felek S. Lumbar spondylodiscitis secondary to Enterobacter cloacae septicaemia after extracorporeal shockwave lithotripsy. Ann Rheum Dis 2001; 60: 989-990.
21. Karamalegos AZ, Diokno AC, Moylan DF. Formation of perinephric abscess following extracorporeal shockwave lithotripsy. Urology 1989; 34: 277-280.
22. Zimhony O, Goland S, Malnick SD, Singer D, Geltner D. Enterococcal endocarditis after extracorporeal shockwave lithotripsy for nephrolithiasis. Postgrad Med J 1996; 72: 51-52.
23. Schaden W. Extrakorporale Stosswellentherapie (ESWT) bei Pseudarthrosen und verzögerter Frakturheilung. Trauma Berufskrankh 2000; 2: S333-S339.
24. Ueberle F, Delius M, Guo L. [Using shockwaves for transfer of molecules in cells]. Biomed Tech (Berl) 2002; 47 Suppl 1 Pt 1: 382-385.

25. Bao S, Thrall BD, Gies RA, Miller DL. In vivo transfection of melanoma cells by lithotripter shockwaves. Cancer Res 1998; 58: 219-221.
26. Stoller ML, Workman SJ. The effect of extracorporeal shockwave lithotripsy on the microbiological flora of urinary calculi. J Urol 1990; 144: 619-621.
27. Kerfoot WW, Beshai AZ, Carson CC. The effect of isolated high-energy shockwave treatments on subsequent bacterial growth. Urol Res 1992; 20: 183-186.
28. Reid G, Jewett MA, Nickel JC, McLean RJ, Bruce AW. Effect of extracorporeal shockwave lithotripsy on bacterial viability. Relationship to the treatment of struvite stones. Urol Res 1990; 18: 425-427.
29. von Eiff C, Overbeck J, Haupt G, Herrmann M, Winckler S, Richter KD, Peters G, Spiegel HU. Bactericidal effect of extracorporeal shockwaves on Staphylococcus aureus. J Med Microbiol 2000; 49: 709-712.
30. Gollwitzer H, Horn C, Henne M, von Eiff C, Gerdesmeyer L. Bakterizider Effekt hochenergetischer extrakorporaler Stosswellen: Ein in vitro Nachweis. submitted .
31. Hoover DG, Metrick C, Papineau AM, Farkas DF, Knorr D. Biological Effects of High Hydrostatic-Pressure on Food Microorganisms. Food Technology 1989; 43: 99-107.
32. Ludwig H, Gross P, Scigalla W, Sojka B. Pressure inactivation of microorganisms. High Pressure Research 1994; 12: 193-197.
33. Arroyo G, Sanz PD, Prestamo G. Response to high-pressure, low-temperature treatment in vegetables: determination of survival rates of microbial populations using flow cytometry and detection of peroxidase activity using confocal microscopy. J Appl Microbiol 1999; 86: 544-556.
34. Buck GE, O'Hara LC, Summersgill JT. Rapid, simple method for treating clinical specimens containing Mycobacterium tuberculosis to remove DNA for polymerase chain reaction. J Clin Microbiol 1992; 30: 1331-1334.
35. Burkhart NW, Crawford J. Critical steps in instrument cleaning: removing debris after sonication. J Am Dent Assoc 1997; 128: 456-463.
36. Scherba G, Weigel RM, O'Brien WD, Jr. Quantitative assessment of the germicidal efficacy of ultrasonic energy. Appl Environ Microbiol 1991; 57: 2079-2084.
37. Bailey MR, Blackstock DT, Cleveland RO, Crum LA. Comparison of electrohydraulic lithotripters with rigid and pressure-release ellipsoidal reflectors. II. Cavitation fields. J Acoust Soc Am 1999; 106: 1149-1160.
38. Delius M, Draenert K, Al Diek Y, Draenert Y. Biological effects of shockwaves: in vivo effect of high energy pulses on rabbit bone. Ultrasound Med Biol 1995; 21: 1219-1225.
39. Huber P, Jochle K, Debus J. Influence of shockwave pressure amplitude and pulse repetition frequency on the lifespan, size and number of transient cavities in the field of an electromagnetic lithotripter. Phys Med Biol 1998; 43: 3113-3128.
40. Maier M, Milz S, Wirtz DC, Rompe JD, Schmitz C. [Basic research of applying extracorporeal shockwaves on the musculoskeletal system. An assessment of current status]. Orthopade 2002; 31: 667-677.
41. Wang CJ, Huang HY, Pai CH. Shockwave-enhanced neovascularization at the tendon-bone junction: an experiment in dogs. J Foot Ankle Surg 2002; 41: 16-22.
42. Wang CJ, Wang FS, Yang KD, Weng LH, Hsu CC, Huang CS, Yang LC. Shockwave therapy induces neovascularization at the tendon-bone junction. J Orthop Res 2003; 21: 984-989.
43. Gollwitzer, Horn, Henne, Gerdesmeyer. [Antibacterial effectiveness of high-energetic extracorporeal shockwaves: an in vitro verification], Z Orthop Ihre Grenzgeb. 2004 Jul-Aug;142(4):462-6.

10

Extracorporeal Shockwave Therapy and Avascular Necrosis of the Femoral Head
Intraosseous Pressure Measurements

J. Hausdorf,[1,2] A. Lutz,[3] M. Maier[4]

Summary

The recently used hip preserving therapy options in avascular necrosis of the femoral head (AVN) mostly end in total hip replacement in the short or medium term. Based on the evidence of bone regeneration on healthy bones, indications for extracorporeal shockwave therapy have been expanded and clinical treatments of femoral head necrosis have been studied. The purpose of this study was to verify if extracorporeal shockwaves weaken by-passed bone and to look for modification of measurable acoustic shockwave parameters inside the femoral head. In this study shockwaves were delivered to the femoral heads of pigs and the intraossary pressure was measured. Depending on intraossary transmission, we could detect measureable pressure signals. The conclusion was to shorten the distance as much as possible when avascular necrosis of the femoral head needs shockwave therapy. However, further in vitro and in vivo investigations have to be done before clinical shockwave application in AVN of the femoral head can be recommended.

---

[1] *Orthopedic Dept. Ludwig-Maximilians-University Munich*
[2] *Institute of Surgical Science, Ludwig-Maximilians-University Munich*
[3] *Dornier MedTech, Wessling*
[4] *Rheumatology Dept. Oberammergau*

Introduction

Aseptic necrosis of the femoral head is defined as a vascularization disorder of the femur head epiphysis. Necrotic degeneration of spongious and compact bones as well as bone marrow were described in AVN[14]. The pathogenesis remains unclear, but increased intraossary thrombogenesis (thrombophilia, hypofibrinolysis) and local ischemia were discussed[5]. A total of 5-10% of total hip replacement is caused by femoral head necrosis[9]. Femoral head necrosis constitutes a highly relevant clinical problem. Usually AVN of the femoral head affects young patients between 30 and 50 years of age[6]. In 70-80% a bilateral occurrence is observed[13].

The therapy in early stages, classified as type I and II according to ARCO classification, is effective in 22% of cases, which was confirmed in Meta analysis of 819 patients[13]. Even with drilling to relieve pressure and increase vascularization, 30-60% of cases finally end in total hip replacement (5, 20, 12). Without any therapeutic intervention, necrosis progression generally takes place within 2 years including significant joint destruction[13]. Due to the joint incongruence, a secondary arthrosis was found in all patients and hip preserving options were no longer feasible.

Until now, only few studies have described the effect of ESWT on AVN of the femoral head. All studies showed a prospective uncontrolled design [16, 11, 17, 8, 15] and the working mechanism recently remains unclear. The ESWT is applied to support local osseous repair processes of the necrosis by induction of osteoneogenesis and angioneogenesis, which is already described[3, 15, 25]. On the other hand, ESWT is to break up the sclerotic border zone - present in the irreversible Stage ARCO II - through intraossary microfragmentation. These local mechanical effects lead to revitalization of the avascular zone. The clinical outcome after ESWT, published in 3 prospective uncontrolled trials, is not evidence-based because of the inhomogeneity of the study design and the different treatment parameters used. But at least all trials conclude that ESWT seems to be effective in the early stages of the avascular necrosis of the femoral head by stimulating repair processes[16, 11, 17, 8, 15].

Regarding the large differences in acoustic properties (soft tissue to bone), the question still remains unanswered: Does a bony or soft tissue environment have significant impact on acoustic energy such that emitted energy decreases to close to undetectable levels inside the femoral head? The following study attempts to shed some light on that issue.

Material and Methods

Measurements were performed using the electrohydraulic XL-1 shockwave generator (Dornier med tech, Wessling, Germany). The unit includes an integrated water bath in which the objects are to be immersed. Focus was localized via laser beam along two planes and water degassed and tempered at 37.5° C. Voltage varied in 2 kV steps from 18 to 26 kV. Each time 15 impulses were applied at a frequency of 1 Hz.

Pressure amplitude was measured with a PCB hydrophone (Serial number 1221). Inside the hydrophone piezocrystals were exposed to acoustic pressure impulses and react by release of small electric impulses when compressed. Compression of the piezocrystal generates electrical signals recorded by an oscilloscope (Waverunner 2 LT 342 from LeCroy, Chestnut Ridge, USA).

Fresh femurs from 100-kg pig cadavers were used as bone material. Carcasses were refrigerated 24 hours at 6° C, then released by the veterinarian. Following careful removal of soft tissue, the material was frozen at -20° C. Prior to the experiment, bones were defrosted in an isotone saline solution (0.9% NaCl).

The PCB hydrophone was placed parallel to the focus axis in all measurements (Figure 1). Placement and positioning were verified by a balancing system. The laser adjustment feature on the unit was used to ensure the exact hydrophone positioning.

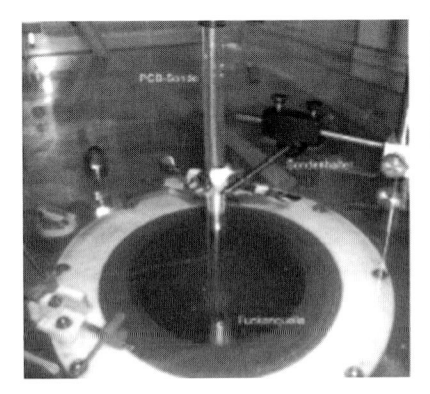

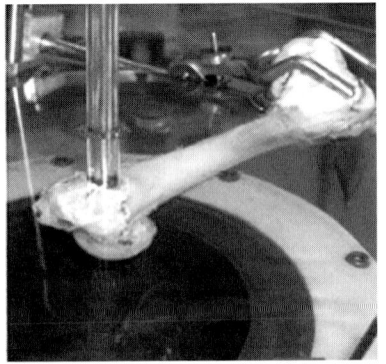

Figure 1. a) Positioning of the PCB-hydrophone in water bath to perform reference measurements. b) Intraosseous positioning of hydrophone.

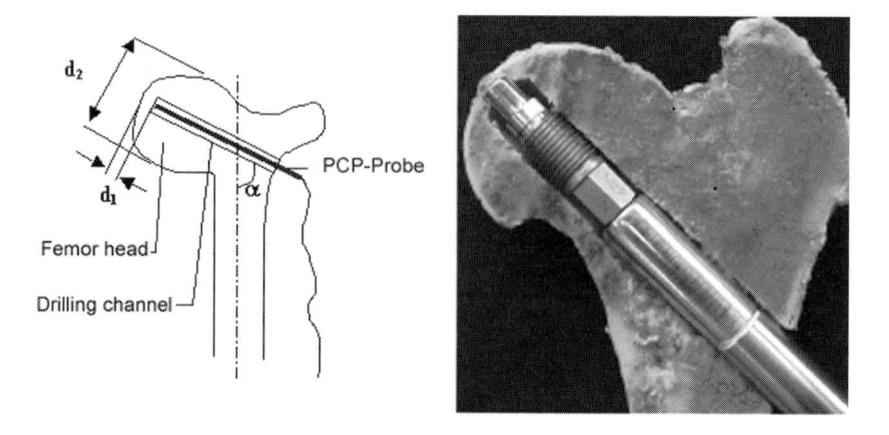

Figure 2. Hydrophone placed inside the femoral head

In order to place the PCB hydrophone inside the femoral head, the femurs (identified as bones 1-3) were drilled as shown in Figure 2. The angle between longitudinal axis of bone and probe was 45 +/- 1°. Drilling was performed as used for core decompression drilling in surgical techniques. Distance D1 shown in Figure 2 refers to the intraossary distances of the shockwave, D2 designates the diameter of the femoral head. The measurements of individual bones are listed in Table 1.

The probe was introduced into the bony channel under water so that the bony drilling channel was completely filled with water. In another measurement, a mid-split femoral head hemisphere was positioned between the shockwave source and hydrophone. Distance between the hydrophone and bone was increased to be sure no mechanical contact could occur during the measurements (Figure 3).

	d1 [mm]	d2 [mm]
bone 1	13	40
bone 2	8	35
bone 3	15	35

Table 1. Bone characteristics

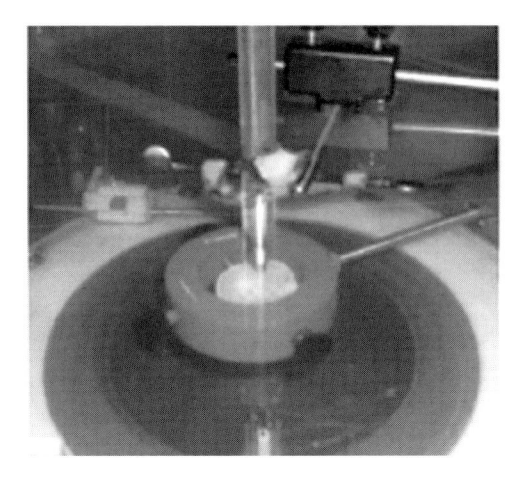

Figure 3. Measurements in split femoral head – absorber measurement

After bone measurements were done, bone was removed and repeated measurements taken with identical parameters were performed as reference measurements.

The results were shown as mean values of each measured sequence. The statistical errors Δx were defined as the product of the standard deviation of each mean value and the t-factor of the t-distribution. Confidence level was defined as 95%.

Results

The reference measurements we conducted demonstrate the effect of voltage and spark wear on pressure amplitude. The results listed in Figure 4 show an increase in pressure amplitude as voltage increases. A comparison between measurements 3 and 5 shows differences in terms of maximum amplitude, the course of pressure gain and error size. The differences result from the use of different sparks. While measurement 5 was conducted with a new device (only 250 impulses delivered), measurement 3 was performed with a used one. Greater wear in measurement 3 effects a lower pressure amplitude at identical voltage and a greater error size when measurements were repeated. In addition, the gradient of the measurement curve decreased with increasing voltage.

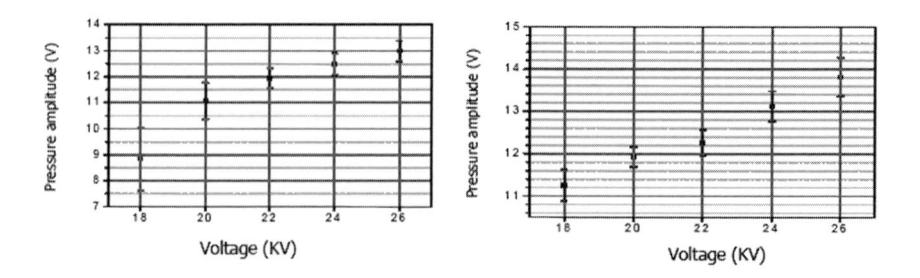

Figure 4. Pressure amplitude in water prior (left) and after (right) spark was changed. Values given as mean and standard deviation (SD).

In order to minimize the effect of electrode wear on the measurement, it is necessary to conduct reference measurements immediately before or after bone measurement.

The pressure amplitude in the bone was measured with different voltages and identical bone thickness d1 as well as with identical voltage and varying bone thickness (Table 2).

The graph in Figure 5 shows the result of the voltage-dependent measurement. With increasing voltage, intraosseous pressure amplitude increases and the pressure related shockwave parameter looks similar to those of reference measurements.

	bone 1 (13 mm)		bone 2 (8 mm)		bone 3 (15 mm)	
voltage [kV]	mean [V]	SFr	mean [V]	SD	mean [V]	SD
18			5,09	0,32		
20	-4,13	0,07	6,08	0,18	-1,55	0,14
22			6,20	0,15		
24			6,73	0,30		
26			7,00	0,18		

Table 2. Pressure amplitude of bone measurements

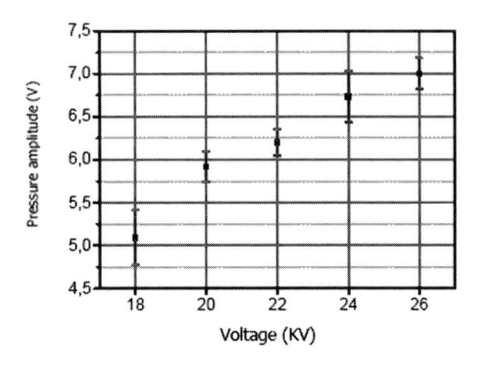

Figure 5. Pressure amplitude in bone (8 mm)

In order to determine a weakening of pressure amplitude in the bone, intraosseous measurements were calculated with reference measurements. Figure 6 shows the absorption of the pressure signal with varying voltage. Weakening through the femoral head varies between 42 and 48%. The measurement was carried out in bone 2.

The effect of bone thickness on absorption is shown in Figure 7. Measurements were performed on bones 1, 2 and 3. Shockwaves were applied with 20 kV. As a result we found an increase of absorption related to bone thickness d1.

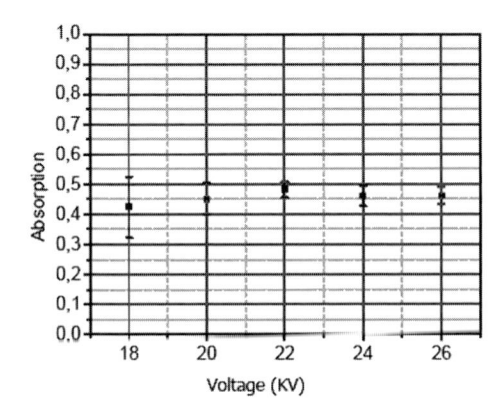

Figure 6. Energy absorption related to voltage (bone 2, 8 mm distance).

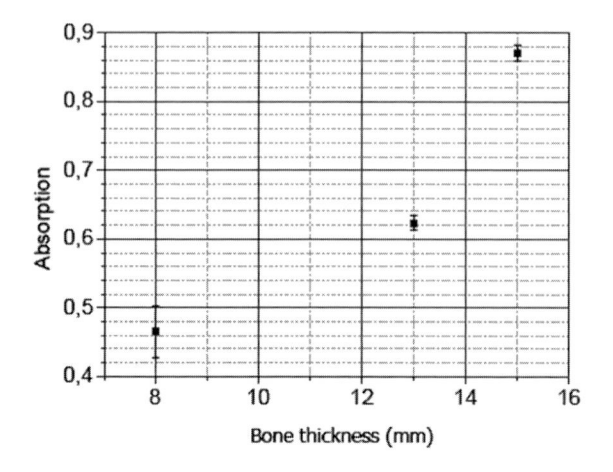

Figure 7. Absorption related to bone thickeness D1.

An average value of 4.52 V (+/- 0.38 V) was found on measurements on the bone slice (10 mm thickeness) used as absorber. This is related to 62% absorption. Based on the absorption measured on bones 1-3, weakening of 45% could be estimated for an intraossary distance of 10 mm.

Discussion

The measuring of absolute pressure and energy values when applying shockwaves as produced in patient tissue is faced with technical difficulties[2].

For absolute measurements of shockwaves, a measuring system which records the complete shockwave impulse is required. From a technical point of view, laser hydrophones mostly fit this requirement but they are difficult to use because of specific technical characteristics. Since laser hydrophones are calibrated in terms of water, absolute values of pressure can be indicated exclusively in water. The fiber hydrophone therefore has to be coupled only via water medium. A water-filled drill channel inside the bone must be created to provide intraosseous measurements. Two specific effects exist: first of all, the bone-related decrease of energy, and further on the partial reflection of shockwaves along the bone/water interface. This causes the primary pressure pulse to be superimposed by reflection effects. In contrast, PCB hydrophones are easier to handle. They are also appropriate for relative measurements of peak pressure but they are limited to determine the course of pressure over time.

Despite these technical limitations, data on pressures and energy flux densities effectively reaching the bone are necessary to adequately set up the shockwave treatment. Accordingly, the authors believe the relative measurements they conducted to be a first step in discussing shockwave parameters in avascular necrosis of the femoral head. Animal experiments and clinical studies should not be conducted until there is evidence that relevant pressures can be detected inside the femoral head. Our findings as well as those from Gerdesmeyer et al. conclude that shockwaves show a signicant and also clinically relevant decrease in energy and pressure. Finally, the spontaneous course of AVN of the femoral head stage I and II according to ARCO remains unclear[3]. Even if no reaction can be achieved in the bone due to excessive weakening of the extracorporeal shockwaves, a clinical and radiological improvement may be achieved which could be misinterpreted as shockwave-related.

Since an earlier study [2] proposed the theory that shockwaves weaken almost completely thus questioning the possibiity to treat femoral head necrosis, an attempt was made to reproduce the results presented so far in a realistic experiment setup.

When considering the weakening of the signal as a function of voltage, the weakening is 42% at 18 kV and 46% at 26 kV. The distance in the bone was 8 mm and nearly 50% reduction of pressure was found. Earlier studies published reduction of 83%[2]. Differences in methodology and study setup may account for such differences in results since not all measurements carried out so far were conducted inside the femoral head.

Measurements on bone slices of different thicknesses show a thickness-related tendency. The longer the distance, the lower the pressure amplitude. Weakening of 45% was found in the 8 mm slice size, 62% in the 13 mm size and 87% when the bone slice dimension was about 15 mm. From this point of view our findings could confirm earlier results [2]—higher weakening when measured outside the bone with intermediate bone piece (measured weakening 62%), compared to intraosseous measurements (estimated weakening 45%), which show a significant reflection of shockwave energy on the bone/water interface.

In summary, it can be concluded that shockwave energy inside the femoral head increases with increasing applied voltage. Absorption appears to be independent of voltage but a clear relation was found between absorption and the intraossary distance traveled by the shockwave.

In clinical use of ESWT in AVN of the femoral head a precise and controlled focus positioning of the shockwaves seems to be unconditionally necessary. Additionally, the necrosis zone has to be exposed as close to the shockwave device as possible to reduce the amount of bony tissue the shockwave has to pass, even if positioning of the patient and necrosis exposure are already very difficult. In vitro studies, animal experiments and placebo-controlled multicentered studies are yet to be undertaken to support the use of shockwaves in AVN of the femoral head. But recently, neovascularisation and osteogenetic effects of shockwaves have been shown for other indications.

Literature

1. Cleveland RO, Lifshitz DA, Connors BA, Evan AP, Willis LR, Crum LA. In vivo pressure measurements of lithotripsy shockwaves in pigs. Ultrasound Med Biol. 1998 Feb;24(2):293-306
2. Gerdesmeyer L, Hauschild M, Ueberle F. ESWT bei Hüftkopfnekrose – Fokusmessungen. 3. Drei-Länder-Treffen der Österreichischen, Schweizer und Deutschen Fachgesell-schaften für Stoßwellentherapie am 21./22.03.03, München. Abstractband p 63.
3. Hausdorf J, Maier M, Delius M Extracorporeal shockwaves induce production of bone growth factors from osteoblasts. Calcified Tissue Int. (2004) 74 (Suppl 1): S50-S51
4. Hofmann S, Kramer J, Leder K, Plenk HJr, Engel A. Osteonekrosen: Pathophysiologie und Magnetresonanztomographie. Orthopäde 1994; 23:16-27
5. Hofmann S, Mazieres B. Osteonekrose: Natürlicher Verlauf und konservative Therapie. Orthopäde 2000; 29:403-410
6. Hopson CN, Siverhus SW Ischemic necrosis of the femoral head. Treatment by core de-compression. J Bone Joint Surg Am. 1988 Aug;70(7):1048-51
7. Jones JP. Intravascular coagulation and osteonecrosis. Clin Orthop 1992; 277:41-53
8. Kramer J, Breitenseher M, Imhof H, Urban M, Plenk HJr, Hofmann S. Bildgebung bei der Osteonekrose. Orthopäde 2000; 29:380-388
9. Langlais F, Fourastier J. Rotation osteotomies for osteonecrosis of the femoral head. Clin Orthop 1997; 343:110-123
10. Lauber S, Ludwig J, Hötzinger H. Hochenergetische extrakorporale Stoßwellentherapie bei Hüftkopfnekrosen. Z Orthop 2000; 138:Oa3-Oa4
11. Lausten GS, Mathiesen B. Core decompression for femoral head necrosis. Prospective study of 28 patients. Acta Orthop Scand. 1990 Dec;61(6):507-11
12. Lausten GS. Non-traumatic necrosis of the femoral head. Int Orthop. 1999;23(4):193-7

13. Leder K, Knahr K Results of medullary space decompression in the early stage of so-called idiopathic femur head necrosis Z. Orthop Ihre Grenzgeb. 1993 Mar-Apr;131(2):113-9
14. Ludwig J, Lauber S, Lauber J, Hötzinger H. Stoßwellenbehandlung der Hüftkopfnekrose des Erwachsenen. Z Orthop 1999; 137:Oa2-Oa5
15. Maier M, Hausdorf J, Tischer T, Milz S, Weiler C, Refior HJ, Schmitz C New bone forma-tion by extracorporeal shockwavesDependence of induction on energy flux density. Orthopade. 2004 Dec;33(12):1401-1410
16. Mont MA, Hungerford DS. Non-traumatic avascular necrosis of the femoral head. J Bo-ne Joint Surg Am 1995; 77 :459-474
17. Mont MA, Hungerford MW. Therapie der Osteonekrose - Grundlagen und Entschei-dungshilfen. Orthopäde 2000; 29:457-462
18. Plenk HJr, Hofmann S, Breitenseher M, Urban M. Pathomorphologische Aspekte und Reparaturmechanismen der Femurkopfosteonekrose. Orthopäde 2000; 29:389-402
19. Röhrig H, Wirtz DC ESWT on therapy of necrosis of the femoral head. 4th Congress of the International Society for Muskuloskeletal Shockwave Therapy (ISMST), 24.05.-26.05.2001, Berlin. Abstract Book, p.52.
20. Russo S, Galasso O, Corrado B. The avascular necrosis of the head femur: Re-sults with shockwave treatment. Sonderausgabe der Orthopädischen Praxis 2000; S.94-95
21. Russo S, Galasso O, Gigliotti S. Shockwave therapy for the treatment of hip necrosis. 2nd Internat Congress of the European Society for Musculoskeletal Shockwave Therapy, 1999, London, Proceedings
22. Stulberg BN, Bauer TW, Belhobek GH Making core decompression work. Clin Orthop. 1990 Dec;(261):186-95
23. Wirtz DC. Nichttraumatische Hüftkopfnekrose. In: Peters K (ed.) Knochenerkrankungen. 2001; Thieme Verlag, Stuttgart
24. Wirtz DC, Zilkens KW, Adam G, Niethard FU. MRT-Kontrollierte Ergebnisse nach core decompression des Hüftkopfes bei aseptischer Osteonekrose und transientem Mark-ödem. Z Orthop 1998; 136:138-146
25. Wang FS, Wang CJ, Chen YJ, Chang PR, Huang YT, Sun YC, Huang HC, Yang YJ, Yang KD Ras induction of superoxide activates ERK-dependent angiogenic transcription factor HIF-1alpha and VEGF-A expression in shockwave-stimulated osteoblasts.
26. J Biol Chem. 2004 Mar 12;279(11):10331-7

11

Extracorporeal Cardiac Shockwave Therapy as a New Therapeutic Option for Ischemic Cardiomyopathy

Takahiro Nishida, M.D. and Hiroaki Shimokawa, M.D.

Background

Prognosis of ischemic cardiomyopathy still remains poor due to the lack of effective treatments. To develop a non-invasive therapy for the disorder, we examined the in vitro and in vivo effects of extracorporeal shockwaves (SW). Shockwaves are well known to induce angiogenesis.

Methods and Results

SW treatment to cultured human umbilical vein endothelial cells significantly up-regulated mRNA expressions of vascular endothelial growth factor and its receptor Flt-1 in vitro. A porcine model of chronic myocardial ischemia was made by placing an ameroid constrictor at the proximal segment of the left circumflex coronary artery, which gradually induced a total occlusion of the artery with sustained myocardial dysfunction but without myocardial infarction in 4 weeks. Thereafter, extracorporeal SW therapy to the ischemic myocardial region (200 pulses/spot for 9 spots at 0.09 mJ/mm^2) was performed (n=8), which induced a complete recovery of left ventricular ejection fraction, wall thickening fraction, and regional myocardial blood flow (RMBF) of the ischemic region in 4 weeks. By contrast, animals that did not receive the therapy had sustained myocardial dysfunction and RMBF (n=8).

These results suggest that extracorporeal cardiac SW therapy is an effective and non-invasive therapeutic strategy for ischemic heart disease.

Introduction

Prognosis of ischemic cardiomyopathy without an indication of coronary intervention or coronary artery bypass grafting still remains poor because medication is the only therapy to treat the disorder[1]. Thus, it is mandatory to develop an effective and non-invasive therapy for ischemic cardiomyopathy.

It has been recently suggested that shockwave (SW) therapy could enhance angiogenesis in vitro[2, 3]. A SW is a longitudinal acoustic wave, traveling with ultrasound speed in water and body tissue. It is a single pressure pulse with a short needle-like positive spike of less than 1 microsecond duration and amplitude up to 100 MPa followed by a tensile part of several microseconds with lower amplitude[4]. A SW is known to exert "cavitation effects" (a micrometer sized violent collapse of bubbles inside the cells) and has recently been demonstrated to induce localized stress on cell membranes that resembles shear stress[4, 5]. We examined the possible beneficial effects of SW therapy on ischemia-induced myocardial dysfunction in a porcine model of chronic myocardial ischemia in vivo[6].

Material and Methods

We treated single-donor human umbilical vein endothelial cells (HUVEC) with 500 pulses of SW at 4 different energy levels (0=control, 0.02, 0.09, 0.18, and 0.35 mJ/mm^2). The cells were stored 24 hours in the same medium before RNA extraction. Equal amounts of mRNA were analyzed by ribonuclease protection assay (RPA).

We put an ameroid constrictor around the proximal LCx in order to gradually induce a total occlusion of the artery in 4 weeks. We applied low energy SW (0.09 mJ/mm^2, approximately 10% of the energy for the lithotripsy treatment) to 9 spots of the ischemic region (200 pulses/spot) guided by an echocardiogram equipped within a specially designed SW generator (Storz Medical AG, Kreuzlingen, Switzerland) (Figure 1A). We were able to focus the SW in any part of the heart under echocardiography guidance (Figure 1B). We performed the SW treatment (n=8) 4 weeks after the implantation of an ameroid constrictor 3 times within one week. We measured left ventricular ejection fraction (LVEF) by left ventriculography, wall thickening fraction by epicardial echocardiography and regional myocardial blood flow by colored microsphere.

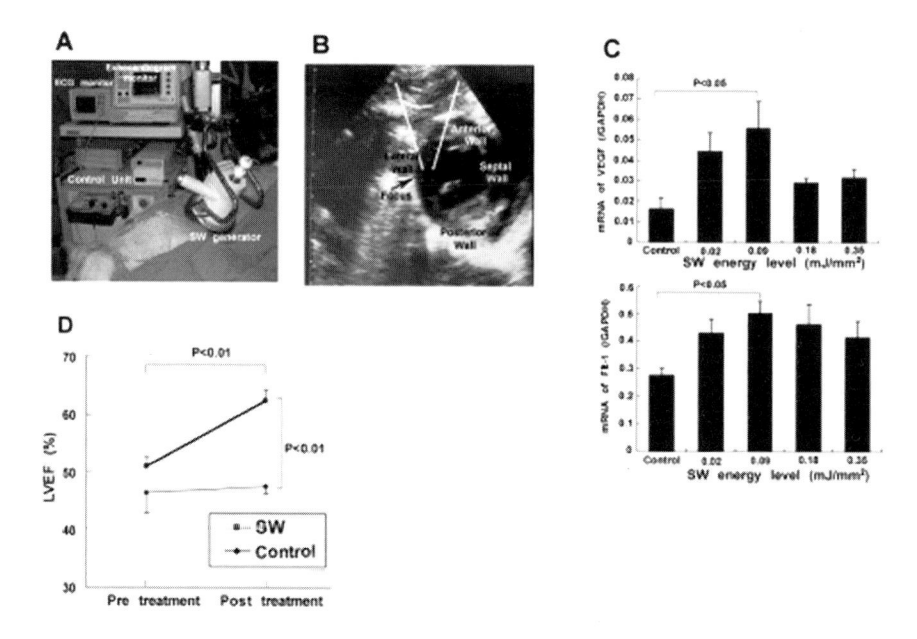

Figure 1. A. The machine is equipped with a SW generator and in-line echocardiography; B. The SW pulse is easily focused on the ischemic myocardium under the guidance of echocardiography (black arrow); C. SW treatment up-regulated mRNA expression of VEGF (A) and Flt-1 (B) in HUVEC in vitro with a maximum effect noted at 0.09 mJ/mm2; D. The SW therapy normalized LVEF in the SW group but not in the control group.

To examine the effect of SW treatment to the ischemic myocardium in vivo, we counted the number of factor VIII-positive cells in the endocardial and epicardial wall in 10 fields of the LCx region.

Total RNA was isolated from rapidly frozen ischemic LV wall (LCx region) after 3 SW treatments were done. Quantification of VEGF and its receptor Flt-1 was performed by amplification of cDNA using an ABI Prism 7000 real-time thermocycler. Western blot analysis for VEGF was also performed in 3 sections from the ischemic LV wall (LCx region). The regions containing VEGF proteins were visualized by ECL Western blotting luminal reagent (Santa Cruz Biotechnology, Santa Cruz, CA). The extent of the VEGF was normalized by that of β-actin.

Results

The effects of SW treatment significantly up-regulated mRNA expressions of VEGF and its receptor Flt-1 in HUVEC with a maximum effect noted at 0.09 mJ/mm^2 (Figure 1C).

Four weeks after the ameroid implantation, LVG demonstrated an impaired LVEF in both groups, while at 8 weeks follow up, LVEF was normalized in the SW group but remained impaired in the control group (Figure 1D).

At 4 weeks, we observed a significant reduction in WTF (%) in both groups (13±2 in the control and 13±3 in the SW group) (Figure 2A). However, at 8 weeks, the SW treatment markedly improved WTF in the SW group (30±3) but not in the control group (9±2) under control conditions (Figure 2A). Under dobutamine-loading conditions, which mimicked exercise conditions, WTF was further reduced at 4 weeks after the ameroid implantation in both groups (16±3 in the control and 18±2 in the SW group), however, at 8 weeks, WTF was again markedly ameliorated only in the SW group (31±2) but not in the control group (16±4) (Figure 2B).

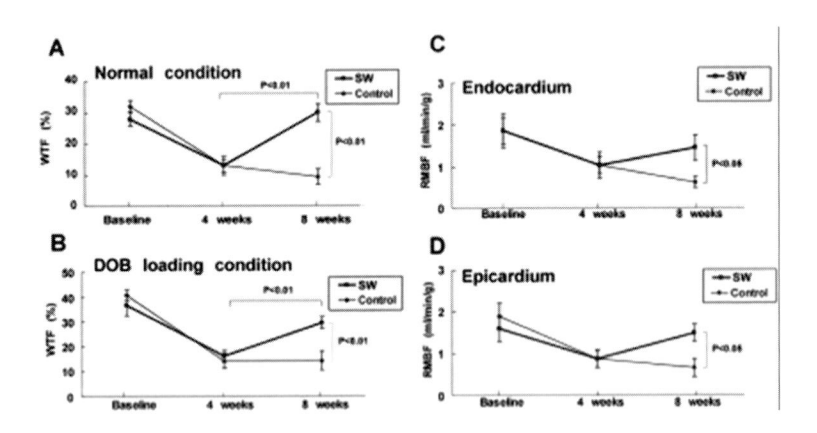

Figure 2. A and B. The SW therapy induced a complete recovery of wall thickening fraction (WTF) of the ischemic lateral wall under control conditions (A) and under dobutamine (DOB) loading conditions (B); C and D. The SW therapy significantly increased regional myocardial blood flow (RMBF) assessed by colored microspheres in both the endocardium (C) and the epicardium (D).

At 4 weeks, RMBF in the endocardium and epicardium (ml/min/g) was equally decreased in both groups (1.0±0.3 and 0.9±0.2 in the control and 1.0±0.2 and 0.9±0.2 in the SW group, respectively). The SW treatment again improved RMBF in the endocardium (0.6±0.1 in the control and 1.4±0.3 in the SW groups, P<0.05) (Figure 2D) as well as in the epicardium (0.7±0.2 in the control and 1.5±0.2 in the SW groups, P<0.05) (Figure 2D).

Quantitative analysis demonstrated that the number of capillaries was significantly higher in the SW group in both the endocardium (840±26 in the control and 1280±45 in the SW group, P<0.05) (Figure 3A) and the epicardium (820±30 in the control and 1200±22 in the SW group, P<0.05) (Figure 3B). RT-PCR analysis and Western blotting demonstrated a significant up-regulation of VEGF mRNA expression (8.0±6 in the control and 32±8 in the SW group, P<0.05) (Figure 3A) and protein expression (2.23-fold increase in the SW group, P<0.05) (Figure 3B) after the SW treatment to the ischemic myocardium in vivo.

Discussion

The new findings of the present study are that extracorporeal cardiac SW therapy enhances angiogenesis in the ischemic myocardium and normalizes myocardial function in a porcine model of chronic myocardial ischemia in vivo. Thus, the present study demonstrates the potential usefulness of extracorporeal cardiac SW therapy as a non-invasive treatment of chronic myocardial ischemia. In the present study, we were able to demonstrate that SW treatment (1) normalized global and regional myocardial functions as well as regional myocardial blood flow of the chronic ischemic region, (2) increased vascular density in the SW-treated region, and (3) enhanced mRNA expression of VEGF and its receptor Flt-1 in HUVEC in vitro and VEGF production in the ischemic myocardium in vivo. Thus, SW-induced up-regulation of the endogenous angiogenic system may offer a novel and promising non-invasive strategy for the treatment of ischemic heart disease.

Advantages of extracorporeal cardiac SW therapy

Recent attempts to enhance angiogenesis in the ischemic organs include gene therapy and bone marrow cell transplantation therapy. The main purpose of gene therapy is to induce over-expression of a selected angiogenic ligand (e.g. VEGF) that leads to angiogenesis in the ischemic region. Bone marrow cell

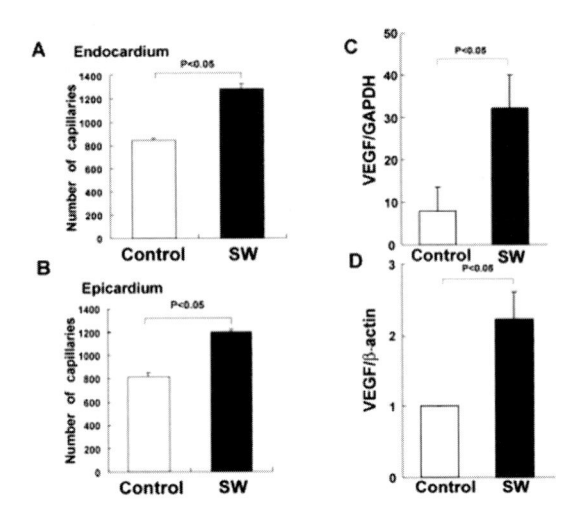

Figure 3. A and B. Capillary density was significantly greater in the SW group (SW) than in the control group (Control) in both the endocardium (A) and the epicardium (B); C and D. SW treatment up-regulated mRNA (C) and protein (D) expressions of VEGF in the ischemic myocardium.

transplantation therapy, which depends on the adult stem cell plasticity, may also be a useful strategy for angiogenesis because endothelial progenitor cells could be isolated from circulating mononuclear cells in humans and shown to be incorporated into neovascularization[7].

A major advantage of extracorporeal cardiac SW therapy over these two strategies is the fact that it is non-invasive and safe without any adverse effects. If necessary, we could treat patients repeatedly (even out-patients) with SW therapy because no surgery, anesthesia, or even catheter intervention is required. Thus, extracorporeal cardiac SW therapy appears to be an applicable and non-invasive treatment for ischemic heart disease.

Mechanisms for SW-Induced Angiogenesis

When a SW hits tissue, cavitation (a micrometer sized violent collapse of bubbles) is induced by the first compression by the positive pressure part and the expansion with the tensile part of a SW[4]. Because the physical forces generated by cavitation are highly localized, a SW could induce localized stress on cell membranes as altered shear stress affects endothelial cells[8]. Although precise mechanisms for the SW-induced biochemical effects remain to be examined, these mechanisms may be involved in the underlying mechanisms for the SW-induced angiogensis. Indeed, Wang et al. reported that SW therapy induces angiogenesis of Achilles tendon-bone junction in dogs[9].

Conclusion

We were able to demonstrate that non-invasive extracorporeal cardiac SW therapy effectively increases regional myocardial blood flow and normalizes ischemia-induced myocardial dysfunction without any adverse effects. Thus, extracorporeal cardiac SW therapy may be an effective, safe and non-invasive treatment for ischemic cardiomyopathy, but prospective controlled trials have to be performed to prove clinical efficacy as well.

Literature

1. Jessup M, Brozena S. Heart failure. N Engl J Med. 2003;348:2007-18.
2. Gutersohn A, Caspari G. Shockwaves upregulate vascular endothelial growth factor m-RNA in human umbilical vascular endothelial cells. Circulation. 2000;102 (Supple):18.
3. Nishida T, Oi K, Tatewaki H, Uwatoku T, Abe K, Kajihara N, Eto M, Morita S, Yasui H, Takeshita A, Shimokawa H. Extracorporeal shockwave therapy induces a complete recovery of ischemia-induced myocardial dysfunction in pigs. Circulation. 2003;108:95-96.
4. Apfel RE. Acoustic cavitation: a possible consequence of biomedical uses of ultrasound. Br J Cancer. 1982;45 (Supple):140-146.
5. Maisonhaute E, Prado C, White PC, Compton RG. Surface acoustic cavitation understood via nanosecond electrochemistry. Part III: Shear stress in ultrasonic cleaning. Ultrason Sonochem. 2002;9:297-303.
6. Nishida T, Shimokawa H, Oi K, Tatewaki H, Uwatoku T, Abe K, Matsumoto Y, Kajihara N, Eto M, Matsuda T, Yasui H, Takeshita A, Sunagawa K. Extracorporeal cardiac shockwave therapy markedly ameliorates ischemia-induced myocardial dysfunction in pigs in vivo. Circulation. 2004;110:3055-61.
7. Asahara T, Murohara T, Sullivan A, Silver M, van der Zee R, Li T, Witzenbichler B, Schatteman G, Isner JM. Isolation of Putative Progenitor Endothelial Cells for Angiogenesis. Science. 1997;275:964-966.
8. Fisher AB, Chien S, Barakat AI, Nerem RM. Endothelial cellular response to altered shear stress. Am J Physiol. 2001;281:L529-L533.

9. Wang CJ, Huang HY, Pai CH. Shockwave-enhanced neovascularization at the tendon-bone junction: an experiment in dogs. J Foot Ankle Surg. 2002;41:16-22.

12

Clinical Application of the EMS Swiss DolorClast®
L. Gerdesmeyer, M. Henne, P. Diehl, H. Gollwitzer, M. Göbel

In general, the following recommendations apply when using the Swiss DolorClast®:

- In all indications, patient biofeedback is used to localize the region of interest. The treatment area is determined by palpating the relevant pain region and a skin marker could be used to verify the previous defined area during the treatment.
- A coupling medium such as ultrasound gel or certain oils (e.g. castor oil) must be used to ensure delivery of the shockwave to the treatment region without a significant loss of enegy between skin and applicator. Disconnection must be avoided.
- Local anesthesics are not recommended and should be administered based on patient demand and indicated and performed by a physician.
- A gradual pressure increasing application of 500 shockwave impulses may be appropriate to patients' pain adaptation. The applied energy should be increased slowly during this initial phase. Clinical applications have shown a significant reduction in pain perception after a brief application period.
- Minor side effects may occur but without clinical relevance. Published minor adverse events were described as local swelling, hematoma, petechial bleeding and pain during the treatment. In general, all side effects disappear in just a few days without the need for specific treatment.
- Based on the consensus of radial shockwave therapy practitioners, treatment parameters were dicussed and defined later on (2002). Decisions were based on technical and physical parameters, clinical experience of the practitioners as well as on published data (listed in Table 1).

Nomenclature and treatment parameters

Medical indication	Synonym	Note	Frequency	Pressure (bar)	Application force	Impulses	Sessions	Applicator	Interval
Plantar fasciitis	Heel pain		8 – 10	2,5 – 4	strong	2.000	3 – 5	15 mm	weekly
Lateral epicondylitis	Tennis elbow		4 – 8	2,5 – 4	light	2.000	3 – 5	15 mm	weekly
Rotator cuff tendinopathy	Shoulder pain, impingement syndrome	If calcification exists, success can be verified by X-ray or ultrasound	4 – 8	2,5 – 4	medium	2.000	3 – 5	15 mm	weekly
Patella tendiopathy	Jumpers knee		6 – 10	2 – 3	medium	2.000	3 – 5	15 mm	weekly
Tibial edge syndrome	Shin splints		6 – 10	1,5 – 2,5	soft	2.000	3 – 5	15 mm	weekly
Iliotibial band friction syndrome			6 – 10	2,5 – 3,5	strong	2.000	3 – 5	15 mm	weekly
Achillodynia		Treatment proximal and/or distal	6 – 10	3 – 4	soft	2.000	3 – 5	15 mm	weekly

Table 1. Nomenclature and treatment parameters

Treatment of tennis elbow (Epicondylopathia humeri radialis)

The following differential diagnoses apply:

- Acute tendon and muscle injuries (near elbow)
- Apophyseal disorders
- Osteochondrosis
- Loose bodies
- Elbow arthrosis
- A vascular bone necrosis (Morbus Panner)
- Fracture of the radius head
- Supinator slit syndrome
- Pronator teres syndrome

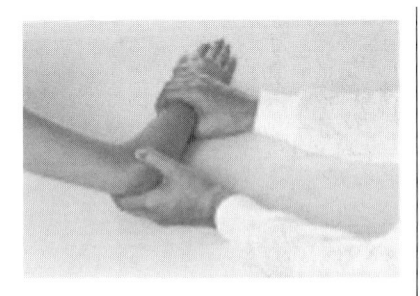

The treatment area is localized by palpation (biofeedback).

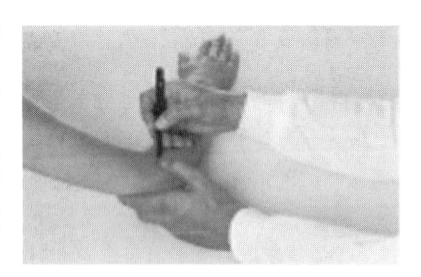

Once the pain area is localized, the skin is marked over the treatment area.

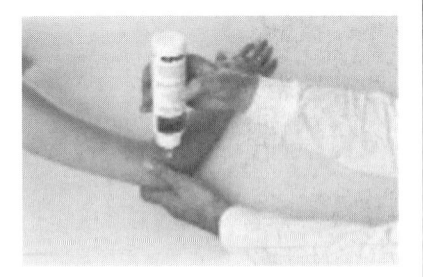

EMS Swiss DolorClast® coupling gel improves delivery.

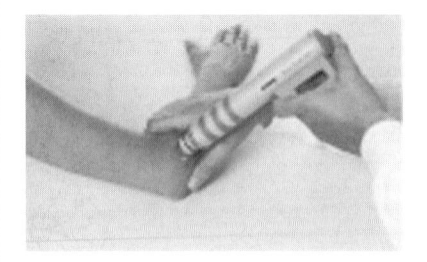

A 15 mm applicator is applied with soft application pressure.

Treatment of heel spur (plantar fasciitis)

The following differential diagnoses apply:

- Tarsal tunnel syndrome
- Calcaneal stress fracture
- Coalition, calcaneo navicular
- Anterior calcaneal stress fracture

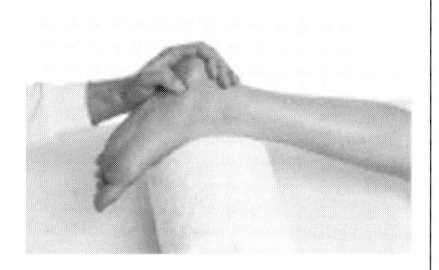

The treatment area is localized by palpation (biofeedback).

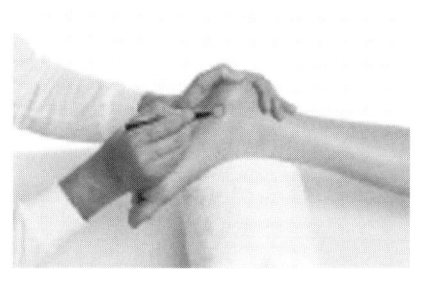

Once the pain area is localized, the skin is marked over the treatment area.

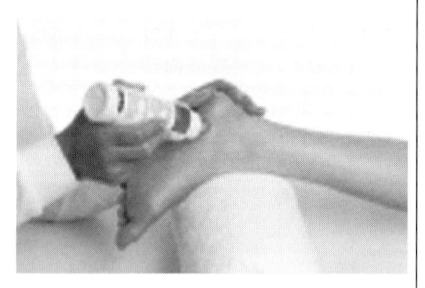

EMS Swiss DolorClast® coupling gel improves delivery.

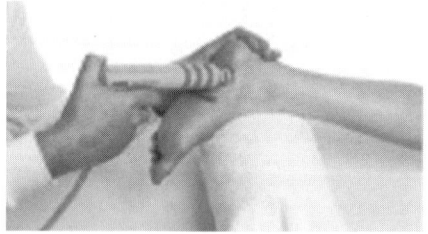

A 15 mm applicator is applied over the treatment area with strong application pressure. Application pressure 4 bar.

Treatment of rotator cuff enthesiopathy

The following differential diagnoses apply:

- Subacromial bursitis
- AC joint arthrosis
- Shoulder joint instability
- Degenerative damage and long biceps tendon disorders
- Frozen shoulder
- Nerval disorders
- Arthrosis of the glenohumeral joint

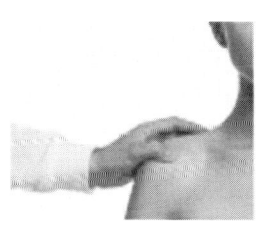

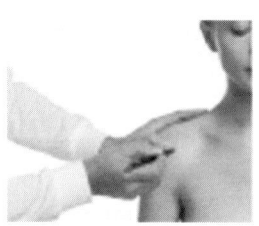

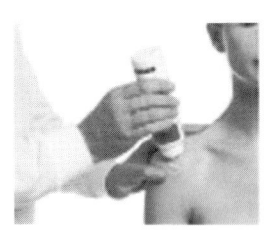

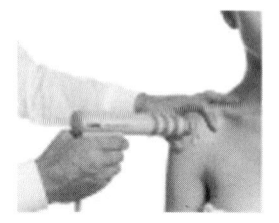

The treatment area is localized by radiology or sonography and by palpation (biofeedback).

During localization the skin is marked over the treatment area.

EMS Swiss DolorClast® coupling gel improves delivery.

A 15 mm applicator is applied over the treatment area with high application pressure. Application pressure 4 bar.

If calcification is present, x-rays or ultrasound should be used for reexamination.

Treatment of patella tip syndrome

The following differential diagnoses apply:

- Femoropatellar cartilage damage and arthrosis
- Bursitis prepatellar or pes anserinus
- Osgood-Schlatter
- Morbus Sinding-Larsson
- Bipartite Patella
- Plica (= med. shelf) syndrome
- Meniscal tears

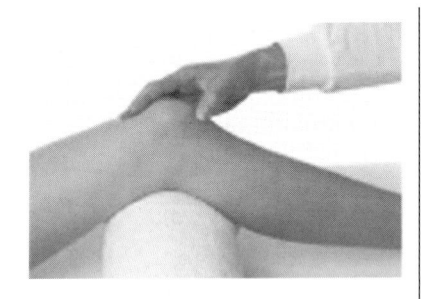

The treatment area is localized by palpation.	Once the pain area is localized, the skin is marked over the treatment area.
EMS Swiss DolorClast® coupling gel improves delivery.	A 15 mm applicator is applied over the treatment area with soft application pressure.

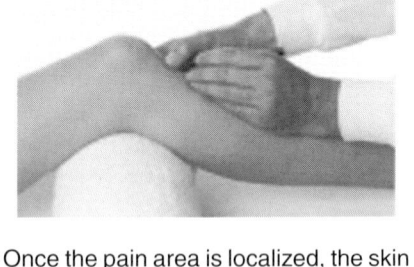

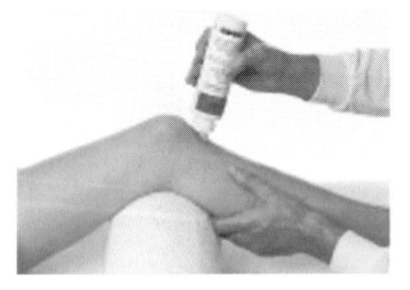

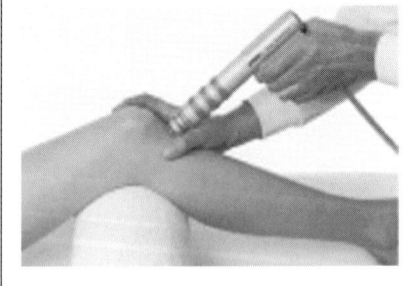

Treatment of tibialis anterior syndrome

The following differential diagnoses apply:
- Tib. post. and flexor hallucis longus lesion
- Arthrosis of the ankle joint
- Osteochondritis dessicans (OCD) of the talus
- Nerve entrapment syndromes
- Tarsal tunnel syndrome
- Muscle hernias
- Arterial vessel disease
- Stress fracture
- Osteomyelitis
- Radiculopathy L4
- Compartment syndrome
- Chronic venous insufficiency

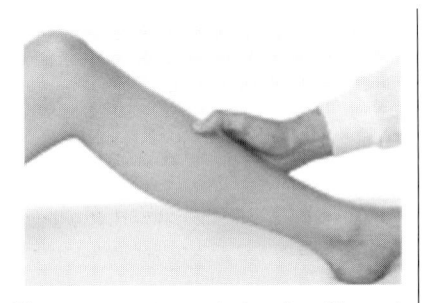

The treatment area is localized by palpation.	Once the pain area is localized, the skin is marked over the treatment area.
EMS Swiss DolorClast® coupling gel improves delivery.	A 15 mm applicator is applied over the treatment area with medium dorsal, soft medial and lateral application pressure.

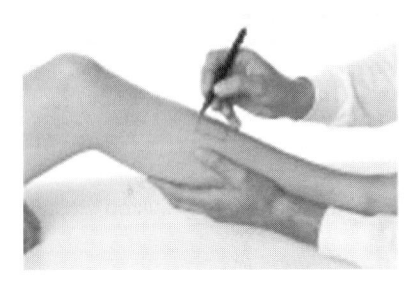

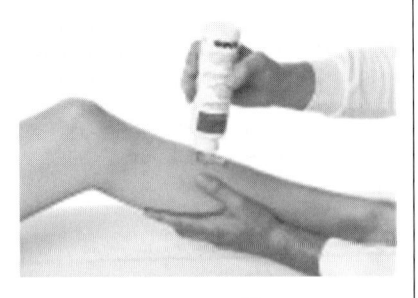

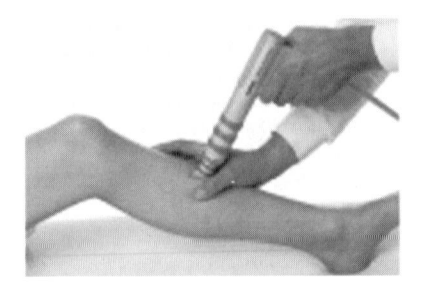

Treatment of achillodynia

The following differential diagnoses apply:
- Posterior ankle cartilage damage
- Bursitis subachilleal
- Partial Achilles tendon ruptures
- Stress fracture (MT III, calcaneus)
- Radiculopathy L5
- Osteochondritis dessicans (OCD) of the talus
- HLA B27 positive (rheumatoid arthritis)
- Tendon insufficiency of the ankle joint
- Os trigonum
- Posterior heel spur
- Snow board ankle

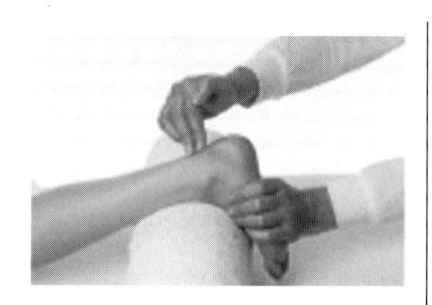

The treatment area is localized by palpation.

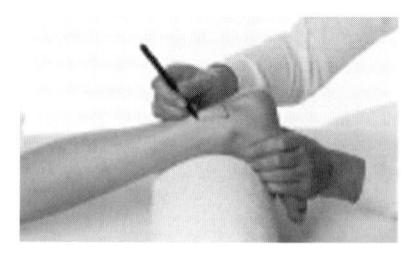

Once the pain area is localized, the skin is marked over the treatment area.

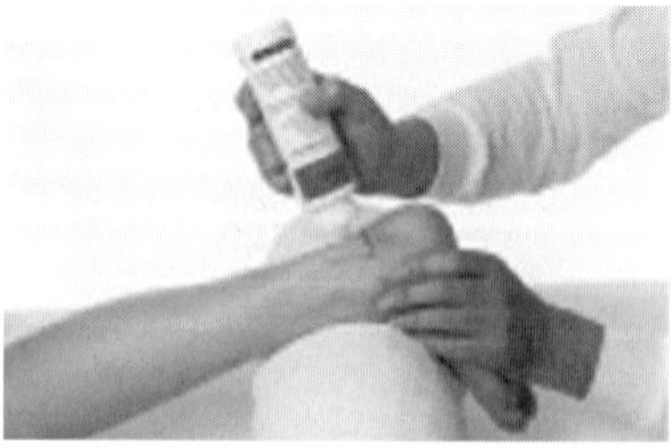

EMS Swiss DolorClast® coupling gel improves delivery.

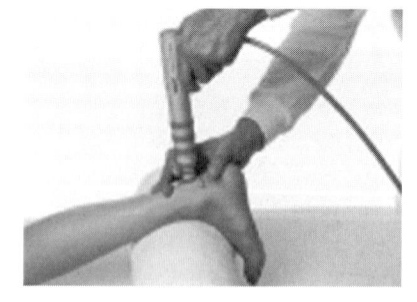

A 15 mm applicator is applied over the treatment area with medium dorsal, medial and lateral application pressure (continuous impulse mode).

Treatment of iliotibial band enthesiopathy

The following differential diagnoses apply:

- Coxarthrosis
- High lumbar radicular or pseudo-radicular syndromes
- Hernia inguinalis or femoralis
- N. cutaneous fem. syndrome
- Stress fracture
- Epihyseolysis capitis femoris
- Hip dysplasia

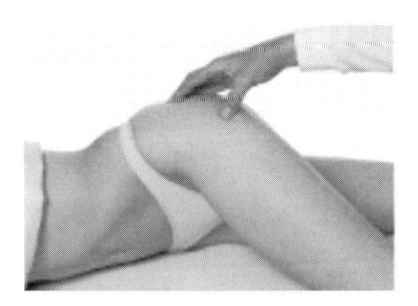

The treatment area is localized by palpation.	Once the pain area is localized, the skin is marked over the treatment area.
EMS Swiss DolorClast® coupling gel improves delivery.	A 15 mm applicator is applied over the treatment area with modeate to strong application pressure. The handpiece is positioned vertically on the skin.

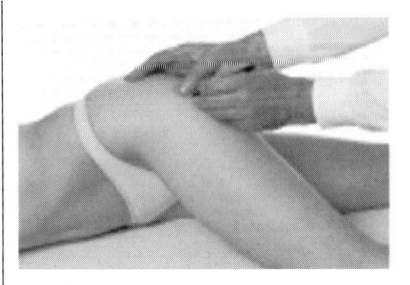

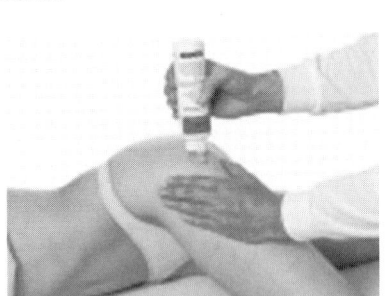

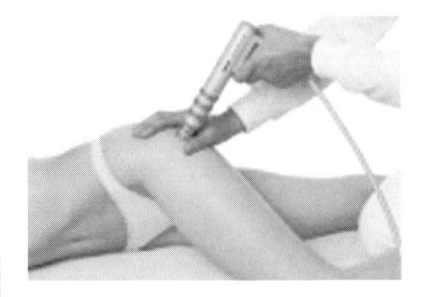

13

Method Swiss DolorClast® (rESWT) – System Components
Thomas Stierle

Meeting the requirements of a modern orthopedic ESWT device

After several years of orthopedic shockwave application using adapted lithotripsy devices, orthopedists realized that commonly used shockwave devices did not meet the requirements of musculoskeletal treatments. Therefore the surgeons directed their following request to their industrial partners:

"It is the consensus that the industry is called up to develop a new generation of shockwave devices. For pain therapy, the following characteristics are needed: small and mobile devices. The applied energy must be easy to adjust as well as variable to applicate. The shockwave head (handpiece) should be mobile. For this purpose the shockwave head must be minimized in size and weight. A patient can always be positioned as usual on a barrow and be treated from above."

(Orthopaedic study group of the German Shockwave lithotripsy society, consensus meeting, 1/28/1995, Tuebingen, published in "Die Stosswelle: Forschung und Klinik," Christian Chaussy, Tuebingen, 1995)

A modern ESWT – device

EMS began researching the effect of pneumatically generated shockwaves on bone tissue as long ago as 1990. With the Swiss LithoClast®, EMS has, for years, been producing a highly effective pneumatically driven device that works in harmony with other extracorporeal lithotripters used in urology. When developing the Swiss DolorClast®, the EMS specialists accepted the above challenge because of their conviction that an ESWT device developed on the basis of the successful Swiss LithoClast® would withstand comparison to conventional ESWT devices in the treatment of pain. With the introduction of the Radial Extracorporeal Shockwave Therapy (rESWT) the Swiss DolorClast® is setting a new standard in Extracorporeal Shockwave Therapy (ESWT).

Operating principle

The EMS device is based on an entirely new concept in the treatment of musculoskeletal soft tissue pain. The Swiss DolorClast® is a modified Swiss LithoClast® device, producing shockwaves in the low to medium-energy range, similar to those used in intracorporeal lithotripsy. Figure 1 illustrates the principle:

A projectile in the handpiece is accelerated at high speed using a precisely controlled compressed air pulse. The projectile is directed with a tolerance of a few micrometers. When the projectile strikes the applicator installed in the handpiece – like the first ball-bearing striking the next ball-bearing – its kinetic energy is converted into mechanical energy.

This energy is transmitted from ball-bearing to ball-bearing or along the applicator, without movement. At the end of the applicator, the shockwave is coupled out into human tissue. To minimize transmission losses (which would occur in the air between applicator-skin-interface) contact gel is used to guide the shockwave.

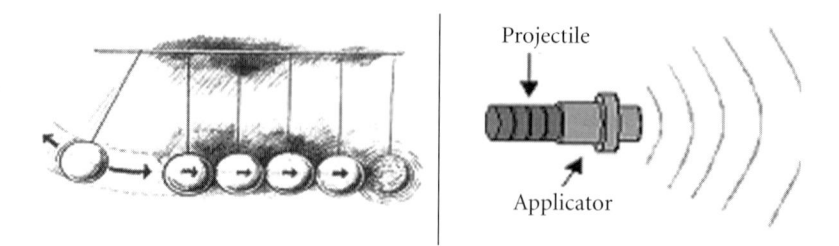

Figure 1. Simplified operating principle: on the left, the ballbearing model; on the right, drawing of a projectile and applicator.

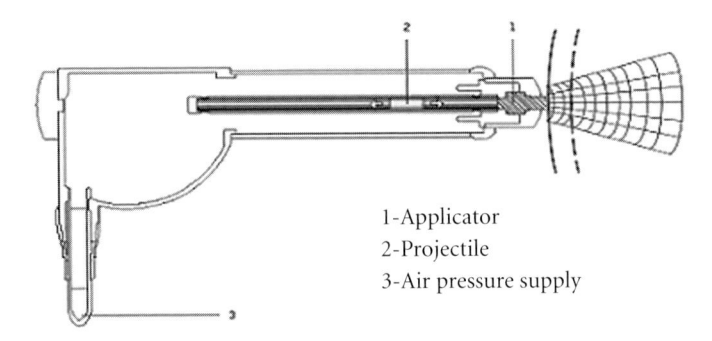

1-Applicator
2-Projectile
3-Air pressure supply

Figure 2. Operating principle of Swiss DolorClast® Handpiece.

Method Swiss DolorClast® - Concept

The indications for pain therapy mostly are superficial, so it seemed natural to forego a complicated technical localization unit, which, for surface application, would have also been pointless.

The shockwave source of the Swiss DolorClast® emits shockwaves from the tip of the applicator. They propagate radially into the body.

The effectiveness of the method has been clinically tested. The handpiece supplied can be used for all indications of the Swiss DolorClast®.

Indication	Distance to skin surface
Rotator cuff tendinopathy (Impingement syndrome)	2 - 3 cm
Lateral and medial Epicondylitis	0.1 - 0.5 cm
Plantar fasciitis	1 - 2 cm
Achilles tendinitis	1 cm
Iliotibial band friction syndrome	2 – 3 cm
Dupuytren's contracture	0.5 cm
Patella tendinitis	1 – 2 cm
Pain caused by myogeloses (trigger points)	ca. 2 cm

Table 1. Location of various indications in pain therapy.

Radial propagation (rESWT)

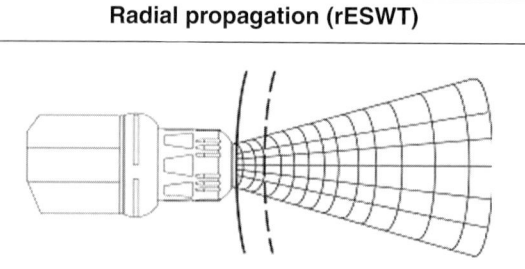

| Energy discharged: | 0,16 mJ/mm^2 |
| Propagation: | Radial |

Figure 3. Propagation of the Swiss DolorClast® shockwave.

Swiss DolorClast® - System components

The EMS Swiss DolorClast® basic system and its components.

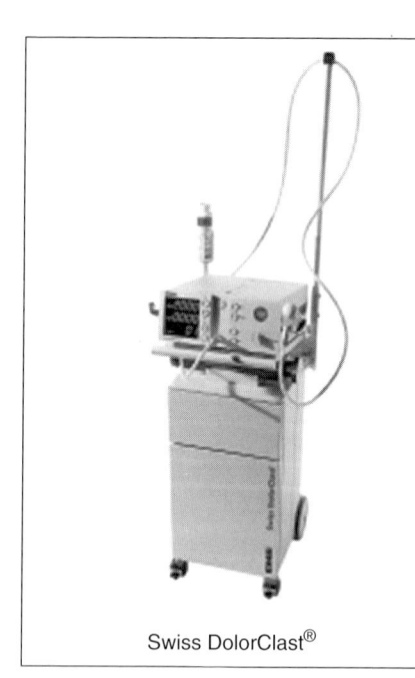

Swiss DolorClast®	EMS Swiss DolorClast® consists of a • Control unit • Handpiece (rESWT) • Foot pedal • Compressor • Gel • Cart The Swiss DolorClast® cart accommodates accessories, e.g. applicators, application gel, instruction manual, foot pedal and compressor.

METHOD SWISS DOLORCLAST® (rESWT) — SYSTEM COMPONENTS   133

Front display of the control unit	The clearly laid out, functional arrangement of the operating and control instruments makes EMS Swiss DolorClast®, easy to use. The desired number of shockwaves, firing rate, and application pressure to be applied can be set effortlessly before or even during treatment.
Foot pedal	Application of the shockwaves can be controlled only by using the foot pedal.
EMS Swiss DolorClast® Handpiece	The EMS Swiss DolorClast® handpiece is designed for broad-surface (radial) energy discharge. The modular construction makes the handpiece easy to clean and sterilize.
EMS Gel	EMS Gel is necessary for an optimized useage of the EMS Swiss DolorClast®. The viscosity of the gel is verified specific for the rESWT therapy.

Swiss DolorClast® - Accessories

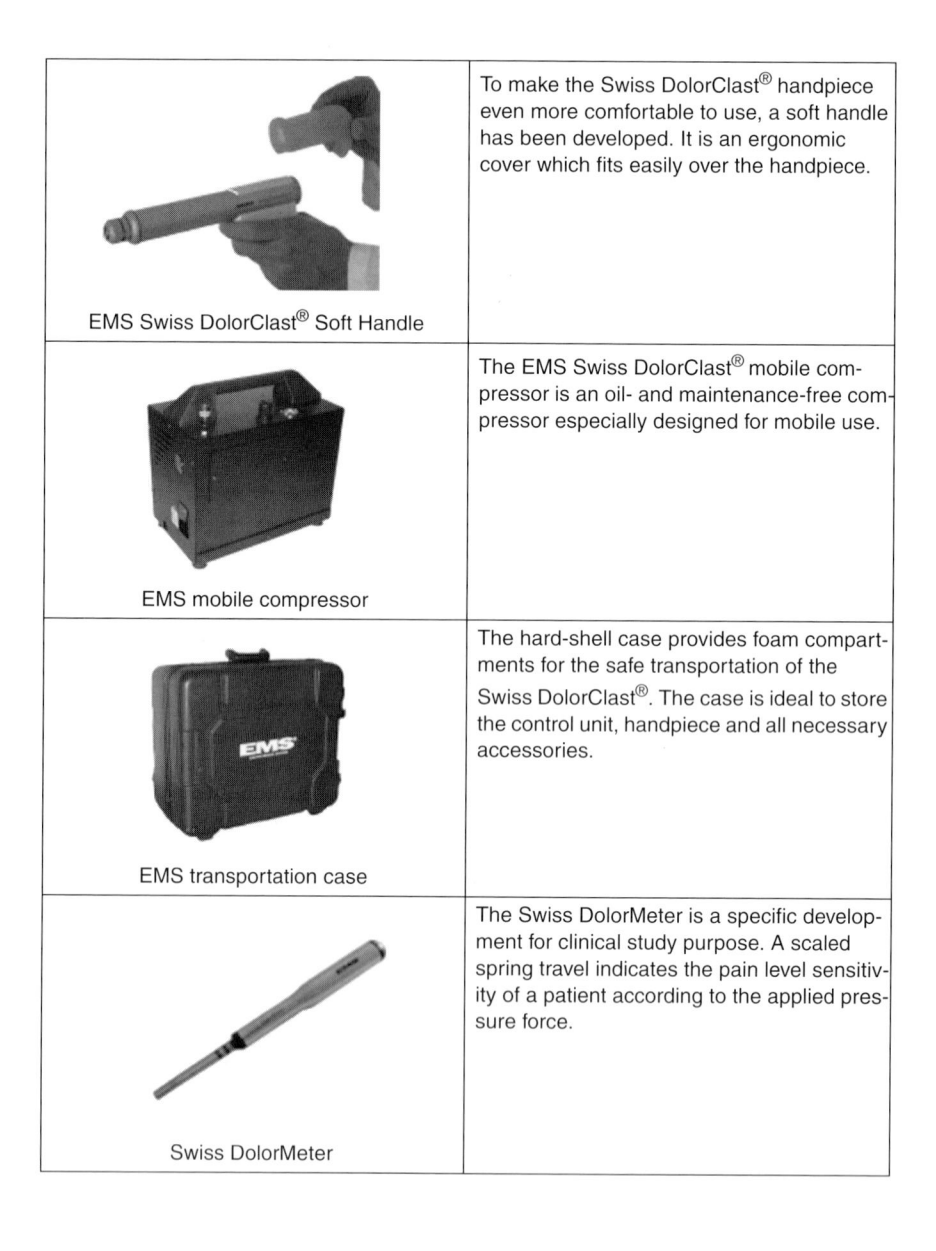

EMS Swiss DolorClast® Soft Handle	To make the Swiss DolorClast® handpiece even more comfortable to use, a soft handle has been developed. It is an ergonomic cover which fits easily over the handpiece.
EMS mobile compressor	The EMS Swiss DolorClast® mobile compressor is an oil- and maintenance-free compressor especially designed for mobile use.
EMS transportation case	The hard-shell case provides foam compartments for the safe transportation of the Swiss DolorClast®. The case is ideal to store the control unit, handpiece and all necessary accessories.
Swiss DolorMeter	The Swiss DolorMeter is a specific development for clinical study purpose. A scaled spring travel indicates the pain level sensitivity of a patient according to the applied pressure force.

METHOD SWISS DOLORCLAST® (rESWT) – SYSTEM COMPONENTS 135

Swiss DolorClast® - Handling

The proper use of the Swiss DolorClast® requires prior knowledge and professional expertise. It is essential that user instructions be read and understood by any practitioner who intends to use the equipment. This applies equally to all associated instruments and tools as well as components and accessories.

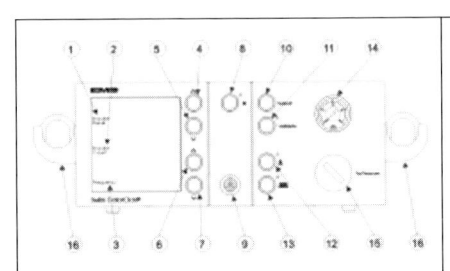

Front of control unit

1. Display for pre-set pulse counts per session
2. Display for reading present pulse count
3. Display for treatment frequency
4. Control to increase pulse count per session
5. Control to decrease pulse count per session
6. Control to increase treatment frequency
7. Control to decrease treatment frequency
8. Standby / ON with control light
9. Connector to handpiece
10. "Select": activate to change pre-set count per session
11. "Validate": conclude pre-setting procedure with control light

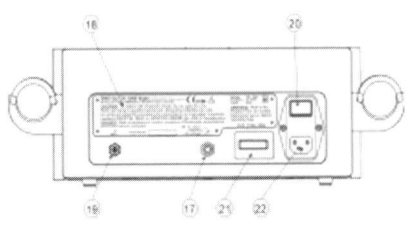

Back of control unit

12. Control with control light for single pulse mode
13. Control with control light for multiple pulse mode
14. Gauge for working pressure (Accuracy 1.6 % at 4 bar)
15. Regulator: adjustment of working pressure
16. Handpiece holder
17. Socket for compressed air supply
18. Manufacturer's identification plate and serial number
19. Socket for foot pedal with nut
20. Main switch on / off
21. Display for total pulse count
22. Main plug and fuse box

Prior to initial operation	The following requirements must be met before initial operation: • The Swiss DolorClast® must be properly connected to an appropriate source of compressed air. • The handpiece must be connected to the handpiece connection (9). • The Swiss DolorClast® foot pedal must be activated (19).
Initial operation	Press key (8) on the front. Standby mode is shown by an illuminated indicator light.
Impulse presetting	Press "Select" key (10). Current impulse count is shown in upper window (1) with blinking digit field. Press "Select" key (10) to switch back and forth between the digits. Press (⋀) key (4) to raise the exact number of impulses necessary for the treatment or press (⋁) key (5) to lower the number. Press "Validate" (11) to confirm the desired impulse count.
Operating mode key	The operator can choose between single impulse mode (12) and continuous impulse mode (13). **Single impulse mode:** Press (⊓) symbol key (12). Indicator light illuminates. A single impulse is released from the handpiece by activating the foot pedal. **Continuous mode:** Press (⊓⊓⊓) key (13). Indicator light illuminates. The handpiece continues to deliver a series of impulses as long as the foot pedal remains activated. As a rule, continuous impulse mode is used during treatment. Single impulse mode is used only to test the unit.
Operating pressure control	A dial (15) is used to set desired operating pressure. Turn clockwise to increase application pressure. A manometer (14) shows the operating pressure.
Setting operating frequency	Press (⋀) (6) to increase frequency, press (⋁) (7) to lower frequency. The lower display (3) shows the exact operating frequency.

General recommendations for device setting:

Preparation	Determine painful area by palpation based on patient biofeedback and mark the treatment area. Important: Apply Swiss DolorClast® coupling gel evenly prior to treatment.
Recommended operating parameters	- Up to 500 introductory impulses - 2000 impulses per session - 3-5 sessions at weekly intervals - 2.5-4 bar operating pressure - 6-10 Hz operating frequency
Recommendations	Apply therapy to the treatment area with circular movements in continuous impulse mode. For patients highly sensitive to pain, begin treatment at 2 bar operating pressure and 6 Hz operating frequency. Analgesic effect appears after 500 impulses. For further treatment steps, use successive increases in operating pressure (bar) and operating frequency (Hz). The generally recommended operating parameters must be reached. Application pressure is to be reduced slightly if the patient is too sensitive to pain.

Literature:

1. EMS SA, Nyon, Switzerland

14

Orthopedic Shockwave Treatment at Urologic Work Stations

M. Hauschild, A. Waizenhöfer, H. Brandner, W. Mittelmeier

Historical Development

Orthopedic shockwave therapy is still a young form of therapy. In 1991 Valchanou was the first to use ESWT for the treatment of pseudarthroses following mere experimental attempts involving the musculoskeletal system.

Shockwave therapy finds its medical origins in urology. The first in vitro lithotripsies were performed in the early '70s. Ten years later, Chaussy was the

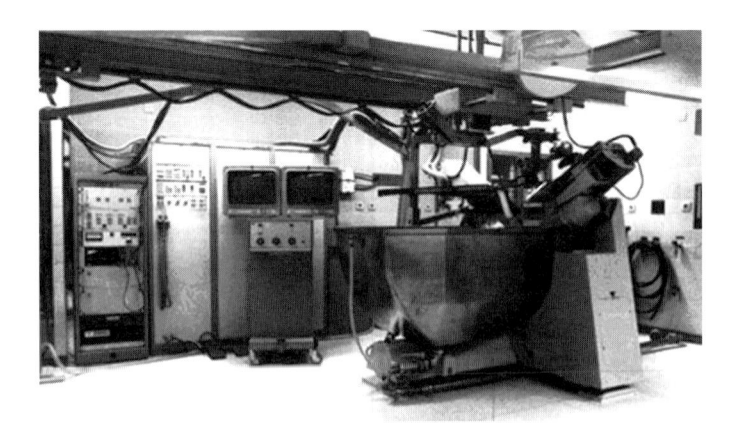

Figure 1. Historic urologic work station for lithotripsy.

first to destroy kidney stones in a patient[5]. Subsequently ESWT evolved to become a standard urologic therapy for the treatment of kidney and ureteral stones. During that time, effects on the musculoskeletal system were considered as a secondary effect.

In terms of orthopedics, the indication for the treatment of pseudarthrosis was followed by expansion of the therapy to treatment of calcific tendonitis of the shoulder by Dahmen in 1992[6]. Such an orthopedic application was based on the transfer of the effects of lithotripsy to the musculoskeletal system. It was believed at that time that the treatment of bones would trigger microfractures with secondary callous formation and osseous healing would be induced. Today, the ESWT mechanism has been shown to induce osteonegenesis and vasculogenesis as well as biochemical reactions. Even the direct disintegration of calcium deposits in calcific tendinosis of the shoulder appears to be of secondary importance overall in terms of functional result.

In the meantime it is believed that the formation of nitric oxide induced by mechanical stimulation and associated synthetases are responsible for the better part of the observed effects[15]. A direct effect on substance P metabolism also appears to be responsible for the analgesic effect[14, 21]. Based on the analgesic effects, firstly decribed by Dahmen, the ESWT indications were expanded to include epicondylitis, heel spur and other chronic insertion endinopathies[6].

With 100,000 treatments per year performed in the mid-nineties, practitioners performed more orthopedic than urologic procedures even though at that time there was no evidence of efficacy in the sense of evidence-based medicine for any musculoskeletal applications. Industry responded to such developments by producing equipment increasingly designed to meet the needs of orthopedists. In terms of mobile work stations, however, the differences were and are minor. The main features for orthopedic equipment were an extended coupling head for the treatment of pathologies near the surface and the integration of a linear scanner for sonographic localization.

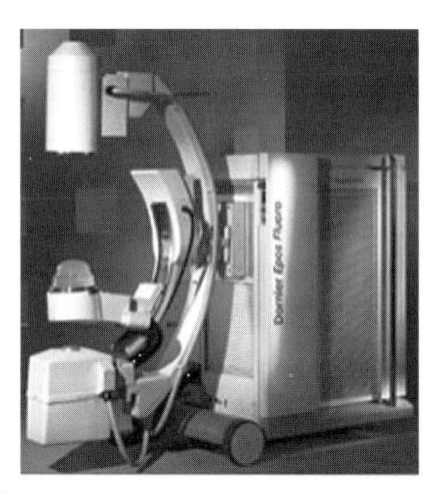

Figure 2. ESWT unit for orthopedic and urologic applications.

Musculoskeletal applications dropped significantly when the Federal Office of Public Health and Insurance removed ESWT from its list of covered therapies due to the lack of evidence of efficacy[7]. This prompted a multitude of studies initiated in order to bring such evidence of efficacy for a wide variety of indications of the musculoskeletal system. In summary, today's findings indicate that such evidence has been brought for the high-energy treatment of calcific tendonitis[9]. Contradictory findings are reported in the literature for some indications but chronic plantar heel pain has recent evidence[10, 17, 3, 4, 19, 20].

With a drop in treatments and a reduction in insurance coverage, institutions with urology and orthopedics departments began to develop synergies partly for monetary reasons; shockwave treatments limited to orthopedics were only profitable for a minority of institutions.

Over the past few years, the following diagnoses have been proven as indications:

- Pseudarthrosis
- Calcific tendonitis

- Heel spur
- Epicondylitis
- (Insertion tendinopathies)

One problem when comparing the published studies on shockwave therapy is the broad range of underlying treatment and physical parameters. Today it is well known that energy flow density, used almost exclusively for a long time, and the subsequent distinction made by Rompe between low, medium and high-energy treatments allow only limited comparison between different equipment[16].

The evidence-based foundation for defining general indication-based treatment parameters is still lacking today.

Murnau Treatment Protocol

In order to make the observed findings comparable, the authors established indication-related application protocols based on their empirical data.

Treatment was focused on pseudarthroses. For each diagnosis we defined certain impulses, amplitude, frequency, application pressure of the coupling head and interval period in the event of repeat treatments.

All treatments were performed with a mobile work station from Dornier Medizintechnik.

The Compact Delta operates based on electromagnetic shockwave emission. Localization is via an isocentric C-arm or an integrated linear scanner. When using the urologic coupling head, pathologies near the surface require a correspondingly long distance between emitter and treatment area. Energy flow density is divided in 9 stages (A-C, 1-6) with a maximum value of 0.96 mJ/mm^2 and can be adjusted within a frequency range of 2-6 Hz. Patients are positioned on a three-dimensional, mobile and almost fully transparent table system.

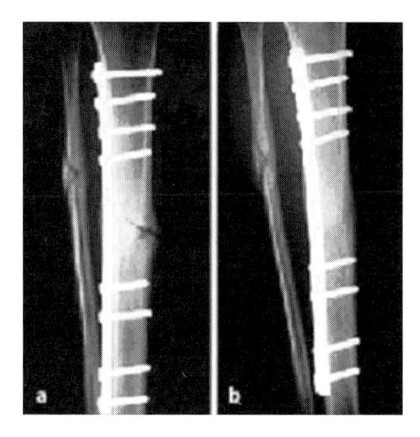

Figure 3. X-ray images of pseudarthrosis before/after treatment.

Indication-Based Application Protocols

Pseudarthrosis

- Amplitude: 5-6
- Fluoroscopic localization: isocentric
- Frequency: 2 Hz
- Impulse count: 2000
- Positioning: prone position, ventral coupling
- Application pressure: 1-2
- Treatment interval: 6 weeks
- Treatment frequency: 3 times
- Analgesic: 150 mg Diclofenac, or analgosedation

Localization is of decisive importance regarding treatment outcome. Using an isocentric C-arm, radiological imaging of pseudoarthrosis in the area of the long bones must be conducted on two planes in order to bring the treatment focus to the region of interest. Our experience shows that the application of maximum high energy flow density correlates with good result. In our opinion this also justifies a combination with short time general anesthesia if no satisfastory

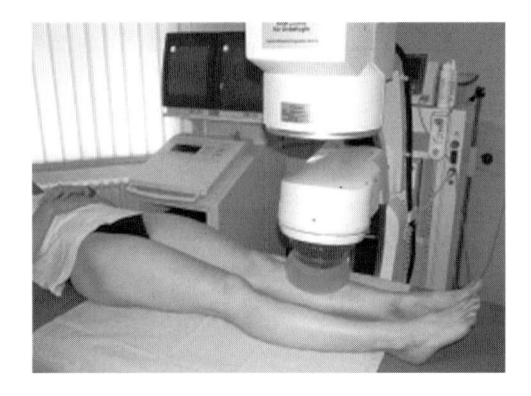

Figure 4. Coupling for pseudarthrosis.

pain relief can be achieved with other analgesic methods. However, a large majority of patients were treated with a very low analgesic of 150 mg Diclofenac taken prior to ESWT. We believe that the existence of pseudoarthroses following several operations among our patients with consecutive local sensitivity disorders accounts for such a low dosage.

Calcific tendinitis

- Amplitude: 3-4
- Fluoroscopic localization: isocentric or sonographic

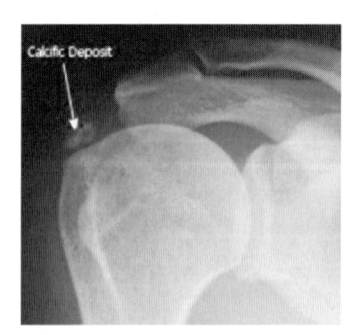

Figure 5. X-ray of calcified shoulder.

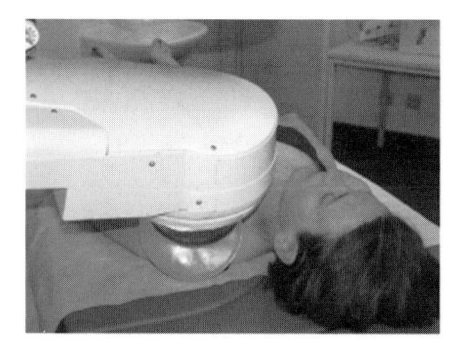

Figure 6. Coupling and positioning for calcified shoulder.

- Frequency: 2 Hz
- Impulse count: 2000
- Positioning: prone position
- Application pressure: 1-2
- Treatment interval: 4 weeks
- Treatment frequency: 3 times
- Analgesic: 150 mg Diclofenac, or local infiltration or analgodesation

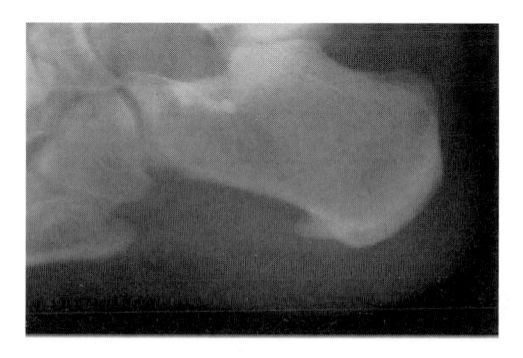

Figure 7. X-ray of plantar heel spur.

Precise clinical examination of the patient as well as radiological classification of the deposit were essential for positive outcome after ESWT. Of decisive importance for the clinical examination is, above all, the evaluation of the functionality of the rotator cuff and the exclusion of accompanying pathologies in order to make a satisfactory assessment of surgery as a potential alternative.

Heel Spur

- Amplitude: B-2
- Localization: clinical pain focus, biofeedback
- Frequency: 2-4 Hz
- Impulse count: 2000
- Positioning: Supine position, coupling to medial foot
- Application pressure: 1-2
- Treatment interval: 2 weeks
- Treatment frequency: 3 times
- Analgesic: 150 mg Diclofenac, or local infiltration

In contrast with modern radial units, which recommend direct plantar coupling, the treatment of heel spur should be medial parallel to the foot sole due to

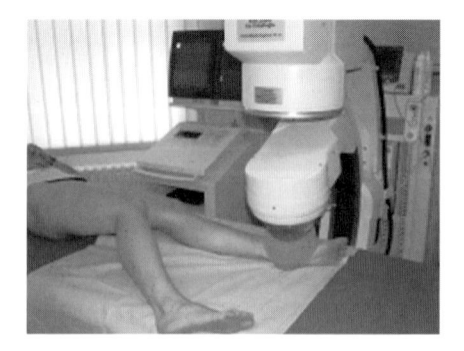

Figure 8. Coupling and positioning for plantar heel spur.

focus size and related depth of penetration. Localization is merely clinical by provoking the typical pressure pain.

Enthesiopathies

Amplitude A-C

- Localization: clinical pain focus, biofeedback
- Frequency: 4 Hz
- Impulse count: 2000
- Positioning: prone or side position, direct coupling via pain focus
- Application pressure: 1-2
- Treatment interval: 1 week
- Treatment frequency: 3 times
- Analgesic: 150 mg Diclofenac, or local infiltration

The treatment of pathologies near the surface with the large unit represents a great challenge because it makes localization via biofeedback significantly more difficult due to the large coupling head and small focus.

The associated treatment of adjacent muscles and any trigger points commonly found in radial units is, comparatively speaking, impossible in the large unit.

Our Own Investigations/Findings

All treatments conducted by our work group were recorded prospectively in accordance with the above mentioned protocols. At the same time, clinical and radiological findings were entered, updated and archived. For the treatment of bone healing disorders, we found a success rate of 85%. When data are limited to actual pseudarthrosis, the rate of bony consolidation is still 74%[2].

These figures coincide largely with those found in the literature. However our results show, in part, significant differences in treatment parameters thus making it impossible to compare recently published data[1, 18].

148 EXTRACORPOREAL SHOCKWAVE THERAPY

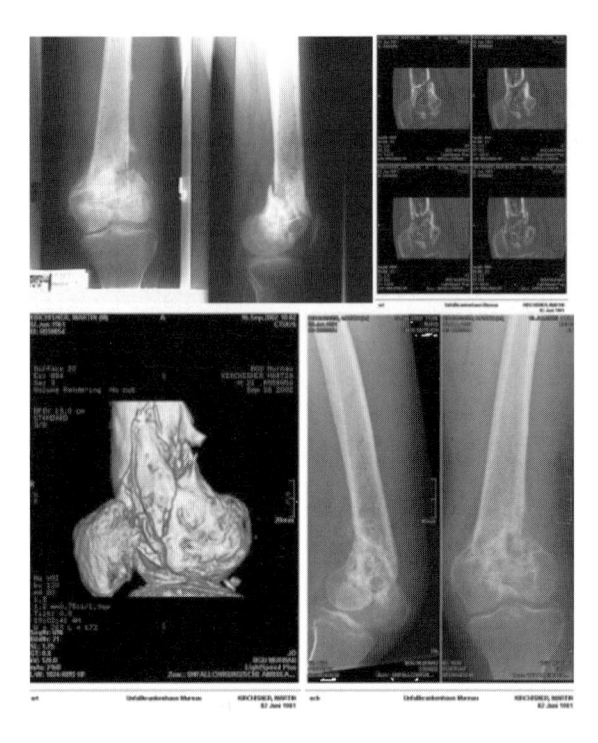

Figure 9. X-ray and CT of fracture of the distal upper thigh before and after shockwave treatment – callus formation.

A large portion of the findings in ESWT is based on experimental studies. Particularly noteworthy in terms of the effects on bones are the studies conducted by Gerdesmeyer et al. in 2002 [8] and Wang et al. in 2002 [22] in addition to those by Maier et al. in 2002[14]. Animal experiments conducted with a large electrohydraulic unit described significant disintegrating effects on the bone. Since bone particles were also found in the lung, the authors also advised against the use of energy density in excess of 0.9 mJ/mm^2 in humans.

Since the treatment of pseudarthroses in accordance with the Murnau protocol routinely involved higher energy flow densities, we began a prospective study in collaboration with our department of internal medicine. In 50 patients no changes in parameters were found that would point to a charge of the cardiovascular or pulmonary system. In our opinion it is furthermore justified that

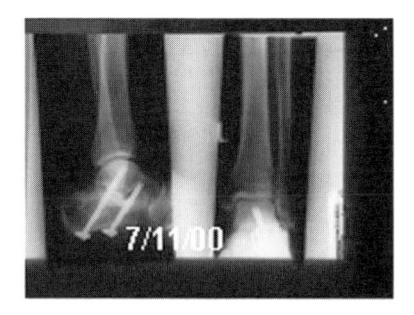

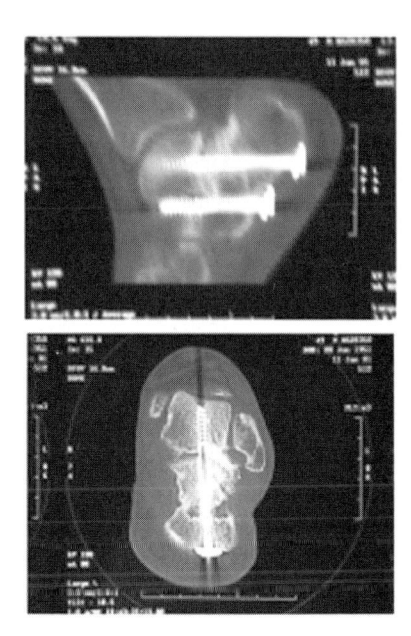

Figure 10. X-ray and CT of USG arthrodesis/pseudarthrosis - poor indication.

the high-energy treatment of bone pathologies represents a method with few side effects[12].

The extreme cases of pseudarthrosis following severe open fractures presented by our study group justify that high-energy shockwave therapy should also be attempted as part of a multimodal treatment concept in such cases[13].

Similar to the results found by Schaden, we also were able to demonstrate that the treatment of pseudarthroses after arthodesis in the areas of OSG and USG shows the poorest results. Prior to the beginning of treatment, CT images may be used to prevent frustrating therapy attempts[11].

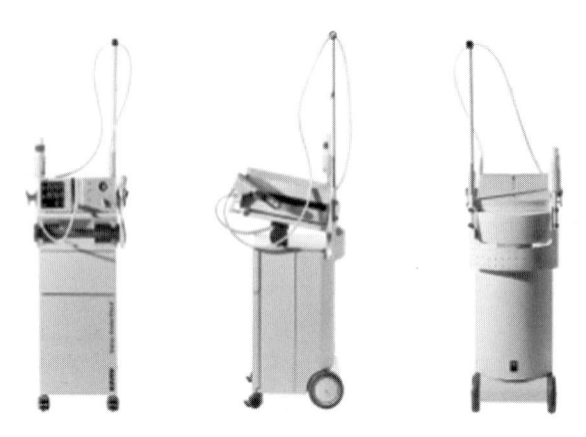

Figure 11. Swiss DolorClast® from EMS for the treatment of enthesiopathies.

Large scale unit vs. Radial Shockwave devices

Basically, units differ in terms of the following:

- Price/size
- Handling
- Energy flow density
- Localization
- Shockwave emission

In other words, a valid comparison is not permitted due to such major differences in concept. We rather look upon the different concepts as meaningful supplements to one another even in terms of treatment indications.

While we believe the prospects of success for the treatment of pseudarthrosis and calcific tendonitis to be greater with the mobile high energetic work station, the radial shockwave is clearly preferable for the treatment of close-to-skin pathologies. Current studies conducted with the Swiss DolorClast® from EMS have shown good treatment results in particular in the case of heel spur and lateral epicondylitis.

There are a number of reasons why radial shockwave therapy will no doubt hold its own in the outpatient arena, not the least of which is to reduce cost. But based on our experience, we also see as before an indication for the use of high-energy ESWT treatments for pseudarthrosis therapy. The high energetic devices used in orthopedics are an indispensable part of extracorporeal shockwave therapy.

Literature

1. Beutler, S., G. Regel, et al. (1999). "[Extracorporeal shockwave therapy for delayed union of long bone fractures - preliminary results of a prospective cohort study]." Unfallchirurg 102(11): 839-47.
2. Brandner H, S. K. (2000). "Extrakorporale Stoßwellentherapie bei Knochenheilungsstörung." Trauma und Berufskrankheit
3. Buchbinder, R., S. Green, et al. (2002). "Shockwave therapy for lateral elbow pain." Cochrane Database Syst Rev(1): CD003524.
4. Buchbinder, R., R. Ptasznik, et al. (2002). "Ultrasound-guided extracorporeal shockwave therapy for plantar fasciitis: a randomized controlled trial." Jama 288(11): 1364-72.
5. Chaussy C, S. E., Jocham D, Brendl W, Forssmann B (1982). "First clinical experiences with extracorporeally induced destruction of kidney stones by shockwaves." J Urol 127: 417-420.
6. Dahmen GP, M. L., Nam VC, Skruodies B (1992). "Extrakoporale Stoßwellentherapie im knochennahen Weichteilbereich an der Schulter." Extr Orthopaedica 11: 25-27.
7. Fritze, J. (1998). "[Extracorporeal shockwave therapy (ESWT) in orthopedic indications: a selective review]." Versicherungsmedizin 50(5): 180-5.
8. Gerdesmeyer, L., S. Schrabler, et al. (2002). "[Tissue-induced changes of the extracorporeal shockwave]." Orthopade 31(7): 618-22.
9. Gerdesmeyer, L., S. Wagenpfeil, et al. (2003). "Extracorporeal shockwave therapy for the treatment of chronic calcifying tendonitis of the rotator cuff: a randomized controlled trial." Jama 290(19): 2573-80.
10. Hammer, D. S., S. Rupp, et al. (2000). "Extracorporal shockwave therapy in patients with tennis elbow and painful heel." Arch Orthop Trauma Surg 120(5-6): 304-7.
11. Hauschild M, B. H. (2002). ESWT after Arthrodesis of the lower ankle joint - necessity of preliminary CT-scan. ISMST, Winterthur, CH.
12. Hauschild M, B. H. (2003). High energy ESWT and possible Lung Embolism - Investigation of BGA, ECG and clinical Parameters. ISMST, Orlando, USA.
13. Hauschild M, B. H. (2003). High energy ESWT for Pseudoarthrosis of a comminuted supracondylar femoral fracture. ISMST, Orlando, USA.
14. Maier, M., S. Milz, et al. (2002). "[Basic research of applying extracorporeal shockwaves on the musculoskeletal system. An assessment of current status]." Orthopade 31(7): 667-77.
15. Mariotto, S., E. Cavalieri, et al. (2005). "Extracorporeal shockwaves: from lithotripsy to anti-inflammatory action by NO production." Nitric Oxide 12(2): 89-96.

16. Rompe, J. D., P. Eysel, et al. (1997). "[Extracorporeal shockwave therapy in orthopedics. Positive results in tennis elbow and calcific tendinitis of the shoulder]." Fortschr Med 115(18): 26, 29-33.
17. Rompe, J. D., C. Riedel, et al. (2001). "Chronic lateral epicondylitis of the elbow: A prospective study of low-energy shockwave therapy and low-energy shockwave therapy plus manual therapy of the cervical spine." Arch Phys Med Rehabil 82(5): 578-82.
18. Schoellner, C., J. D. Rompe, et al. (2002). "[High energy extracorporeal shockwave therapy (ESWT) in pseudarthrosis]." Orthopade 31(7): 658-62.
19. Speed, C. A., D. Nichols, et al. (2002). "Extracorporeal shockwave therapy for lateral epicondylitis—a double blind randomised controlled trial." J Orthop Res 20(5): 895-8.
20. Speed, C. A., D. Nichols, et al. (2003). "Extracorporeal shockwave therapy for plantar fasciitis. A double blind randomised controlled trial." J Orthop Res 21(5): 937-40.
21. Wang, F. S., C. J. Wang, et al. (2002). "Superoxide mediates shockwave induction of ERK-dependent osteogenic transcription factor (CBFA1) and mesenchymal cell differentiation toward osteoprogenitors." J Biol Chem 277(13): 10931-7.
22. Wang, F. S., K. D. Yang, et al. (2002). "Extracorporeal shockwave promotes growth and differentiation of bone-marrow stromal cells towards osteoprogenitors associated with induction of TGF-beta1." J Bone Joint Surg Br 84(3): 457-61.

Treatment Result of rESWT (Swiss DolorClast®) with the Use of a Focused Handpiece A Pilot Study

J. Schöll, H. Lohrer

Introduction

For some 10 years extracorporeal shockwave therapy has been proven for the treatment of chronic insertion tendopathies[2, 4, 8]. In the meantime, numerous studies are available which show good treatment results of extracorporeal shockwave therapy even based on criteria of evidence-based medicine (prospective-controlled, randomized studies). This statement also applies to radial extracorporeal shockwave therapy [11] introduced in 1998 and embraced today by far by the largest number of users. Accordingly, the ESWT is the best treatment method for chronic heel insertion diseases compared to surgery or other conservative therapy concepts[12].

Standard indications of the musculoskeletal system today are fasciitis plantaris, epicondylitis humeri radialis and calcific tendonitis of the shoulder[3].

The different treatment parameters (energy generation, energy density, dosage, treatment frequency) and especially possible differences between radial and focused shockwave application continue to be the subject of scientific debates.

In studies conducted so far, a comparison between the results of treatments with focused and radial (unfocused) extracorporeal shockwaves showed no difference in the treatment of fasciitis plantaris [10] and calcific tendonitis as well[1].

Today, a focused handpiece is available for the pneumatically generated extracorporeal shockwaves (EMS Medical GmbH of Konstanz, Germany).

From January to July 2002, The Institute for Sports Medicine in Frankfurt am Main evaluated this handpiece as part of a pilot study on 41 patients with standard indications (16 with calcific tendonitis, 20 with fasciitis plantaris and 5 with epicondylitis humeri radialis).

Material and methods

The 41 patients suffering from calcific tendonitis, fasciitis plantaris or epicondylitis humeri radialis (27 women and 14 men, mean age 53.3 ± 12.8 years) with mean pain interval of 23.3 ± 30.0 months were enrolled. At least two unsuccessful conservative treatment methods must have been performed previously.

The treatment consisted of 3 sessions at weekly intervals with 2000 low-energy focused impulses (no local anesthesics). Treatment pressure was 3 bar for calcific tendonitis and fasciitis plantaris and 2 bar for lateral epicondylitis. Examinations were conducted prior to the treatments as well as 3 weeks after therapy completion.

Quality of life, ability to work and sports activity were selected as criteria of efficacy.

The objective criteria was pain threshold for semiobjective assessment by using the DolorMeter pain measurement component[6, 11]. In addition, pain during routine daytime activities (ADL) as well as pain during first steps in the morning was evaluated in post treatment studies by using the Visual Analog Scale (VAS).

Results

Calcific tendinitis of the shoulder (calcific tendinitis)

Sixteen patients (9 women and 7 men age 53,2 ± 7,2 years) with calcified tendonitis fit the inclusion criteria and took part in the study. When asked about quality of life before treatment, 15 patients (93.75%) scored themselves as

	Baseline	After ESWT	Significance
Morning pain	5.0 ± 2.8 VAS	1.9 ± 1.8 VAS	P < 0.01
ADL pain	6.1 ± 2.1 VAS	2.5 ± 2.1 VAS	P < 0.01

Table 1. VAS treatment results for calcific tendinitis of the shoulder.

"unsatisfactory," one patient (6.25%) with "satisfactory." After completion of the treatment, 2 patients (12.5%) ranked the obtained quality of life as "very good," 8 patients (50%) as "good," 4 patients (25%) as "satisfactory" and only 2 patients (12.5%) as "unsatisfactory."

When questioned about the capacity to work prior to treatment, 3 patients (18.75%) answered "not able to work" and 10 patients (62.5%) were "able to work." Three patients (18.75%) were retired. Following the treatment, only one patient (6.25%) was "unable to work" while 12 patients (75%) were "able to work."

The question about sports activity was answered by 5 patients (31.25%) as "impossible." In another 5 patients (31.25%) sports activity was "limited but possible" and 6 patients (37.5%) practiced no sport. Following the treatment 4 patients (25%) were capable of sports "without limitation" and 6 patients (37.5%) said their sports activity was "limited but possible."

Pain during first steps in the morning as well as pain during activities of daily living decreased successively and were found significantly lower after intervention compared to the baseline (Table 1).

The pain threshold as measured with the DolorMeter rose significantly from 1.3 ± 0.5 N before treatment to 3.3 ± 0.9 N ($p < 0.01$).

Heel spur (fasciitis plantaris)

Twenty patients (15 women and 5 men age 52.0 ± 16.2 years) with fasciitis plantaris/heel spur could be enrolled after fulfilling all inclusion criteria.

	Baseline	After Treatment	Significance
Morning pain	2.8 ± 2.8 VAS	1.5 ± 2.0 VAS	P = 0.01
ADL pain	5.5 ± 2.4 VAS	3.0 ± 2.4 VAS	P < 0.01

Table 2. VAS treatment results for fasciitis plantaris

The question about quality of life was answered prior to treatment by 11 patients (55%) as "unsatisfactory," by 8 patients (40%) as "satisfactory" and by one patient (5%) as "good." After the treatment quality of life was ranked by 3 patients (15%) as "very good," by 5 patients (25%) as "good," by 10 patients (50%) as "satisfactory" and 2 patients (10%) as "unsatisfactory."

"Able to work" status was reported for 13 patients (65%), and 7 patients (35%) were retired. Since no patients were recorded as "not able to work" prior to treatment, these data remained unchanged after the treatment.

Before the treatment, sports activity was "impossible" for 6 patients (30%) and "limited but possible" for 4 patients (20%). Two patients (10%) were able to practice sports "without limitation" but the extremity was not exposed to the effort. Eight patients (40%) practiced no sports. Following the treatment, 5 patients (25%) were able to practice sports "without limitation," 6 patients (30%) were able to practice sports in a "limited but possible" fashion and one patient was unable to practice sports. Morning pain without exertion as well as pain during the ADL decreased successively and significantly after ESWT (Table 2).

The pain threshold as measured with the DolorMeter rose significantly from 2.1 ± 0.5 N before treatment to 3.5 ± 1.1 N ($p < 0.01$).

Tennis elbow (epicondylitis humeri radialis)

Five patients (3 women and 2 men age 58.8 ± 9.8 years) with tennis elbow took part in the study.

The question about quality of life before the treatment was answered by 4 patients (80%) as "unsatisfactory" and by one patient (20%) as "very poor."

	Baseline	After Treatment	Significance
Morning pain	2.3 ± 2.1 VAS	0.7 ± 0.8 VAS	P > 0.05
ADL pain	7.8 ± 1.9 VAS	5.0 ± 2.7 VAS	P > 0.05

Table 3. VAS treatment results for lateral epicondylitis

After the treatment, 2 patients (40%) judged the quality of life as "good," 1 patient (20%) as "satisfactory" and only 2 patients (40%) as "unsatisfactory."

One patient (20%) was "unable to work" prior to the treatment, one patient (20%) was "able to work" and 3 patients (60%) were retired. After the treatment this ratio remained unchanged.

Prior to ESWT, 2 patients (40%) said sports activity was "limited but possible," and 3 patients (60%) said the question did "not apply." Following the treatment, one patient (20%) was able to practice sports "without limitation" and one patient (20%) remained able to practice sports in a "limited but possible" fashion.

Average values for morning pain as well as pain during ADL did not change significantly (Table 3).

The pain threshold as measured with the DolorMeter did not rise significantly. It rose from 1.8 ± 0.4 N before treatment to 2.0 ± 1.0 N (p > 0.05).

Discussion

Treatments with the focussed applicator show good results in patients with calcified tendonitis of the shoulder and heel spur. When evaluating quality of life after the treatment 87.5% of patients scored themselves as satisfactory and excellent. In only 2 patients (12.5%) the quality of life remained unsatisfactory. In the treatment of heel spur, 90% of patients qualified their condition as satisfactory to excellent, 2 patients (10%) considered the outcome as unsatisfactory. The pain syndrome improved significantly in both groups.

Upon completion of the study, patients evaluated the outcome as excellent in 10 cases (24.4%), good in 15 cases (36.6%), satisfactory in 6 cases (14.6%) and unsatisfactory in 10 cases (24.4%).

This study is comparable in terms of treatment result to conventional focused shockwave units as well as treatment results with radial shockwave therapy. This statement applies to the results shown in the literature [7, 9] as well as our own results[5, 10, 11]. The treatment for tennis elbow showed no statistically relevant improvement. The result is probably affected by the insufficient sample size and statistic power.

The treatment was well tolerated by all patients and no local anesthesics were used. No clinically relevant side effects occurred.

Further studies need to be performed to verify these results through a controlled and randomized approach.

Summary

According to this pilot study, the focussed applicator could be used in calcific tendonitis of the shoulder and heel spur. The applicator we used is not recommended for tennis elbow.

Literature

1. Gremion G, Augros R, Gobelet Ch, Leyvraz P-F (2000): Wirksamkeit der extrakorporalen Stoßwellentherapie bei der Calcific tendinitis der Schulter. Schweizerische Zeitschrift für Sportmedizin und Sporttraumatologie 48: 8-11
2. Haupt G, Katzmeier P: Anwendung der hochenergetischen extrakorporalen Stoßwellentherapie bei Pseudarthrosen, Calcific tendinitis der Schulter und Ansatztendinosen (Fersensporn, Epicondylitis). In: Chaussy Ch, Eisenberger F, Jocham D, Wilbert D (Hrsg.): "Die Stoßwelle - Forschung und Klinik". Attempto Verlag, Tübingen, 1995: 143-146
3. Heller K-D, Niethard FU (1998): Der Einsatz der extrakorporalen Stoßwellentherapie in der Orthopädie – eine Metaanalyse. Z Orthop 136: 390-401
4. Lohrer H, Schöll J, Alt W, Hirschmann M (1998): Die extrakorporale Stoßwellentherapie. Leistungssport 28: 42-44
5. Lohrer H, Schoell J, Arentz S, Froelich T, Straub T, Penninger E, Diesch R, Haupt G (2001): Effectiveness of radial shockwave Therapy (RESWT) on tennis elbow and plantar fasciitis. Book of Abstracts. CASM/ACMS annual symposium and sport medicine Conference, Calgary/CAN

6. Lohrer H, Schöll J (2001): Anterior knee pain in athletes. Book of abstracts. 6th Annual Congress of the European College of Sport Science: 64
7. Rompe J-D, Küllmer K, Vogel J, Eckardt A, Wahlmann U, Eysel P, Hopf C, Kirkpatrick CJ, Bürger R, Naffe B (1997): Extrakorporale Stoßwellentherapie - Experimentelle Grundlagen, klinischer Einsatz. Der Orthopäde 03: 215-228
8. Rompe J-D (1997): Extrakorporale Stoßwellentherapie – Grundlagen, Indikation, Anwendung. Chapmann & Hall GmbH, Weinheim
9. Schleberger R, Williger J (1997): Orthopädische Stoßwellentherapie (ESWT) am Stütz- und Bewegungsapparat. Kontraste 2: 38-45
10. Schöll J, Lohrer H (2000): Radiale Stoßwellentherapie des Fersensporns. Orthopädie Mitteilungen 2: A 14
11. Schöll J, Lohrer H (2001): Fasciitis plantaris – eine Indikation zur Stoßwellentherapie. Orthopädie Schuhtechnik 7-8: 66-70
12. Sistermann R, Katthagen B-D (1998): Komplikationen, Nebenwirkungen und Kontraindikationen der Anwendung mittel- und hochenergetischer extrakorporaler Stoßwellen im orthopädischen Bereich. Orthopädie 136: 175-181

Results of Radial Shockwave Treatment of Sports-Induced Diseases (Achillodynia, Patella Tip Syndrome and Tibialis Anterior Syndrome)

J. Schöll, H. Lohrer, S. Arentz

Summary

This prospective pilot study was conducted to assess the effects of radial extracorporeal shockwaves on chronic achillodynia, patella tip syndrome and tibialis anterior syndrome. Forty patients with chronic therapy-resistant achillodynia, 45 patients with chronic therapy-resistant patella tip syndrome and 17 patients with chronic therapy-resistant tibialis anterior syndrome received rESWT for 3-5 sessions. The results show significant pain relief (at rest, pressure and exertion) as well as an increase of pain threshold. The long term outcome showed further improvement up to one year. Radial extracorporeal shockwave therapy is a promising therapeutic option even for sports-related degenerative diseases. Further controlled and randomized studies are required to confirm these findings.

Introduction

Achillodynia, patella tip syndrome and tibialis anterior syndrome are well known as sports-induced degenerative diseases. The natural course primarily seems to be chronic and progressive.

A large number of therapeutic options exist, but most of them do not have an evidence based approach. Regarding infiltration techniques in chronic achillodynia with corticoid substances, a potential risk of iatrogen-induced tendon rupture is well known.

From a pathological-anatomical point of view, we consider achillodynia to be a combination of paratendinosis and tendinosis of the Achilles tendon. These components are more or less marked[32]. Repetitive microtrauma and insufficient regeneration as well as local inflammatory changes in the paratendinum trigger the initially latent process of Achilles tendon degeneration[16]. The tendon 2-7 cm proximal of the calcanear insertion area is the most affected region. Achillodynia itself is characterized by stress-dependent local pain associated with pressure dolence and swelling of the Achilles tendon[19].

The issue of Achilles tendon injuries has recently once again come to be important in sports medicine. Within the German national track and field team a total of 21 out of 70 athletes suffered relevant Achilles tendon injuries during the 2000 Olympic Games in Sydney. Four of these athletes have undergone surgery since then, 10 patients underwent significant long term sport restrictions. Achillodynia is a typical sports injury induced by running. James et al. reported in 1978 achillodynia in 11% of running-induced sports injuries[15]. Endogenous causes (e.g. hyperuricemia) are rare. Anomalies of the lower extremity and previous tendineous lesions bring about increased pronation. For that reason the Achilles tendon is exposed to increased torsion[38].

As a typical insertion tendopathy, patella syndrome, so called jumper´s knee injury, features histologically mucoid denegeration, fibrinoid necroses, microruptures and regeneration at the tendon/bone junction[18]. The jumper´s knee is known as one of the most common insertion tendopathies. Becker & Krahl in 1978 reported patella pathologies in about 37.8% of all tendopathies in athletes[4]. We observed 7.4% of all patients suffering from jumper´s knee in our own Institute for Sports Medicine. Already among 14 to 18 year-old basketball players, the prevalence of patella tip syndrome is 7%, but prevalence increases with age[8]. Martens et al. in 1982 discussed volleyball and football as a predictive factor because 2/3 of the patients participated in these sport activities[28]. Orava & Leppilahti in 1999 found insertion endopathies of the lig. patellae most often (44%) in the differential diagnosis in patients with "anterior knee pain[30]." One third of all patients report time-out periods of more than 6 months[7]. In terms of jumper's knee, the pathology is mostly located close to the tip of the patella (79%). In 16% of the jumper´s knee patients, pain was found at the patella base, in 3% at the tuberositas tibiae and in 2% along the entire lig. patellae[30].

In a prospective study conducted with sports students an incidence of 13.8% was found within a two year period[40].

Repetitive jumps, particularly vertical ones, seem to be a significant predictive factor in patella tip syndrome.

The medial tibialis anterior syndrome is characterized by a load dependent local pain at the tibialis anterior in the middle and lower third. An exudative hypertrophic tenosynovitis is correlated to the tibialis posterior tendon [16] and frequently caused by intensive running and most often by sudden load peaks. Forefoot runners are more affected than heel runners[25].

Tibialis anterior syndrome occurs in 2.5% of top athletes[20]. Among active track and field athletes, the medial tibialis anterior syndrome is the third most common sports injury after achillodynia and stress fractures[22]. Endurance athletes are more often afflicted by tibialis anterior syndrome.

The efficacy of extracorporeal shockwave therapy to treat different chronic insertion endopathies has often been documented in controlled randomized and prospective studies [23, 34, 35] even though no consensus has been reached so far on the energy to be applied, on the number of shockwaves or on treatment frequency. Considered today as standard indications in the musculoskeletal system are fasciitis plantaris, epicondylitis humeri radialis, pseudarthrosis and calcific tendonitis of the shoulder[14]. The different treatment modalities (energy generation, energy flux density, dose and treatment frequency) continue to be the subject of scientific debate. Until now comparative studies of treatments with focused and radial extracorporeal shockwaves show no difference for fasciitis plantaris [36] or calcific tendonitis of the shoulder[12]. Apart from our own publication [26], clinical studies of the effect of ESWT for achillodynia, patella tip syndrome and tibialis anterior syndrome have not been published. In experiments conducted on rabbits Rompe et al. showed dose-dependent effects of extracorporeal shockwaves on the Achilles tendon[33]. High energies (> 0.6 mJ/mm^2) lead to injuries, necroses and edema.

Objective of the study

This study is designed as a prospective trial to investigate the effect of rESWT on sports-induced enthesiopathies such as chronic achillodynia, chronic patella tip syndrome and chronic tibialis anterior syndrome.

Patients, material and methods

Between September 1998 and October 2000, 102 subjects (40 with achillodynia, 45 with patella tip syndrome and 17 with tibialis anterior syndrome) have fulfilled all inclusion and exclusion criteria. They were enrolled in the outpatient orthopedic clinic of the Institute for Sports Medicine in Frankfurt am Main.

The patients of the study groups were on average 35.8 ± 10.5 years old for achillodynia, 24.2 ± 9.8 years old for patella tip syndrome and 21.2 ± 4.6 years old for tibialis anterior syndrome. For the athletes suffering from achillodynia, the mean height was 178.5 ± 7.5 cm and the mean weight was 75.9 ± 12.6 kg. In the athlete group suffering from patella tip syndrome, their height was 179.1 ± 8.9 cm and their weight was 73.7 ± 13.7 kg. Athletes with tibialis anterior syndrome were 172.7 ± 8.9 cm tall and weighed 57.7 ± 8.0 kg. All patients of the study groups were active athletes. In the achillodynia and tibialis anterior syndrome groups running sports were predominant. Patients with patella tip syndrome were primarily affected by jumps (Table 1).

Prior to enrollment, at least two of the conservative standard therapies such as targeted sole inserts, physical and rehabilitation therapy, bandages, local infiltrations and radiation were performed without success (Table 2).

After one year, 33 patients (82.5%) with chronic achillodynia, 40 patients (88.9%) with patella tip syndrome and 15 patients (88.2%) with chronic tibialis anterior syndrome could be re examined (Table 3).

Sports	Achillodynia	Jumper´s knee	Tibialis anterior syndrome
Jogging	8	3	0
Middle distance	5	1	3
Long distance	5	0	4
Soccer	4	6	2
Long jump	4	2	0
Handball	4	1	2
Tennis	3	6	3

Sports	Achillodynia	Jumper´s knee	Tibialis anterior syndrome
Triathlon	2	1	0
Bike racing	2	0	0
Volleyball	1	8	0
Decathlon	1	1	1
Gym	1	0	0
Basketball	0	11	0
Ballett	0	3	0
High jump	0	1	2
Total	40	45	17

Table 1. Demographic data of patients enrolled in the rESWT trial.

Prior treatment	Achillodynia	Jumper´s knee	Tibialis anterior syndrome
Physiotherapy	31	26	11
Massage	15	13	7
Electrotherapy	30	30	10
Medication (oral)	14	12	7
Eternal ointment	8	9	3
Tape	11	21	2
Infiltration (without cortsone)	22	13	3
Infiltration (with cortisone)	8	2	3
Inserts	7	7	3
Cast	6	7	1
Acupuncture	4	1	0
Soft tissue radiotherapy	1	0	0
Operation	5	2	1

Table 2. Treatments proir to the rESWT study.

	Baseline	Weeks after rESWT			
		1	4	12	26	52
Achillodynia	40	40	39	33	33	33
Jumper´s knee	45	45	45	42	40	40
Tibialis anterior syndrome	17	17	17	15	15	15

Table 3. Patients examined from 1 to 52 weeks after rESWT.

Achillodynia and jumper´s knee were defined as an exertion-dependent and pressure-pain related injury of the Achilles tendon[21]. A thickening of the tendon had to be shown.

The tibialis anterior syndrome was defined as an exertion-dependent and pressure pain injury to the medial tibialis anterior. This injury could not be localized presisely but had to extend over at least 5 cm in the middle and lower third of the tibialis anterior. X-rays had to exclude tibia stress fracture.

The sagital diameter of the Achilles tendon and the ligamentum patellae as well as the central echogenity was documented by ultrasound prior to rESWT. The mean thickness of the Achilles tendon was 7.5 ± 2.0 mm and the mean thickness of the ligamentum patellae was 6.7 ± 2.5 mm. Following the treatment, no significant loss in tendon thickness was found.

Exclusion criteria were defined as systemic predispositions (hyperurikemia, positive HLA B 27, positive rheuma factors), distal Achilles tendopathies, subachillary bursitides, heel-adjacent pain syndrome imitating achillodynia, intraarticular knee joint injuries (in particular associated chondropathic injuries), instabilities of the patella and stress fractures of the tibia.

The treatment was performed with the Swiss DolorClast®. The applicator (handpiece) was pressed upon the treatment area up to the first ring with application pressure categorized as "medium." As the patient adjusted to the shockwave-induced pain, the applied energy was increased during the treatment from 2 to 4 bar. Analgesia of the treatment zone was not necessary.

Therapy was delivered in five sessions at one-week intervals (Figures 1-3). Two thousand impulses per treatment session were applied. Treatment frequency was 6 Hz.

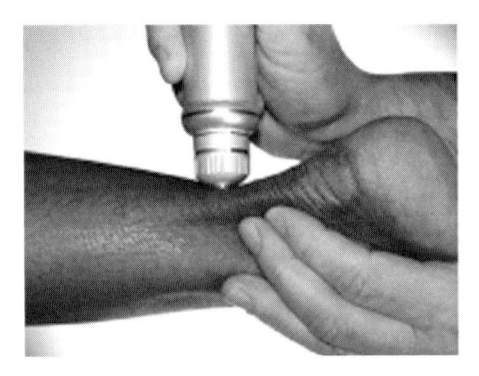

Figure 1. rESWT of Achillodynia.

In all diagnoses, based upon clinically evaluated maximum pain threshold, the pain area was treated in a linear meanderlike and circular fashion (biofeed back).

An exam was performed before each treatment. Follow-up exams were performed 1, 4, 12, 26 and 52 weeks following the end of the treatment.

For a sports-specific evaluation criteria, we chose the pain-free period patient was able to practice sports (shown in minutes). We also verified the pressure related pain sensation measured by the standardized visual analog scale (VAS).

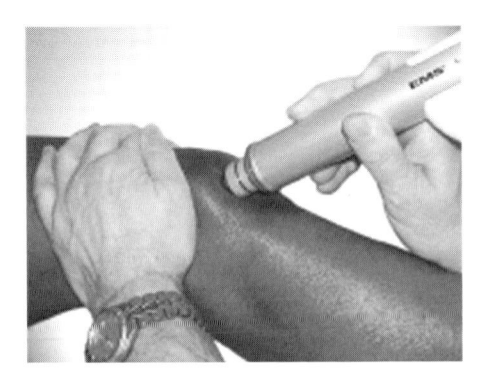

Figure 2. rESWT of the jumper´s knee.

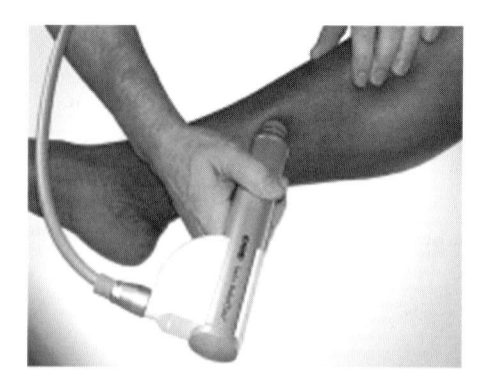

Figure 3. rESWT of the tibialis anterior syndrome.

We used the Dolormeter as a semi-objective measuring tool. It provides for a standardized application of defined pressure (Figure 4).

It allows evaluation of the threshold of local pain tolerance (in Newton) as well as the subjective pain response (VAS) on a defined pressure of 30 Newton.

Results

After rESWT we observed an excellent clinical outcome (Table 4). The baseline value for pain at rest before rESWT was 1.7 ± 2.5 VAS for achillodynia, 1.6 ± 2.4 VAS for patella tip syndromey and 1.7 ± 1.9 VAS for tibialis anterior syndrome. One week after rESWT patients with achillodynia improved to 0.4 ±- 1.0 VAS (p ≤ 0.01). The group with patella tip syndrome reached 0.8 ± 1.7 VAS (p ≤ 0.05) one week after treatment completion. Patients with tibialis anterior

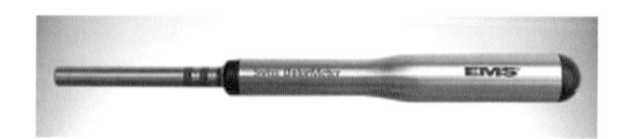

Figure 4. The EMS Dolormeter for standardized local pain measurement.

syndrome reached 0.6 ± 1.7 VAS (p≤ 0.05) one week after the last rESWT. The follow-up exam twelve weeks after the last rESWT showed 0.1 ± 0.3 VAS for achillodynia (p ≤ 0.01), 0.3 ± 0.7 VAS for patella tip syndrome (p ≤ 0.01) and 0.5 ± 1.6 VAS for tibialis anterior syndrome (p ≤ 0.01). At the end of the observation period of one year, patients with achillodynia had improved to 0.1 ± 0.3 VAS (p ≤ 0.01), those with patella tip syndrome improved to 0.3 ± 0.7 VAS (p ≤ 0.01) and those with tibialis anterior syndrome were down to 0.1 ± 0.2 VAS (p ≤ 0.01).

Prior to treatment, the pain threshold determined by the DolorMeter was 14.1 ± 6.6 N in achillodynia patients, 15.1 ± 7.4 N in patella tip syndrome patients and 16.1 ± 7.1 N in tibialis anterior syndrome patients. One week after the last rESWT, patients with achillodynia improved to 27.5 ± 10.9 N (p ≤ 0.01), patients with patella tip syndrome showed 28.7 ± 14.0 N (p ≤ 0.01) and those with tibialis anterior syndrome improved to 29.1 ± 12.3 N (p ≤ 0.01). The 12 week exam threshold was 38.4 ± 11.8 N in achillodynia (p ≤ 0.01), 32.9 ± 15.6 N in patella tip syndrome (p ≤ 0.01) and 32.9 ± 11.2 N in tibialis anterior syndrome. After 1 year, patients with achillodynia had improved to 41.9 ± 11.6 N (p ≤ 0.01), those with patella tip syndrome showed 35.3 ± 15.0 N (p ≤ 0.01) and patients with tibialis anterior syndrome also improved to 40.5 ± 10.4 N (p ≤ 0.01).

Prior to the treatment, the pressure pain determined by the DolorMeter at 30 N and VAS was 6.7 ± 3.2 VAS for achillodynia, 5.5 ± 2.9 VAS for patella tip

Achillodynia						
	Baseline	Weeks after rESWT				
		1	4	12	26	52
Pain at rest (VAS)	1.7±2.5	0.4±1.0**	0.3±1.3**	0.1±0.3**	0.1±0.2**	0.1±0.3**
Pain threshold (Newton)	14.1±6.6	27.5±10.9**	31.2±13.4**	38.4±11.8**	43.3±9.1**	41.9±11.6**
Local pressure (30 N, VAS)	6.7±3.2	2.6±3.6**	1.8±3.4**	0.7±1.8**	0.5±1.8**	0.9±2.6**
Pain during exercise (VAS)	7.8±1.7	2.2±2.5**	1.3±2.2**	0.5±1.1**	0.4±1.0**	0.7±1.6**
Pain-free running interval (min.)	14.4±18.5	63.0±37.0**	75.4±38.1**	87.5±35.2**	96.7±34.7**	90.0±43.0**

Jumper's knee

	Baseline	Weeks after rESWT				
		1	4	12	26	52
Pain at rest (VAS)	1.6±2.4	0.8±1.7*	0.6±1.6**	0.3±0.7**	0.3±0.7**	0.3±0.7**
Pain threshold (Newton)	15.1±7.4	28.7±14.0**	30.6±14.5**	32.9±15.6**	34.6±15.5**	35.3±15.0**
Local pressure (30 N, VAS)	5.5±2.9	2.3±3.0**	2.2±3.0**	2.1±2.9**	1.9±2.9**	1.7±2.6**
Pain during exercise (VAS)	5.5±2.3	2.8±3.0**	2.5±2.9**	2.3±2.8**	1.9±2.4**	1.9±2.5**
Pain-free running interval (min.)	10.4±15.0	54.3±50.9**	57.0±48.9**	62.8±49.2**	71.2±49.1**	70.3±48.7**

Tibialis anterior syndrome

	Baseline	Weeks after rESWT				
		1	4	12	26	52
Pain at rest (VAS)	1.7±1.9	0.6±1.7*	0.6±1.7*	0.5±1.6**	0.5±1.7**	0.1±0.2**
Pain threshold (Newton)	16.1±7.1	29.1±12.3**	31.8±11.6**	32.9±11.2**	36.3±11.9**	40.5±10.4**
Local pressure (30 N, VAS)	6.2±2.8	2.4±3.3**	2.3±3.5**	1.7±2.8**	1.5±2.8**	0.9±1.9**
Pain during exercise (VAS)	7.8±1.7	1.8±3.1**	2.2±3.0**	1.9±2.9**	1.6±2.8**	0.9±1.9**
Pain-free running interval (min.)	11.2±14.4	62.9±48.9**	72.9±47.5**	91.3±48.8**	91.3±48.8**	105.0±34.8**

Table 4. Outcome after rESWT (* = $P \leq 0.05$; ** = $P \leq 0.01$).

syndrome and 6.2 ± 2.8 VAS for tibialis anterior syndrome. One week following the treatment series, patients with achillodynia improved to 2.6 ± 3.6 VAS (p ≤ 0.01), patients with patella tip syndrome to 2.3 ± 3.0 VAS (p ≤ 0.01) and patients with tibialis anterior sybdrome to 2.4 ± 3.3 VAS (p ≤ 0.01). Twelve weeks after rESWT, 0.7 ± 1.8 VAS was found in patients suffering from achillodynia (p ≤ 0.01), 2.1 ± 2.9 VAS in patients with patella tip syndrome (p ≤ 0.01) and 1.7 ± 2.8 VAS in patients with tibialis anterior syndrome (p ≤ 0.01). At the end of the observation period of 1 year, achillodynia improved to 0.9 ± 2.6 VAS (p ≤ 0.01), patella tip syndrome to 1.7 ± 2.6 VAS (p ≤ 0.01) and tibialis anterior syndrome to 0.9 ± 1.9 VAS.

The pain during sports actvities prior to treatment was 7.8 ± 1.7 VAS for achillodynia, 5.5 ± 2.3 VAS for patella tip syndrome and 7.8 ± 1.7 VAS for tibialis anterior syndrome. One week after the last rESWT, patients with achillodynia improved to 2.2 ± 2.5 VAS (p ≤ 0.01), the group with patella tip syndrome reached 2.8 ± 3.0 VAS (p ≤ 0.01) and the tibialis anterior syndrome group reached 1.8 ± 3.1 VAS (p ≤ 0.01). Twelve weeks after the last rESWT, the scores were 0.5 ± 1.1 VAS for achillodynia (p ≤ 0.01), 2.3 ± 2.8 VAS for patella tip syndrome (p ≤ 0.01) and 1.9 ± 2.9 VAS for tibialis anterior syndrome (p ≤ 0.01). At the end of the follow up period of 1 year, patients with achillodynia had improved to 0.7 ± 1.6 VAS (p ≤ 0.01), patients with patella tip syndrome showed 1.9 ± 2.5 VAS (p ≤ 0.01) and the tibialis anterior syndrome group was scored at 0.9 ± 1.9 VAS (p ≤ 0.01).

The pain-free running interval at baseline as identified by the patients themselves was 14.4 ± 18.5 minutes for achillodynia, 10.4 ± 15.0 minutes for patella tip syndrome and 11.2 ± 14.4 minutes for tibialis anterior syndrome. One week after tha last rESWT, patients with achillodynia had improved to 63.0 ± 37.0 minutes (p ≤ 0.01). In the group with patella tip syndrome a pain-free interval of 54.3 ± 50.0 minutes (p ≤ 0.01) was reached. One week after treatment completion, the tibialis anterior syndrome group showed a pain-free interval of at least 62.9 ± 48.9 minutes, (p ≤ 0.01). The follow-up exam twelve weeks after the treatment showed a pain-free interval increase up to 87.5 ± 35.2 minutes for achillodynia (p ≤ 0.01), up to 62.8 ± 49.2 minutes for patella tip syndrome (p ≤ 0.01) and up to 91.3 ± 48.8 minutes for tibialis anterior syndrome (p ≤ 0.01). At the end of the observation period of 1 year, patients with achillodynia had improved to 90.0 ± 43.0 minutes (p ≤ 0.01), patients with patella tip syndrome to 70.3 ± 48.7 minutes (p ≤ 0.01) and patients with tibialis anterior syndrome to 105.0 ± 34.8 minutes (p ≤ 0.01).

Overall, 60% of patients with achillodynia, 40% of patients with patella tip syndrome and 58.8% of patients with tibialis anterior syndrome were found to be pain-free one year after the last rESWT (Figure 5). Improvement was recorded by 12.5% of patients with achillodynia, 24.4% of patients with patella tip syndrome and 17.7% of patients with tibialis anterior syndrome. In 27.5% of patients with achillodynia, 35.6% of patients with patella tip syndrome and 23.5% of patients with tibialis anterior syndrome the pain was unchanged 12 month after the last rESWT compared to baseline.

Discussion

Neither in terms of conservative treatment nor in terms of surgery for chronic degenerative injuries to the Achilles tendon (achillodynia), ligamentum patellae (patella tip syndrome) and tibialis anterior syndrome, the treatment options were evidence based[29, 9, 25]. In terms of nomenclature for chronic tendon damage associated with running and jumping, concensus is still lacking[27]. Even the precise pathology remains unclear[17]. Today, a degenerative-microtraumatic genesis is discussed but histologically relevant inflammatory cells have never been described on a relevant scale[16].

Studies determining the natural course of these diseases are not available[31].

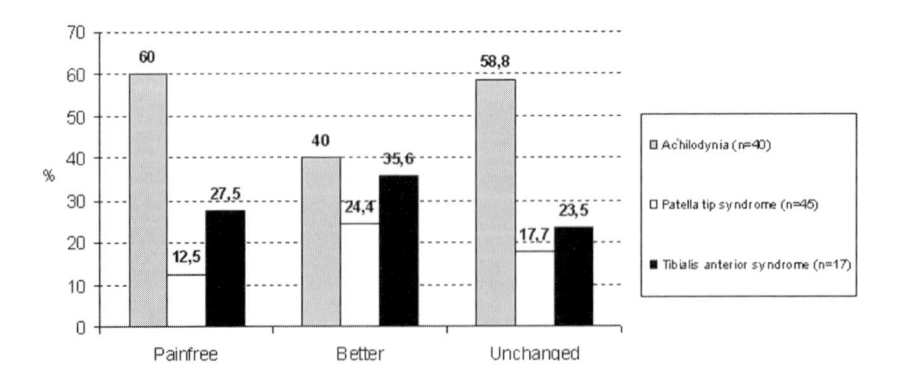

Figure 5. Overall outcome 1 year after the last rESWT.

From a diagnostic point of view, achillodynia is to be limited to the free course of the tendon some 2-7 cm above its insertion zone. It must be differentiated from other achillary (distal insertion endopathy, dorsal heel spur, bursitis subachillea) and periachillary pain syndromes[21].

Studies on the conservative therapy of achillodynia report from 41 to 67% excellent results[6, 1]. For surgery, Tallon et al. report an average success rate of 77.4% in a literature review[39]. These authors point especially to a low methodical quality of the published studies. Studies with greater methodological deficits show comparatively better results.

For the treatment of patella tip syndrome, Cook and Khan reported ten randomized studies for the conservative treatment but no randomized studies for surgery[9]. These authors conclude that neither a specific conservative nor a special operative method for treating this injury can be recommended.

Achillodynia and patella tip syndrome feature histologically mucoid degeneration fibrinoid necroses, microruptures and regeneration[16].

Tibialis anterior syndrome is an exudative hypertrophic tenosynovitis of the tibialis posterior tendon[16]. Specific data on the efficacy of conservative forms of treatment for medial tibialis anterior syndrome have not been published. Our own experience indicates that surgery is required. Good results are shown in retrospective, non-controlled design[25].

The efficacy of extracorporeal shockwave therapy in different chronic insertion tendopathies has been documented repeatedly in the literature through controlled, randomized and prospective studies[23, 11, 34, 35]. In other studies the efficacy of ESWT was not demonstrated because of some study limitations[5, 13].

Local anesthesia was not necessary in this study. In the meantime, it was demonstrated that local anesthesia has a negative impact on treatment success[3].

Today, standard indications of the musculoskeletal system are fasciitis plantaris, epicondylitus humeri radialis and calcific tendonitis of the shoulder[14]. The various treatment modalities (energy generation, energy density, dosage and treatment frequency) continue to be a subject of scientific debate. A comparison of treatments with the focused and radial (unfocused) extracorporeal shockwave for fasciitis plantaris shows no difference[36]. Achillodynia, patella tip syndrome and tibialis anterior syndrome are sports-induced, chronic injuries that are different from insertion endopathies such as fasciitis plantaris. Compared to results of conservative and surgical options, the results of this pilot study must be evaluated as good, especially since at least two conservative pretreatment methods failed. The success rate after one year (pain-free or improvement over 50%) is 72.5% for Achillodynia, 67.4% for patella tip syndrome and 76.5% for tibialis anterior syndrome and is hardly any different from the average success rate of 77.4% found by Tallon et al. following surgery (77.4%)[39].

The study was limited by the uncontrolled study design. Therefore the results cannot be considered as sufficiently certain on the basis of the criteria of evidence-based medicine. Controlled and randomized studies have to be performed to confirm these finings.

Literature

1. Angermann, P, Hovgaard, D (1999): Chronic achilles tendinopathy in athletic individuals: results of nonsurgical treatment. Foot Ankle 20: 43-46
2. Arndt, K.-H. (1976): Achillessehnenruptur und Sport. Barth Verlag, Leipzig
3. Auersperg, V, Labek, G, Ziernhoeld, M, Poulios, N, Rompe, J-D, Boehler, N (2003): Lokalanaesthesie beeinflusst das Ergebnis der N-ESWT an der plantaren Fasciitis. In: Maier M, Gillesberger, F (Hrsg): Kongressband des 3. Drei-Länder-Treffens der Österreichischen, Schweizer und Deutschen Fachgesellschaften. München.
4. Becker, W, Krahl, H (1978): Die Tendopathien. Thieme Verlag, Stuttgart
5. Buchbinder, R, Green, S, White, M, Barnsley, L, Smidt, N, Assendelft, WJ (2002): Shockwave therapy for lateral elbow pain. The Cochrane database of systematic reviews (1), p: CD003524.
6. Clement, DB, Taunton, JE, Smart, GW (1984): Achilles tendinitis and peritendinitis: Etiology and treatment. Am J Sports Med 12: 179-184
7. Cook, JL, Khan, KM, Harcourt, PR, Grant, M, Young, DA, Bonar, SF (1997): A cross sectional study of 100 athletes with jumper's knee managed conservatively and surgically. Br J Sports Med 31: 332-336
8. Cook, JL, Khan, KM, Kiss, ZS, Purdam, CR, Griffiths, L (2000): Prospective imaging study of asymptomatic patellar tendinopathy in elite junior basketball players. J Ultrasound Med 19: 473-479
9. Cook, JL, Khan, KM (2001): What is the most appropriate treatment for patellar tendinopathy? Br J Sports Med 35: 291-294
10. Franke, K (1980): Traumatologie des Sports. Stuttgart, Thieme, 1980
11. Gerdesmeyer, L, Wagenpfeil, S, Haake, M, Maier, M, Loew, M, Wörtler, K, Lampe, R, Seil, R, Handle, G, Gassel, S, Rompe, J-D (2003): Extracorporeal shockwave therapy for the treatment of chronic calcifyung tendonitis of the rotator cuff: a randomized controlled trial. JAMA: The Journal of the American Medical Association, Vol. 290 (19), p:2573-80

12. Gremion, G, Augros, R, Gobelet, Ch, Leyvraz, P-F (2000): Wirksamkeit der extrakorporalen Stosswellentherapie bei der Calcific tendinitis der Schulter. Schweizerische Zeitschrift für Sportmedizin und Sporttraumatologie 48: 8-11
13. Haake, M, Huenerkopf, M, Gerdesmeyer, L, Koenig, IR (2002): Extrakorporale Stosswellentherapie (ESWT) bei epicondilytis humeri radialis – Eine Literaturübersicht. Der Orthopäde, Vol. 31 (7), p: 623-632
14. Heller, K-D, Niethard, FU (1998): Der Einsatz der extrakorporalen Stosswellentherapie in der Orthopädie – eine Metaanalyse. Z Orthop. 136: 390-401
15. James, SL, Bates, BT, Osternig, LR (1978): Injuries to runners. Am J Sports Med 6: 40-50
16. Józsa, L, Kannus, P (1997): Human tendons. Anatomy, physiology and pathology. Human Kinetics. 1-576
17. Khan, KM, Cook, JL (2000): Overuse Tendon Injuries: Where Does the Pain Come From? Sports Medicine and Arthroscopy Review 8: 17-31
18. Krahl, H. (1980): Jumper's Knee" – Ätiologie, Differentialdiagnose und therapeutische Möglichkeiten. Orthopäde 9: 193-197
19. Lohrer, H. (1991): Seltene Ursachen und Differentialdiagnosen der Achillodynie. Sportverl Sportschad 5: 182-185
20. Lohrer, H. (1995): Sport orthopaedics in athletics – an analysis of the current situation. NSA (New Studies in Athletics) 10 (4): 11-21
21. Lohrer, H. (1996): Die Achillodynie – Eine Übersicht Sport u. orthop Sporttraumatol 12: 36-42
22. Lohrer, H., W. Alt, A. Gollhofer (1999): Sportschuhe – Design versus Biomechanik? Sonderheft Orthopädieschuhtechnik: 13-16
23. Lohrer, H, Schoell, J, Arentz, S, Froelich, T, Straub, T, Penninger, E, Diesch, R, Haupt, G (2001): Effectiveness of radial shockwave Therapy (rESWT) on tennis elbow and plantar fasciitis. Book of Abstracts. CASM/ACMS annual symposium and sport medicine Conference, Calgary/CAN
24. Lohrer, H, Schöll, J (2001): Anterior knee pain in athletes. Book of abstracts. 6th Annual Congress of the European College of Sport Science: 64
25. Lohrer, H. (2002): Überlastungsschäden. In C. J. WIRTH (Hg): Fuß: Das Standardwerk für Klinik und Praxis. Stuttgart – New York, Thieme, 2002
26. Lohrer, H, Schoell, J, Arentz S.(2002): Achillodynie und Patellaspitzensyndrom – Ergebnisse der Behandlung austherapierter, chronischer Fälle mit radialen Stosswellen. Sportverletzung Sportschaden 2002;16; 108-114
27. Maffuli, N, Khan, KM, Puddu, G (1998): Overuse Tendon Conditions: Time to Change a Confusing Terminology. Arthroscopy 14: 840- 843
28. Martens, M., Wouters, P, Brussens, A, Mulier, JC (1982): Patellar tendinitis: Pathology and results of treatment. Acta Orthop Scand 53: 445-450
29. McLauchlan, GJ, Handoll, HH (2001): Interventions for treating acute and chronic Achilles tendinits. Cochrane Database Syst Rev (2) pCD000232
30. Orava, S, Leppilahti, J (1999): Overuse injuries of tendons in athletes. In: Jakob, RP, Fulford, P, Horan, F, Hrsg.; European Instructional Course Lectures 4: 128-131
31. Paavola; M, Kannus; P, Paakkala, T, Pasanen, M; Järvinen, M (2000): Long-Term Prognosis of Patients With Achilles Tendinopathy. Am J Sports Med 28: 634-642
32. Puddu, G., Ippolito, E., Postacchini, F.(1976): A classification of Achilles tendon disease. Am J Sports Med 4: 145-150
33. Rompe JD; Kirkpatrick CJ; Kullmer K; Schwitalle M; Krischek O (1998): Dose-related effects of shockwaves on rabbit tendo Achillis. A sonographic and histological study. J Bone Joint Surg (Br) 80:546-552

34. Rompe, J.D., CH. Hopf, B. Nafe, R. Bürger (1996): Low energy extracorporal shockwave therapy for painful heel: a prospective controlled single-blind study. Arch. Orthop. Trauma Surg. 115:75-79
35. Rompe, J.D., CH. Hopf, K. Küllmer, J. Heine, R. Bürger, B. Nafe (1996): Low-energy extracorporal shockwave therapy for persistent tennis elbow. Int Orthop 20:23-27
36. Schöll, J, Lohrer, H (2000): Radiale Stosswellentherapie des Fersensporns. Orthopädie Mitteilungen 2/2000: A 14
37. Schöll, J, Lohrer, H (2001): Fasciitis Plantaris – eine Indikation zur Stosswellentherapie. Orthopädie Schuhtechnik, 7/8, 2001, 66-70
38. Segesser, B., Nigg, B.M. (1980): Insertionstendinosen am Schienbein, Achillodynie und Überlastungsfolgen am Fuß – Ätiologie, Biomechanik, therapeutische Möglichkeiten. Orthopäde 9: 207-214
39. Tallon, C, Coleman; BD, Khan, KM, Maffuli; N (2001): Outcome of Surgery for Chronic Achilles Tendinopathy. Am J Sports Med 29: 315-320
40. Witvrouw, E, Bellemans, J, Lysens, R, Danneels, L, Cambier, D (2001): Intrinsic Risk Factors for the Development of Patellar Tendinitis in an Athletic Population. Am J Sports Med 29: 190-195

Efficacy of Radial Shockwave Therapy for Calcific Tendinitis of the Rotator Cuff - A Prospective Study

Petra Magosch, Sven Lichtenberg, Peter Habermeyer

Introduction

Calcific tendonitis as a common cause of shoulder complaints occurs most often at age 30 to 50. In asymptomatic shoulders, the prevalence of calcific tendonitis is reported between 3% and 20%[1, 26, 31]. Bosworth suspected that 30-45% of asymptomatc patients become symptomatic in the future. The prevalence in patients with shoulder pain is reported between 7% and 54%[7, 8, 26, 31]. Women are affected more often than men with 51-65% suffering from the right shoulder. A bilateral occurrence is observed between 9% and 40% of the cases. In 82-94.5%, the calcific deposit is located close to the supraspinatus tendon[1, 3]. The deposit itself is placed within a zone of hypovascularity. The etiology of calcific tendonitis has not yet been determined. Mechanical, vascular and biochemical factors are discussed. Local increases in pressure bring about a reduction in blood supply and hypoxia of the tendon tissue followed by degeneration of the tendon cells.

Calcific tendonitis shows a phase-like course [30] as shown in Table 1.

The time frame for the spontaneous course of calcific tendonitis varies among individuals and is reported from a few months to several years[21]. Bosworth reports the annual resorption rate to be at 6.4%[1]. Rupp et al. described 32% complete or more than 50% resorption in type I or II Gärtner deposits[26].

Stage 1 Precalcific stage	Calcification without ossification close to the insertion area of the rotator cuff, appearance of metaplasia of chondrocyts.
Stage 2 Calcific stage with formation, rest and resorption phase	Calcific deposits generated by transformed tendocyts with carbonate apatite crystals. No further calcification during the restphase of the deposit. Resorption phase indicated by neovascularitation and initial resorption of the deposit without any reason followed by local swelling and increase of pressure. Spontaneous rupture of the deposit and severe pain syndrome occur.
Stage 3 Postcalcific stage and resorption	Creeping substition of the deposit ending in Restitutio ad integrum.

Table 1. Stages of Calcific Tendinitis[30].

Wolk and Wittenberg [33] reported a 5 year resorption rate of 67% and Noel and Brantus [22] described 30% completely resorbed and 39.5% partially resorbed calcified deposits within a period of 6 months to 19 years.

But recently, the spontaneous cause of the so-called self-limiting disease remains unknown.

Noel and Brantus [22] described an incidence of 10% for postcalcification tendonitis. In 1995 Gärtner [3] proposed a radiologic phase distribution which corresponds to the spontaneous course (Table 2) (Figure 1a-c).

Mole et al. [20] classified the radiologic changes of the calcified deposit in relation to predominant pain symptomatics (Table 3).

Bosworth [1] categorized calcified deposits according to size by the largest diameter in the x-ray image (Table 4).

Type I	Sharp margins, homogeneous structure, low transparency (precalcific stage)
Type II	Sharp margins but higher transparency, more inhomogeneous (calcific stage)
Type III	Smooth margins, cloudly structure, high transparency (postcalcific stage)

Table 2. Classification according to Gärtner[3].

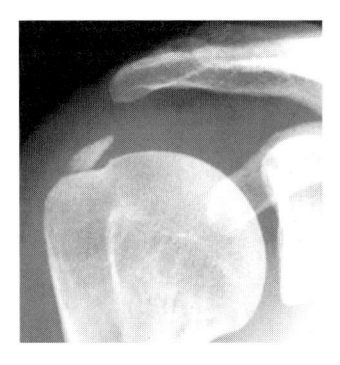

EFFICACY OF RADIAL SHOCKWAVE THERAPY FOR CALCIFIC TENDINITIS   179

Figure 1a.   X-ray of a type I Gärtner deposit.

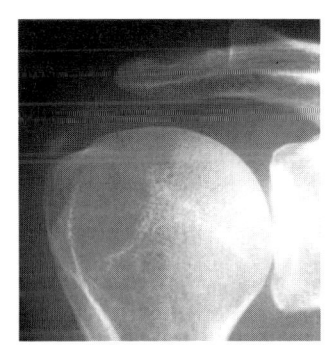

Figure 1b.   X-ray of a type II Gärtner deposit.

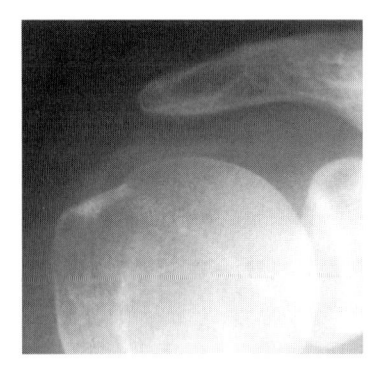

Figure 1c.   X-ray of a type III Gärtner deposit.

Precalcific stage	High density, increasing in size, painful
Calcific stage	High density chronic pain syndrome
Postcalcific stage	Spontaneous resorption of the deposit, inhomogeneous structure, night pain, associated with local bursitis

Table 3. Cassification according to Molé[20].

The size of the calcified deposit, however, does not correlate to the duration or intensity of the clinical complaints[3].

In its clinical course, a distinction is to be made between an acute and a chronic phase[3].

The acute phase begins with sudden, very sharp pains over a period of 2-3 weeks. The shoulder shows hyperalgesia perhaps with swelling and overheating. The patient complains particularly about night pain. Afterwards the pain gradually lessens until it completely disappears. But discomfort often remains for months (postcalcification tendonitis).

Macroscopically, a chalky emulsion is observed which consists of poorly crystalized carbonate apartite. The crystals are resorbed into the tendon or spontaneous rupture into the bursa subacromialis/subdeltoidea occurs (resorption phase). Histology shows a phagocytary resorption of the crystals with hyperemia. By x-ray, deposits were classified as transparent, smooth margins and cloudy structure. They have to be classified as type III according to Gärtner.

The chronic phase of calcific tendonitis is marked by slowly increasing pain which radiates to the insertion area of the deltoid muscle or the upper arm. Patients complain about night pain which prevents them from sleeping. Pain intensity often varies over years.

Type I	< 0.5 cm
Type II	0.5-1.5 cm
Type III	> 1.5 cm

Table 4. Classification according to Bosworth[1].

Upon inspection, the shoulder looks normal and moves freely. No specific clinical findings were available for the chronic phase of calcific tendonitis.

The x-ray shows a partly sharply defined homogeneous dense calcified deposit with unsharply limited and cloudy areas (Gärtner type II). The size of the calcified deposit does not correlate to the discomfort[3].

Calcific tendonitis does not predispose a patient to a rotator cuff lesion. Vice versa, calcium identified in the X-ray does not completely rule out a rupture[10]. Also there is no correlation with degenerative changes in the rotator cuff or osseous subacromial impingement[15].

The initial therapy for symptomatic calcific tendonitis has to be done conservatively by administering oral analgesics/antiinflammatories. In persistent cases, subacromial injection of local anesthetic with or without cortisone is indicated. If intervention does not achieve pain relief, then it is time for extracorporeal shockwave therapy. Again, if pain persists even after such therapy, then calcium deposits may be removed by arthroscopy.

In 1993 Loew used high- and low-energy extracorporeal shockwaves for the treatment of calcific tendonitis[17].

Despite many experimental and clinical studies on ESWT of calcific tendonitis, a consensus of treatment parameters could not be defined regarding energy flux density, number of impulses to be applied or number of treatments[17, 29]. Also, individual anatomic conditions, application technique as well as the type of equipment used have impact on treatment and outcome after ESWT. The principle of shockwave generation does not seem to have significant impact but an excellent study has shown the superiority of high energetic application[4]. This is in part due to the fact that, until now, complete acoustic fields have not been measured under in vivo conditions[4].

Since 2000, a pneumatically generated low-energy radial shockwave with an energy flux density of up to 0.16 mJ/mm^2 in focus has been in use. The principle of ballistically generated shockwaves consists of an extreme acceleration of a projectile through air pressure delivered to an applicator which administers the energy impulse to the tissue.

Unlike conventional shockwave generation principles, the focus of the EMS Dolorclast® applicator is located at the tip of the applicator. The ballistically generated shockwave radiates out from the applicator tip with a penetration depth of 3.5 cm without focus on the shockwave area in the tissue whereby pressure and energy density decrease by the third power of the penetration depth in the tissue. Therefore rESWT appears to be unsuitable for the treatment of calcific tendonitis of the rotator cuff[32]. The objective of radial shockwave therapy for calcific tendonitis is not induction of calcium deposit integration but rather the relief from pain.

The objective of this prospective study is to evaluate the efficacy of ballistic rESWT as a conservative therapeutic option in chronic calcific tendonitis (Gärtner type I and II) of the rotator cuff of the shoulder for pain relief and for its effects on calcium deposits.

Material and Methods

Between 2000 and 2002, 35 patients (23 men, 12 women) with an average age of 47.5 years (33 to 73 years) suffering from chronic calcific tendonitis were enrolled in the prospective study. In 22 subjects the right shoulder was affected (in 13 patients, the left one).

Inclusion criteria were defined as unsuccessful conservative treatment with a minimum pain history of 6 months and deposits classified as Gärtner type II and sized as type II or III according to Bosworth. Obese patients, patients with arthrosis of the AC joint as well as of the glenorhumeral joint and patients with associated rotator cuff rupture were excluded from the study.

Prior to the shockwave treatment, a clinical exam was followed by an x-ray diagnosis of calcific tendonitis in 3 planes (true-ap, axial and y-view). In all patients, rotator cuff ruptures were excluded by MRI.

The average complaint time was 28 months (6 to 120 months). The deposit was localized in the supraspinatus tendon (loco typico) in 33 patients and in the infraspinatus tendon in 2 patients. Type II calcium deposit size was found in 29 patients and 6 patients were scored as type III calcium deposit size according to Bosworth with an average size of 16.6 mm (7 to 37 mm). The mean acromiohumeral distance was 10.4 mm (7 to 13 mm).

The rESWT was administered using the Swiss DolorClast® with energy flux density of 0.16 mj/mm^2 to the patient lying down with a 30 to 45° internal rotation without local anesthesics. The shockwave applicator was placed over the area of maximum pressure pain as indicated by the patient. Two thousand impulses with a working pressure of 2.0 bar and a working frequency of 8 Hz were applied with medium application pressure. All patients got three treatments at intervals of 7 to 10 days.

Side effects such as skin irritations, petechia, hematoma or swelling were not observed in any patient.

During the treatment phase, no physiotherapeutic therapies were done and patients were advised to avoid any overhead sports movements up to 1 week following the last rESWT. The first follow-up exam (4 weeks after the last shockwave application) was followed by additional physiotherapeutic treatments through manual therapy and warm packing.

All patients (100%) received clinical and radiologic follow-up exams 4 weeks, 3 months, 6 months and 12 months after the last rESWT. Functional results were documented with unweighted constant scores. The force was measured with isobex in 90° abduction in the scapula plane. A standardized x-ray exam was conducted in 3 planes (true-ap, axial, y-view).

Statistical data analysis was done with StatView (Abacus Concepts Inc., Berkeley, CA). The T-test for linked samples was conducted for a change in shoulder function, the Chi^2 test for a change in subjective pain symptoms and disintegration of the deposit as well as the Spearmans Rank correlation for the correlation between change in pain symptoms and disintegration of the deposit.

Results

A significant ($p<0.0001$) functional improvement was found in constant scores from an average of 68.5 points (46.2 to 80.6 points) out of maximum 100 points at baseline to 80.5 points (58.3 to 96.1 points) 4 weeks after the treatment. When considering the individual categories of pain, daily activity, freedom of movement and strength, a significant relief from pain ($p=0.0037$) was found 4 weeks after the treatment with a point gain from an average of 6.9 points (1-12 points) out of maximum 15 points prior to rESWT to 10 points (0 to 15 points) after treatment. A significant improvement ($p<0.0001$) in daily activities (ADL) was found from 10.4 points (1 to 18 points) out of maximum 20 points up to 16 points (7 to 20 points). A significant improvement (p=0.02) in freedom of movement was found from 36 points (26 to 40 points) out of maximum 40 points up to 38 points (36 to 40 points). Finally, an average increase in strength of 1.3 kg was found (p=0.2). Later on, the constant score remained approximately the same 3 months after the treatment with an average of 74.7 points (46.7 to 95.8 points; p=0.9), 6 months after treatment with an average of 78.9 points (46.7 to 100 points; p=0.5) and 1 year after rESWT with an average of 79.7 points (62.6 to 100 points; p=0.9).

Four weeks after shockwave therapy, 25.7% of patients were pain free, 54.3% achieved a decrease in pain, 14.2% were found to be unchanged and 5.7% of patients reported an increase of pain. Another significant improvement (p<0.0001) in pain symptoms (n=35) occurred 3 months after the treatment: 50% of patients were pain free, 14.3% reported less pain, 30.7% remained unchanged and 10.7% reported worse pain. Even 6 months following rESWT (n=34) another significant reduction in pain (p=0.003) was observed. At the 6-month follow-up exam, 59.3% of patients were pain free, 25.9% reported improvement and 14.8% of patients suffered the same pain symptoms. No patient reported any exarcerbation of pain. Twelve months after the last treatment (n=32) 80.8% of patients were pain free and 19.2% reported less pain. No patient reported unchanged pain symptoms (Figure 2).

Four weeks after the treatment, x-ray control revealed no calcium deposits in 17.6% of the patients. In 20.5%, a disintegration of the calcium deposit was found

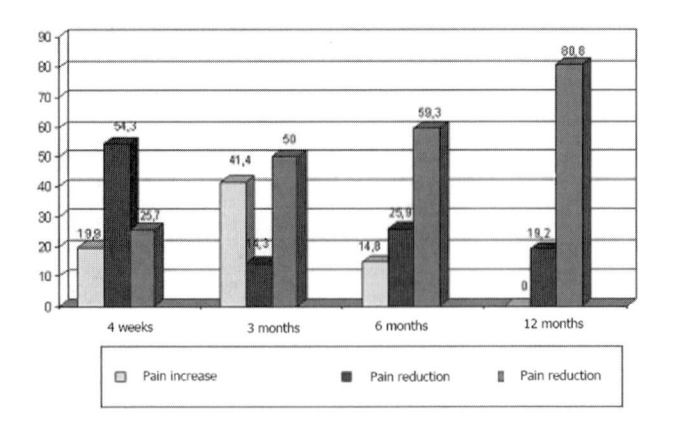

Figure 2. Pain scoring after rESWT.

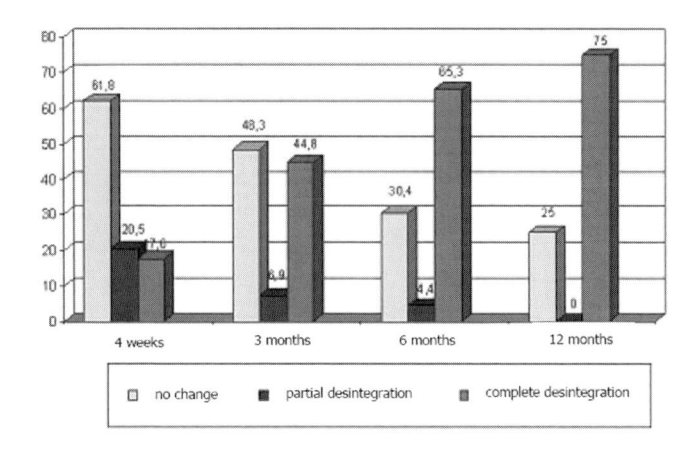

Figure 3. Change of deposit after rESWT.

with a change from Gärtner type II to III in 4 cases and a reduction in calcium deposit at identical stage in 3 cases. In 61.5% of the patients, the calcium deposit was unchanged. Three months following rESWT, no more calcium deposits were found in 44.8% of patients, a disintegration of the deposit with unchanged stage was found in 6.9% of patients, and the calcium deposit was found to be unchanged in 48.3% of the patients.

After 6 months, 30.4% of the patients showed an unchanged calcium deposit, 4.4% of patients (1 patient) showed a disintegration of the calcium deposit without change in diameter and 65.3% of the patients showed no calcium deposit anymore.

After 12 months, we found a complete resorption of the deposit in 75% of the patients and an unchanged deposit in 25%.

At each follow-up exam up to 6 months, a significant disintegration ($p<0.0001$) of the calcium deposit was found. Even 12 months after rESWT, a clear change in calcium deposit took place ($p=0.0507$) (Figure 3).

At each follow-up point, a positive correlation (Spearman Rank Correlation) between change in pain and change in calcium deposit was observed. Four weeks after rESWT, the correlation was 0.523 ($p=0.0031$) and 3 months after rESWT we found a correlation of 0.71 (p=0.0002). After 6 months, the correlation was 0.959 (p<0.0001) and after 12 months the correlation was 0.83 (p<0.0001) between change in pain symptoms and change in calcium deposit.

Within the first 4 weeks after the third shockwave treatment, 2 patients reported an exacerbation of calcific tendonitis with massively painful calcium disintegration. The pain symptoms during this acute phase could be controlled only with local infiltration of a local anesthetic with a corticoid and oral opiod medication. In 1 of the 2 patients this exarcerbation occurred 1 week after treatment. At the 4-week control point, a significant reduction in pain was already reported and the calcium deposit (13 mm diameter before the treatment) was already resorbed. In 1 patient, the exacerbation occurred 4 weeks after the last treatment. At the 4-week follow-up, the patient showed unchanged pain symptoms and unchanged calcium deposit in x-rays (23 mm diameter). Painful resorption of the calcium deposit occurred 3 days after the 4-week follow-up. Three months after the treatment, this deposit was no longer found in the x-ray. By this time the patient had already become completely pain-free.

Up to 8 months following rESWT, a total of 3 patients (8.5%) with unchanged pain symptoms and unchanged calcium deposit underwent an arthroscopic calcium deposit removal.

Discussion

Loew used extracorporeal shockwaves for the first time to treat calcific tendonitis of the shoulder. In a prospective study, he described significant successes in 55% and 65% of patients with one or two applications of 2000 impulses of medium energy (21 kV) versus one single application of 2000 impulses of low energy (18 kV)[12]. In the meantime a few clinical studies on high-energy shockwave therapy of calcific tendonitis of the rotator cuff are now available which document a significant pain-relieving effect associated by improved shoulder function as well as disintegration of calcium deposits[13, 23, 25].

In 20 patients with a 12-month pain history and ineffective conservative therapy, Loew et al. performed two electrohydraulically generated high-energy shockwave applications of 2000 impulses each to achieve pain relief/reduction in 75% of the cases. He also reported improved shoulder function 3 months after the last ESWT. The constant score of 69 points improved and calcium deposit integration occured in 95% of cases[13]. When delivering 2000 low-energy impulses of rESWT 3 times, we obtained a reduction in pain in fewer cases (64.3%). Three months after the treatment, the functional results of our study are comparable to a constant score of 74.7 points. The disintegration of calcium deposits in 51.7% of cases 3 months after rESWT is significantly below the success rate for high-energy ESWT.

Six months after a single treatment with 1500 impulses of electromagnetically generated high-energy shockwaves (EFD 0.28 mJ/mm^2), Rompe et al. found among 40 patients (pain history of 25 months, suffering from calcific tendonitis) a decrease of pain as well as an improved shoulder function. Constant score was reported of 76.9 points in 60% of patients and a disintegration of the calcium deposit was found in 72.5% of the cases[23]. Six months after rESWT we observed a reduction in pain or complete pain relief in 85.2% of patients. The constant score was 78.9 points and a slightly lower calcium deposit disintegration rate of 69.7% was observed.

In another prospective study conducted on 100 patients with an average pain history of 28 months (at least 12 months) and a calcium deposit size of at least 10 mm, Rompe et al. reported an excellent outcome 12 months after ESWT. They performed a single application of 1500 impulses of a high-energy shockwave (EFD 0.28 mJ/mm^2) with an application frequency of 2 Hz. Three weeks later, a significant improvement in constant scores was observed. Within one year the constant score increased from 43 points to 78 points. In 57% of the patients, a disintegration of the calcium deposit was observed radiologically. A complete resorption was achieved in 19%[24]. Within 12 months, low-energy rESWT achieved comparable functional results in our study (constant score of 79.7 points) whereby we observed a clearly higher resorption rate of 75%.

By changing only the energy flux density (from 0.06 mJ/mm^2 to 0.28 mJ/mm^2), Rompe et al. studied the effect of energy flux density on the therapy results for calcific tendonitis. A significantly higher partial or complete calcium deposit disintegration of 64% was found after 6 months in the high-energy patient group than in the low-energy treated group (50%). Functionally, the group treated with high energy shockwaves achieved a significantly higher constant score (88 points) than the low-energy patient group (71 points). The authors, however, pointed out the advantage of low-energy shockwave therapy regarding the absence of plexus anesthesia in patients with cardiac or pulmonary disorders[25].

A prospective randomized study involving 50 patients receiving 3 treatments of 5000 impulses of low-energy shockwaves or a single delivery of 5000 impulses of high-energy shockwaves allowed Seil et al. to conclude that the results of one session of high-energy shockwave treatment were comparable to the outcome after repetitive low-energy shockwave treatments. Six months after ESWT, the low-energy group reached a constant score of 77.5 points and the high-energy group, a constant score of 79.4 points. X-rays revealed that complete or partial resorbtion of the calcium deposit was found in 32% of low-energy treated patients. The rate was 48% in the high-energy treated therapy group[29].

In a randomized prospective study with 3 different treatment protocols, Loew et al. documented that the subjective, functional and radiologic results after shockwave treatment are energy- and dose-dependent. To this effect, they studied 171 patients with a pain history of at least 12 months, a Gärtner type I or II calcium deposit with size of at least 1.5 cm. Patients were randomized into different treatment groups: a control group without treatment, a single session with 2000 impulses of a low-energy shockwave (EFD 0.1 mJ/mm^2), a single session with 2000 impulses of a high-energy shockwave (EFD 0.3 mJ/mm^2), two treatments with 2000 impulses each of high-energy shockwave (EFD 0.3 mJ/mm^2). Three months after the treatment, the patients without therapy achieved a constant score of 47.8 points. The patients who received low-energy shockwave therapy showed a constant score of 51.6 points, the patient group who received a single high-energy treatment showed a constant score of 63.7 points and patients who received two sessions of high-energy therapy showed a constant score of 68.5 points. A decrease in pain 3 months after the therapy was reported by 30% of low-energy treated patients, by 60% of patients treated with high energy in one session and by 70% of patients treated with high energy in two sessions. X-rays revealed a disintegration of the calcium deposit in 20% of low-energy treated patients, in 55% of patients treated in one high-energy session and in 60% of patients treated with two high-energy sessions. After 6 months Loew et al. found a disintegration of calcium deposit in 47% of patients treated in one high-energy session and in 77% of patients treated in two high-energy sessions. The constant score was 67.7 points for patients treated once with high energy and 69.6 points for patients treated in two high-energy sessions. A reduction of pain was achieved after 6 months in 45% of patients treated in a single high-energy session and in 53% of patients with two high-energy sessions[17].

The subjective, functional and radiologic results of the group treated in one low-energy session (pain reduction of 30%, constant score of 51.6 points and disintegration rate of 20% 3 months after the treatment) was clearly below the functional and radiological result of our study. The patient groups showed simlar characteristics. We applied 3 sessions of low-energy therapy with 2000 impulses each. At least we can conclude that therapy success is dose and energy related.

Dahmen et al. [2] treated calcific tendonitis of the shoulder with low-energy shockwaves. All patients experienced a reduction in pain and an improvement in mobility of the shoulder joint even though x-rays revealed no changes in the calcium deposit. This observation was confirmed in our study within the first 4 weeks following low-energy shockwave treatment. Though 28 of 35 patients reported a reduction in pain or relief from pain, x-rays revealed no change in calcium deposit in 21 patients. Three, 6 and 12 months after rESWT our study showed a close correlation between change in pain symptoms and radiologically-confirmed disintegration of the calcium deposit.

Maier et al. [18] demonstrated that the size of the calcium deposit or its morphology before treatment does not affect the functional result of low-energy shockwave therapy. They treated 65 shoulders in 4 sessions each with 2000 impulses of a low-energy shockwave at 2 Hz. After an average follow-up of 18.2 months, a significant functional improvement of the treated shoulder was found in 78% of the cases.

Due to the radial expansion of the ballistic shockwave, pressure and energy density decrease by the third power of the penetration depth into the tissue. This caused Gerdesmeyer et al. [5] to conclude that ballistically generated low-energy shockwaves are rather unsuitable for the treatment of calcific tendonitis of the shoulder as a pathological change in deeper layers. The results of our prospective study appear to contradict this assumption even though it must be noted that obese patients were excluded from our study and that the mechanical mechanism of radial low-energy shockwaves has not been determined with certainty. When comparing the results of our study with the results of low-energy shockwaves generated electrohydraulically, electromagnetically or piezoelectrically, the principle underlying the generation of shockwaves seems to be irrelevant. Even the apparent induction of calcium deposit integration through low-energy radial shockwaves generated ballistically runs counter to our expectations based on current experimental findings.

Today, many animal experiments and clinical studies are available for high- and medium-energy electromagnetic, electrohydraulic and piezoelectric shockwaves. However, some different molecular mechanisms are discussed to explain the effects of shockwave therapy.

Positive effects in different diseases confirm the assumption that different mechanisms are at work. [24]

In vitro studies showed that high-energy shockwaves may induce nerve action potential [28], providing for the release of substance P from non-myelinized nerve fibers. Substance P may bring about the peripheral induction of neurogenic inflammation [11], plasmaextravasion [34] and a stimulation of different cell proliferations. [6] The initial rise in substance P concentration in the area of shockwave focus with subsequent persistent drops in concentration may explain the ESWT-induced initial pain irritation with subsequent persistent analgesis (19).

In biological tissues, the extracorporeal shockwave is credited not only with subordinate thermal and chemical effects but also with a mechanical action proportionate with the size of the difference in impedance at interfaces between different tissues. [9, 14] Since pressure and energy density decrease in the tissue by the third power of the depth of penetration of the radial shockwave, a mechanical effect as well as cavitation phenomena of the ballistically generated shockwave seems rather unlikely in calcific tendonitis.

Within the first 4 weeks and through 12 months, low-energy rESWT brings about a significant reduction in pain and appears to induce a resorption of the calcium deposit, while a significant improvement in shoulder function is obtained only within the first 4 weeks. When comparing the clinical and radiological results 6 months and 12 months after one session of high-energy shockwave therapy with the results 6 months and 12 months after three sessions of low-energy shockwave therapy for calcific tendonitis, both therapy options seem to obtain comparable results. This seems to indicate that the success rate correlates more likely to the energy rather than to the principle of shockwave generation itself.

The clinical and radiological results of our study have to be verified by prospective controlled trials.

Literature

1. Bosworth B. M.. Calcium deposits in the shoulder and subacromail bursitis: A survey of 12122 shoulders. JAMA 1941; 116: 2477-2482.
2. Dahmen GP, Meiss L, Nam VC, Skruodies B. Extrakorporale Stosswellentherapie (ESWT) im knochennahen Weichteilbereich an der Schulter. Extracta Orthop 1992; 15: 25-28.
3. Gärtner, J., A. Heyer. Calcific tendinitis der Schulter. Orthopäde 1995; 24: 284-302.
4. Gerdesmeyer L, Schräbler S, Mittelmeier W, Rechl H. Gewebeinduzierte Veränderungen der extrakorpolaren Stosswelle. Orthopäde 2002: (31): 618-622.
5. Gerdesmeyer L, Maier M, Haake M, Schmitz C. Physikalisch-technische Grundlagen der extrakorporalen Stosswellentherapie (ESWT). Orthopäde 2002; 31: 610-617.
6. Goto T, Yamaza T, Kido MA, Tanaka T. Light- and electron-microscopic study of the distribution of axons containing substance P and the localization of neurokinin-1 receptor in bone. Cell Tissue Res 1989: 293:87-93.
7. Harmon HP. Methods and results in the treatment of 2580 painful shoulders. With special reference to calcific tendinitis and the frozen shoulder. Am J Surg 1958; 95: 527-544.
8. Hedtmann, A, Fett H. Die sog. Periarthropathia humeroscapularis. Klassifizierung und Analyse anhand von 1266 Fällen. Z Orthop 1989: 127:643-649.
9. Howard D, Sturtevant B. In vitro study of the mechanical effects of schock-wave lithottripsy. Ultrasound Med Biol 1997; 23: 1107-1122.
10. Hsu H, Wu J, Jim Y, Chang C, Lo W, Yang D. Calcific tendinitis and rotator cuff tearing: a clinical and radiographic study. J Shoulder Elbow Surg 1994; 3: 159-164.
11. Levine JD, Clark R, Devor M, Helms C, Moskowitz MA, Basbaum AI. Intraneuronal substance P contributes to the severity of treated arthritis. Science 1984; 226: 547-549.
12. Loew M. Die Wirkung extrakorporal erzeugter hochenergetischer Stosswellen auf den klinischen, röntgenologischen und histologischen Verlauf der Calcific tendinitis der Schulter-eine klinische und experimentelle Studie. Habilitationsschrift der Ruprecht-Karl-Universität Heidelberg 1994.
13. Loew M, Jurgowski W, Mau HC, Thomsen M. Treatment of calcifying tendinitis of rotator cuff by extracoporeal shockwaves: A preliminary report. J Shouder Elbow Surg 1995; 4(2): 101-106.
14. Loew M, Jurgowski W, Thomsen M. Effect of extracorporeal shockwave therapy on calcific tendinitis of the shoulder. A preliminary report. Urologe 1995; 34: 49-53.
15. Loew M., D. Sabo, M. Wehrle, H. Mau. Relationship betwwem calcifying tendinitis and subacromial impingement: A prospective radiography and magnetic resonance imaging study. J Shoulder Elbow Surg 1996; 5: 314-319.
16. Loew M. Stosswellenbehandlung bei Erkrankungen an der Schulter und Ellenbogen-Mythen und Wirklichkeit. DVSE Mitteilungsblatt 1997: 5-7.
17. Loew M, Daecke W, Kusnierczak D, Rahmanzadeh M, Ewebeck V. Shockwave therapy is effective for chronic calcifying tendinitis of the shoulder. J Bone Joint Surg 1999; 81-B (5): 863-867.
18. Maier M, Stäbler A, Lienemann S, Köhler S, Feitenhansl A, Dürr HR, Pfahler M, Refior HJ. Shockwave application in calcifying tendinitis of the shoulder-prediction of outcome by imaging. Arch Orthop Trauma Surg 2000; 120: 493-498.

19. Maier M, Milz S, Wirtz DC, Rompe JD, Schmitz C. Grundlagenforschung zur Applikation extrakorporaler Stosswellen am Stütz- und Bewegungsapparat. Orthopäde 2002: 31: 667-677.
20. Molé D, Gonzalves M, Roche O, Sccarlat M. Introduction to calcifying tendinitis. In: Gazielly DF, Gleyze P, Thomas D (eds): The Cuff. Elsevier, Paris 1997
21. Molé D, Roche O, Gonzalves M. Tendinites calcifiantes de la coiffe desrotateurs:traite ment arthroscopique. Société Francaise d'Arthroscopie:Arthroscopie. Elsevier, Paris, 1999; pp 324-329.
22. Noel E, Brantus JF. Les tendinopathies calcifiantes de la coiffe des rotateurestraitement médical. Compe-Rendu des Journées Lyonnaises de l'épaule, Lyon, France, April 1993: 199-213.
23. Rompe JD, Rumler F, Hopf C, Nafe B, Heine J. Extracorporal shockwave therapy for calcifying tendinitis of the shoulder. Clin Orthop 1995; 321: 196-201.
24. Rompe JD, Küllmer K, Vogel J, Eckhardt A, Wahlmann U, Eysel P, Hopf C, Kirkpatrick CJ, Bürger R, Nafe B. Extrakorporale Stosswellentherapie – Experimentelle Grundlagen, klinischer Einsatz. Orthopäde 1997; 26: 215-228.
25. Rompe JD, Bürger R, Hopf C, Eysel P. Shoulder function after extracorporal shockwave therapy for calcific tendinitis. J Shouder Elbow Surg 1998; 7(5): 505-509.
26. Rüttimann, G.. Über die Häufigkeit röntgenologischer Veränderungen bei Patienten mit typischer Periarthritis humeroscapularis und bei Schultergesunden. Inaufuraldissertation, Juris, Zürich 1959.
27. Rupp S, Seil R, Kohn D. Calcific tendinitis der Rotatorenmanschette. Orthopäde 2000; 29: 852-867.
28. Schelling G, Delius M, Gschwender M, Grafe P, Gambihler S. Extracoreal shockwaves stimulate fraog sciatic nerves indirectly via a cavitation-mediated mechanism. Biophysical J 1994: 66:133-140.
29. Seil R, Rupp S, Hammer DS, Ensslin S, Gebhardt T, Kohn D. Extracororeal schockwave therapy in calcific tendinitis of the rotator cuff: comparison of different treatment protocols. Z Orthop Ihre Grenzgeb 1999; (4): 310-315.
30. Uhthoff, H. K., J. F. Löhr. Calcifying tendinitis. In: C. A. Rockwood, F. A. Matsen (eds). The shoulder. Saunders, Philadelphia, pp 989-1008, 1998.
31. Welfling, J.. Die Entfächerung der sog. Periarthritis der Schulter. Orthopäde 1981; 10:187-190.
32. Wess O. Stosswellen versus Druckwellen. Stuttgart, New York: Thieme 2001.
33. Wölk T, Wittenberg RH. Kalzifizierendes Subacromialsyndrom-Klinische und sonographische Ergebnisse unter nicht-operativer Therapie. Z Orthop 1997; 135: 451-457.
34. Zochodne DW. Epineural peptides: a role in neuropathic pain? Can J Neurol Sci 1993; 20: 69-72.

rESWT in Heel Spur (Fasciitis Plantaris)

Gerald Hupt[1]
Rupert Diesch,[2] Thomas Straub,[3] Emil Penninger,[3] Thomas Frölich,[4]
Jakob Schöll,[5] Heinz Lohrer,[5] Dr. Theodor Senge[6]

Introduction

The overall prevalence of fasciitis plantaris is about 15%. Lateral x-ray exams on caucasians revealed plantar and/or dorsal heel spurs in 15.7% whereby both legs were affected in 11%[32]. The incidence rises with age and is comparable for different continents such as Europe, Africa and America[2].

The primary symptom is pain, frequently associated with restrictions in range of motion (ROM)[3, 9, 14]. A multitude of conservative treatments have been described[30, 40, 41]. These include ultrasound [10, 37], Iontopheresis [16] and low-energy laser [12] in addition to physical therapy, steroid injections and non-steroid antiphlogistics, however without evidence brought today of their efficacy. Operative therapy is recommended only following failure of conservative action[1].

---

[1] *Urological clinic and policlinic - University of Cologne*
[2] *Private practice, Friedrichshafen*
[3] *Private practice, Dingolfing*
[4] *Private practice, Stuttgart*
[5] *Sportsmedicine Institute of Frankfurt*
[6] *Urological clinic – Uniersity of Bochum, Herne*

The introduction of extracorporeal shockwaves for the treatment of urolithiasis has revolutionized renal calculi therapy. Additional applications focus on other calculi such as gallstones, pancreatic stones and salivary duct stones[28, 34, 35]. Since 1986 we have tested the effect of shockwaves on the healing of wound and bone fractures in experimental models and were first to demonstrate the osteogenetic potential of shockwaves[21-23]. This led to the therapy of pseudarthroses with shockwaves. Finally, soft tissue diseases such as calcific tendonitis of the shoulder, epicondylitis lateralis and medialis and fasciitis plantaris have also been treated increasingly in recent years[7, 15, 31].

Apart from the conventional generation of shockwaves, these can also be produced ballistically (Lithoclast) and were first used in urology (for endoscopic stone fragmentation). These processes are significantly more economical. Our own studies on soft tissue and bones of rabbits and monkeys showed that the results of treatment with ballistically produced radial shockwaves coincided with those obtained following therapy with focused extracorporeal shockwaves. Accordingly, one can state that the shockwaves produced by either method are comparable in terms of their biological effect. This study examines the effect of radial shockwaves on fasciitis plantaris.

Materials and Methods

All shockwave treatments were performed with the Swiss DolorClast® (Figure 1), a modified device compared to the Swiss LithoClast®, which is a unit for

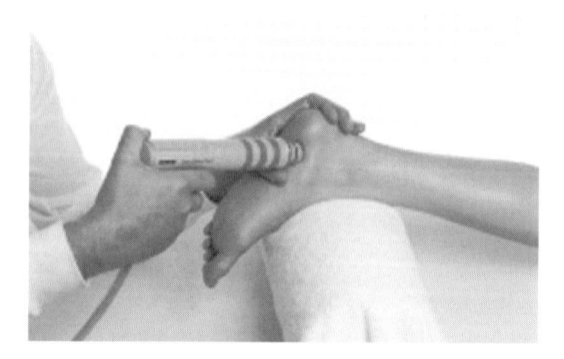

Figure 1. Therapy of the Fasciitis plantaris.

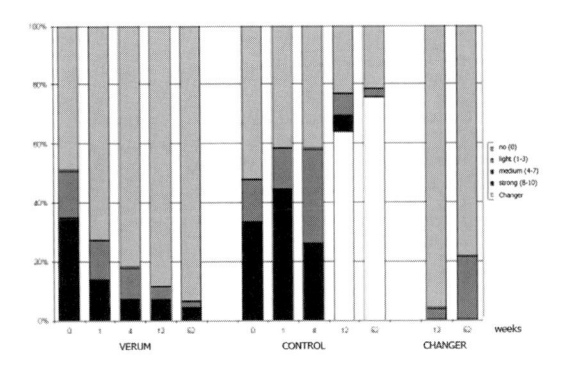

Figure 2. Pain at night.

the endoscopic treatment of calculi[27, 42]. The modifications were based on animal studies conducted on rabbits and rhesus monkeys[19]. In plantar heel pain, the tip of the applicator was positioned at the point where the greatest pain was reported via patient feedback (Figure 2). Shockwaves were delivered via a customary medium (ultrasound gel).

Patients

One hundred and three consecutive patients with chronic fasciitis plantaris were examined as part of a multicentric, prospective, randomized and placebo-controlled study. Patients were enrolled if they reported a pain history of at least 6 months with at least 2 different failed attempts at a conservative treatment indicating the need for surgery. Exclusion criteria were defined as poor health condition (Karnofsky index < 70), a specific intervention within the last two weeks, pregnancy, disturbance in coagulation, tumors in the area to be treated and systemic diseases which could be interpreted as possible causes of pain in differential diagnostics (e.g. collagenosis, rheumatic diseases).

Patients were randomized at a 1:1 ratio into a verum or sham group. While both groups obtained identical treatments, the test set-up was modified in the control group so that no shockwaves would be transmitted. Up to 3 treatments were conducted without local anesthesia. Local anesthesia was administered only in exceptional cases when pain was no longer tolerable. Follow-up exams were conducted after 1, 4, 12 and 52 weeks.

	Total	Verum group	Control group
Age (years)	50.4 ± 11.7	50.4 ± 11.3	50.6 ± 12.3
Female	77	39	38
Male	26	16	10
Right position	49	27	22
Left position	54	28	26
Pain duration (months)	24.0 ± 27.5	23.7 ± 27.4	24.6 ± 28.1

Table 1. Demographic data.

If pain persisted after 4 weeks in patients from the control group, blinding was terminated and admission to the treatment group was authorized.

Questionnaires were filled out by the treating orthopedist or surgeon and forwarded anonymously to the study center for statistical evaluation (SPSS).

Results

One hundred and three patients were admitted to the study. Fifty five patients were randomized into the verum group, 48 into the control group. Demographic data (Table 1) as well as symptoms and initial findings (Table 2) show homogeneity at baseline.

Treatments were performed at an initial pressure of 4 bar with 2000 shockwaves. Local anesthesia was required for 5 patients (9%) in the verum group and 3 patients (6%) in the control group. Local symptoms could be observed immediately following treatment (Table 3), but they disappeared after 1 week.

Eighty-four patients were examined up to 52 weeks after the last rESWT. Night pain, pain at rest and walking improved significantly in the treatment group compared to placebo (Figures 3-5). In fact, an increasing improvement throughout the entire follow-up period could be observed. In the control group no significant change between initial findings and follow-up could be found. Patients who dropped out of the control group 4 weeks after rESWT due to persistent pain received an unblinded active treatment. They finally achieved results similar to the primary treatment group.

	Total	Verum group	Control group
Night pain	32.0	36.4	27.1
Restriction in daily life	95.1	92.7	97.9
Restriction in sports	66.0	74.5	56.3
Restriction in occupation	52.4	58.2	45.8
Maximum walking time	0.0	0.0	0.0
Restricted	57.3	49.1	66.7
Not restricted	14.6	16.4	12.5
Start-up pain	23.3	27.3	18.8
Redness	1.0	0.0	2.1
Overheating	1.9	0.0	4.2
Swelling	6.8	3.6	10.4
Scars	1.0	1.8	0.0
Injection sites	1.0	1.8	0.0
Skewfoot	21.4	20.0	22.9
Splayfoot	35.9	30.9	41.7
Flatfoot	39.8	34.5	45.8
Pes equinocavus	2.9	0.0	6.3

Table 2. Pathology and findings giving as percent (%).

	Total	Verum group	Control group
Irritation	48.5	76.4	37.5
Petechial bleedings	9.7	18.2	0.0
Hematoma	2.9	5.5	0.0
Swelling	20.4	34.5	4.2
Pain	18.4	32.7	2.1

Table 3. Postoperative adverse events (%).

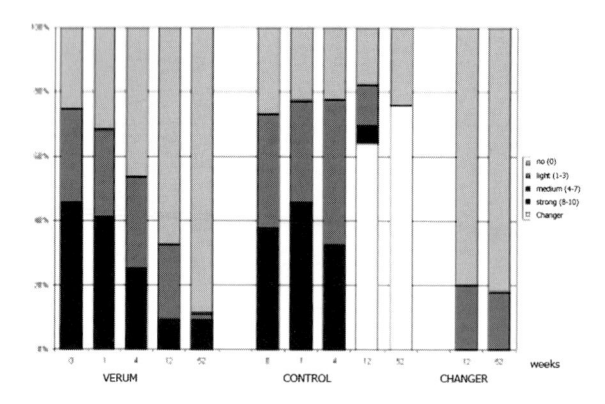

Figure 3. Rest pain.

Limitations in walking time and daily activities in the verum group were persistent in 36% and 34% respectively. Limitations in sports and profession, were persistent in 52% and 50%, even though the extent of the limitation had decreased significantly. Comparative values for the control group are above 70%.

The majority of patients would repeat the treatment after 1 week. This remained unchanged in the verum group. In the control group this value drops down after 4 weeks and once again after 12 weeks (Figure 5). This observation

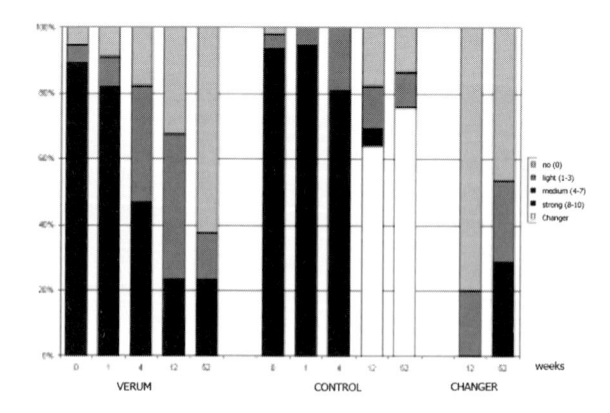

Figure 4. Walking pain.

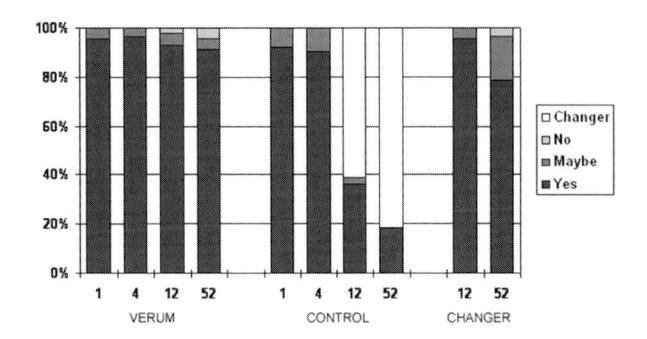

Figure 5. Acceptance of reapplication.

correlates with the patients' satisfaction. After 12 weeks, over 90% of patients report an improvement and more than 60% are even completely satisfied. In the control group, this is documented as 10% (Figure 6).

No clinically relevant side effects were found, but minor petechial bleeding and swelling were reported.

Discussion

In the past 30 years, the effects of many physical factors on the healing processes of bone and soft tissue have been studied. With the consideration of

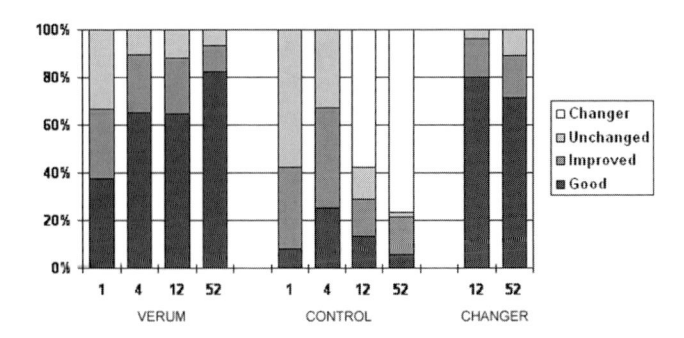

Figure 6. Patient satisfaction.

extracorporeal shockwaves for the treatment of urolithiasis, a new physical medium was introduced to medicine[4, 5]. Shockwaves are able to generate effects without any surgery. These shockwave were used in urolithiasis. As of 1985 gall stones and pancreatic and salivary duct calculi were treated with shockwaves also[28, 34, 35]. Common to all these therapies is a fragmentation of the calculi by the shockwaves.

Shockwaves were used for the first time in 1986 for the purpose of stimulating healing processes rather than fragmenting stones. Low energetic shockwaves were known to stimulate wound healing but high energetic shockwaves did not. These findings were observed in superficial skin wounds in pigs[20]. In addition, shockwaves were shown to have an osteogenetic effect, which led to the use of shockwaves in the treatment of pseudarthrosis[11, 15, 17, 18, 22, 24, 25, 36, 38, 39]. The positive effects on wound healing were no longer used until recent studies have shown again these effects. The wound healing effect is discussed further within the chapter written by Wolfgang Schaden and Richard Thiele.

In the case of fasciitis plantaris, for a long time almost no multicentric, controlled studies have examined conservative or operative processes. In the meantime, several excellent prospective randomized placebo-controlled studies on the effect of focused ESWT have been published, some with partially contradictory results[43, 44, 45]. Therefore, an evaluation of the efficacy of focused ESWT is not conclusively possible but it is certain that a conservative therapy of ESWT is indicated prior to surgery. The recent reviews have shown the evidence of shockwaves on chronic plantar heel pain.

This study reports for the first time on the effect of radial ESWT (rESWT) for the treatment of heel spur. The patients enrolled in this trial had at least two unsuccessful conservative therapies and the pain duration was longer than 6 months. This corresponds to a negative selection.

The subjective success rates of conventional extracorporeal shockwave therapy are shown as 50 to 75% painfree or significant pain reduction[6, 8, 29, 33]. Radial shockwave therapy obtains comparable success rates. The well known placebo effect, which is device associated, was controlled by a sham rESWT group. The essential difference and advantage compared to conventional focused shockwave therapy is: rESWT is easy to administer, no imaging is required, no local anesthesics are required and the cost is significantly reduced. In case of failed rESWT, surgical options remain possible.

The side effects of radial therapy are similar to those of focused ESWT such as transitory pain, petechial bleeding or subcutaneous hematomata in up to 4% of the patients[26]. However, local skin symptoms are clearly more frequent in radial therapy which is easy to explain because of the high energy close to the tip of the applicator. After 1 week, no more side effects were found and no neurological disorders occurred. Local irritation therefore does not appear to reach clinical relevance.

The use of shockwaves in orthopedics remains controversial and continues to be documented by insufficient studies[13].

A multitude of shockwave studies have been published but only few prospective randomized controlled studies are available. Nevertheless, this therapy for fasciitis plantaris has been found to be effective and is not to be classified as "lifestyle" therapy. The high recommendation by patients and physicians supports the clinical evidence that ESWT is effective, much more than any surgical or injection technique.

The radial shockwave therapy examined in our study appears to be clinically effective without side effects. Therefore it is reasonable to use the rESWT for the treatment of chronic fasciitis. In addition, rESWT provides for a very economical treatment when compared to conventional shockwave processes.

Literature

1. Anderson, R.B., M.D. Foster: Operative treatment of subcalcaneal pain. Foote Ankle (US) 9(1989) 317-323
2. Banadda, B.M., O. Gona, D.M. Ndlovu, R. Vaz: Calcaneal spurs in a black African population. Foot Ankle 13(1992) 352-354
3. Baxter, D.E., C.M. Thigpen: Heel pain: operative results. Foot Ankle 5(1984) 16-25
4. Chaussy, C., Extracorporeal shockwave lithotripsy. 1982, Basel: Karger.
5. Chaussy, C., F. Eisenberger, K. Wanner, F. Forssmann, W. Hepp, E. Schmiedt, W. Brendel: The use of shockwaves for the destruction of renal calculi without direct contact. Urol. Res. 4(1976) 175
6. Dahmen, G.P., R. Franke, V. Gonchars, K. Poppe, S. Lentrodt, S. Lichtenberger, S. Jost, J. Montigel, V.C. Nam, G. Dahmen: Die Behandlung knochennaher Weichteilschmerzen mit Extrakorporaler Stosswellentherapie (ESWT), Indikation, Technik und bisherige Ergebnisse. In: Chaussy, C., F. Eisenberger, D. JochamD. Wilbert (Hrsg.): Die Stosswelle - Forschung und Klinik, Attempto Verlag, Tübingen (1995) 175-186.

7. Dahmen, G.P., L. Meiss, V.C. Nam, B. Skruodies: Extrakorporale Stosswellentherapie (ESWT) im knochennahen Weichteilbereich an der Schulter. Extracta Orthopaedica 11(1992) 25-27
8. Diesch, R., G. Haupt: Extracorporeal shockwaves in the treatment of pseudarthrosis, calcific tendinitis of the shoulder and calcaneal spur. In: Siebert, W.M. Buch (Hrsg.): Springer Verlag, Berlin Heidelberg New York (1997) 131-135.
9. DuVries, H.L.: Heel spur (calcaneal spur). A.M.A. Arch. Surg. 74(1957) 536
10. Ebenbichler, G., K.L. Resch: Kritische Überprüfung des therapeutischen Ultraschalls. Wien. Med. Wochenschr. 144(1994) 51-53
11. Ekkernkamp, A., A. Bosse, G. Haupt, A. Pommer: Der Einfluß der extrakorporalen Stosswellen auf die standardisierte Tibiafraktur am Schaf. In: Ittel, T., G. SieberthH. Matthiass (Hrsg.): Aktuelle Aspekte der Osteologie, Springer, Berlin Heidelberg New York (1992) 307-310.
12. Ernst, E., V. Fialka: Low-dose Lasertherapie: eine kritische Prüfung der klinischen Wirksamkeit. Schweiz. Med. Wochenschr. 123(1993) 949-954
13. Fritze, J.: Extrakorporale Stosswellentherapie (ESWT) in orthopädischer Indikation: Eine ausgewählte Übersicht. Versicherungsmedizin 50(5) (1998) 180-185
14. Furey, J.G.: Plantar fasciitis: the painful heel syndrome. J. Bone Joint Surg. 75-A(1975) 672-673
15. Graff, J., Die Wirkung hochenergetischer Stosswellen auf Knochen und Weichteilgewebe. 1989, Bochum: Habilitationsschrift, Ruhr-Universität Bochum.
16. Grossi, E., G.C. Monza, S. Pollavini, L. Bona: NSAID ionisation inthe management of soft tissue rheumatism: role played by the drug, electrical stimulation and suggestion. Clin. Exp. Rheumatol. 4 (1986) 265-267
17. Haist, J.: Die Osteorestauration via Stosswellenanwendung. Eine neue Möglichkeit zur Therapie der gestörten knöchernen Konsolidierung. In: Chaussy, C., F. Eisenberger, D. JochamD. Wilbert (Hrsg.): Die Stosswelle - Forschung und Klinik, Attempto Verlag, Tübingen (1995) 157-161.
18. Haist, J., D. Steeger, U. Witzsch, R.A. Bürger, U. Haist: The extracorporeal shockwave therapy in the treatment of disturbed bone union. 7th Int. Conference on Biomedical Engineering, Singapore (1992) 222-224
19. Haupt, G., Behandlung von Harnsteinen, Knochen und Weichgewebe mit ballistischer Energie: Leistungsfähigkeit und Systemerweiterung einer neuen minimal-invasiven Therapietechnik. 1997: Ruhr-Universität Bochum.
20. Haupt, G., M. Chvapil: Effect of shockwaves on the healing of partial-thickness wounds in piglets. J. Surg. Res. 49(1990) 45-48
21. Haupt, G., A. Ekkernkamp, M. Chvapil, A. Haupt, B. Gerety: Der Einfluß extrakorporaler Stosswellen auf die Knochenbruchheilung. Hefte zur Unfallheilkunde 220(1991) 524
22. Haupt, G., A. Haupt, A. Ekkernkamp, B. Gerety, M. Chvapil: Influence of shockwaves on fracture healing. Urology 39(1992) 529-532
23. Haupt, G., A. Haupt, B. Gerety, M. Chvapil: Enhancement of fracture healing with extracorporeal shockwaves. J. Urol. 143(1990) 230A
24. Haupt, G., A. Haupt, T. Senge: Die Behandlung von Knochen mit extrakorporalen Stosswellen - Entwicklung einer neuen Therapie. In: Chaussy, C., F. Eisenberger, D. JochamD. Wilbert (Hrsg.): Stosswellenlithotripse, Aspekte und Prognosen, Attempto Verlag, Tübingen (1993) 120-126.
25. Haupt, G., P. Katzmeier: Anwendung der hochenergetischen extrakorporalen Stosswellentherapie bei Pseudarthrosen, Calcific tendinitis der Schulter und Ansatztendinosen (Fersensporn, Epicondylitis). In: Chaussy, C., F. Eisenberger, D.

JochamD. Wilbert (Hrsg.): Die Stosswelle - Forschung und Klinik, Attempto Verlag, Tübingen (1995) 143-146.

26. Haupt, G., A. Menne, M. Schulz: Medizinisches Instrument zum Erzeugen und Weiterleiten von extrakorporalen nicht fokussierten Druckwellen auf biologisches Gewebe. Patentanmeldung (1997)

27. Haupt, G., R. Olschewski, S. Hartung, T. Senge: Comparison of laser and ballistic systems by in vitro lithotripsy with a standardized stone model. J. Endourol. 7(1993) S62

28. Iro, H., H. Schneider, C. Födra, G. Waitz, N. Nitsche, H.H. Heinritz, J. Benninger, C. Ell: Shockwave lithotripsy of salivary duct stones. Lancet 339(1992) 1333-1336

29. Krischek, O., J.-D. Rompe, B. Herbsthofer, B. Nafe: Symptomatische niedrigenergetische Stosswellentherapie bei Fersenschmerzen und radiologisch nachweisbarem plantaren Fersensporn. Z. Orthop. 136(1998) 169-174

30. Labelle, H., R. Guibert, N. Newman, M. Fallaha, C.-H. Rivard: Lack of scientific evidence for the treatment of lateral epicondylitis of the elbow. J. Bone. Joint. Surg. 74-B(1992) 646-651

31. Loew, M., W. Jurgowski: Erste Erfahrungen mit der Extrakorporalen Stosswellen-Lithotripsie (ESWL) ind der Behandlung der Tendinosis calcarea der Schulter. Z. Orthop. 131(1993) 470-473

32. Riepert, T., T. Drechsler, R. Urban, H. Schild, R. Matern. Häufigkeit, Altersabhängigkeit und Geschlechtsverteilung des Fersensporns. Analyse der Röntgenmorphologie bei 1027 Patienten der mitteleuropäischen Population. Rofo Fortschr. Geb. Rontgenstr. Neuen Bildgeb. Verfahr. 162(1995) 502-505

33. Rompe, J.D., K. Küllmer, P. Eysel, H.M. Riehle, R. Bürger, B. Nafe: Niedrigenergetische extrakorporale Stosswellentherapie ESWT beim plantaren Fersensporn. Orthop. Praxis 32(1996) 271-275

34. Sauerbruch, T., M. Delius, G. Paumgartner, J. Holl, O. Wess, W. Weber, W. Hepp, W. Brendel: Fragmentation of gallstones by extracorporeal shockwaves. New Engl. J. Med. 314(1986) 818-822

35. Sauerbruch, T., J. Holl, M. Sackmann, R. Werner, R. Wotzka, G. Paumgartner: Disintegration of a pancreatic duct stone with extracorporeal shockwaves in a patient with chronic pancreatitis. Endoscopy 19(1987) 207-208

36. Schleberger, R.: Anwendung der extrakorporalen Stosswelle am Stütz- und Bewegungsapparat im mittelenergetischen Bereich. In: Chaussy, C., F. Eisenberger, D. JochamD. Wilbert (Hrsg.): Die Stosswelle - Forschung und Klinik, Attempto Verlag, Tübingen (1995) 166-174.

37. Stratford, P.W., D.R. Levy, S. Gauldie, D. Miseferi, K. Levy: The evaluation of phonophoresis and friction message as treatments for extensor carpi radialis tendinitis: a randomized controlled trial. Physiotherapy Canada 41(1989) 93-99

38. Sukul, K., E.J. Johannes, E. Pierik, G. van Eijck, M. Kristelijn: The effect of high energy shockwaves focused on cortical bone: an in vitro study. J. Surg. Res. 54(1993) 46-51

39. Valchanou, V.D., P. Michailov: High energy shockwaves in the treatment of delayed and nonunion fractures. Internat. Orthopaedics (SICOT) 15(1991) 181-184

40. Verhaar, J., G. Walenkamp, A. Kester, H. van Mameren, T. van der Linden: Lateral extensor release for tennis elbow. A prospective long-term follow-up study. J. Bone Joint Surg. 75-A(1993) 1034-1043

41. Wittenberg, R., S. Schaal, G. Muhr: Surgical treatment of persistent elbow epicondylitis. Clin. Orthop. 278(1992) 73-80

42. Zhong, P., G.M. Preminger: In vitro comparison of different modes of intracorporeal shockwave lithotripsy. J. Urol. 153(1995) S47

43. Rompe JD, et al. Shockwave application for chronic plantar fasciitis in running athletes – a prospective, randomized, placebo- controlled trial. Am J Sports Med 2003; 31:268-275
44. Buchbinder R, Ptasznik R, Gordon J, Buchanan J, Prabaharan V, Forbes A: Ultrasound-guided extracorporeal shockwave therapy for plantar fasciitis. A randomized controlled trial. JAMA 288: 1364-1372, 2002
45. Haake M, Buch M, Schoellner C, Goebel F: Extracorporeal shockwave therapy for plantar fasciitis: randomised controlled multicentre trial. British Medical Journal 327: 1-5, 2003

rESWT- A New Method for the Treatment of Lateral Epicondylitis

Gerald Haupt[1]
Rupert Diesch,[2] Thomas Straub,[3] Emil Penninger,[3] Thomas Frölich,[4]
Jakob Schöll,[5] Heinz Lohrer,[5] Theodor Senge[6]

Introduction

More than 130 years ago Runge published his "Etiology and treatment of the forearm spasm[1]." Just 10 years ago Morris introduced the term "lawn tennis elbow[2]." Prevalence is described between 1% and 3%[3, 4]. Epicondylitis is associated with severe pain and restriction in range of motion (ROM). More than 50% of patients consult an orthedic surgeon[4]. Surgery is performed in less than 12%[5]. ESWT is well known to achieve excellent or good results in 79% and 89% of patients respectively. Dahmen described the first shockwave therapies in muscular pain disorders. He used large units with focused shockwaves from urologic departments[6]. During the last decade an alternative ESWT option was designed, namely radial Extracorporeal Shockwave Therapy or rESWT using the Swiss DolorClast® device[7]. We have studied the effect on lateral epicondylitis.

---

[1] Urological clinic and policlinic - University of Cologne
[2] Private practice, Friedrichshafen
[3] Private practice, Dingolfing
[4] Private practice, Stuttgart
[5] Sportsmedicine Institute of Frankfurt
[6] Urological clinic – Uniersity of Bochum, Herne

Materials and Methods

One hundred and sixteen consecutive patients with epicondylitis lateralis were examined as part of a multicentric, prospective, randomized and placebo-controlled study. We enrolled patients with a pain history of at least 6 months and at least 2 different failed attempts with a conservative treatment. In all cases surgery was indicated. The exclusion criteria we used were defined as poor health (Karnofsky index < 70), a specific epicondylitis related intervention within 2 weeks prior to ESWT, pregnancy, disturbance of coagulation, tumor, and systemic diseases which could be feasible to generate tennis elbow like pain (e.g. collagenosis, rheumatic diseases).

Patients were randomized into a verum or sham ESWT group. Both groups obtained identical treatments but the placebo group received modified treatment set up to be sure that no energy passes the applicator. Patients were totally blocked from shockwaves. Up to 3 treatments were conducted without local anesthesics except in a few cases if pain was not acceptable. Follow-up exams were conducted 1, 4, and 12 weeks after intervention.

In the placebo or control group, if pain persisted 4 weeks after ESWT, blinding was broken and patients were offered the opportunity to cross over into the active unblinded ESWT group.

Questionnaires were filled out by the treating orthopedist or surgeon and forwarded anonymously to the study center for statistical evaluation (SPSS).

Results

Fifty-five patients were randomized to the placebo group and 61 were randomly assigned to active treatment. Demographic data (Table 1) as well as symptoms and initial findings (Table 2) did not show any statistical difference.

Treatments were performed with 2000 shockwaves at application pressure of 4 bar. Local anesthesia was required in only 11 patients (20%) of the verum group and in 1 patient (1.6%) of the control group. Local symptoms could be observed immediately following the treatment (Table 3), without clinical relevance, and they disappeared completely after 1 week.

	Total	Verum group	Control group
Age (years)	46.2 ± 9.4	47.4 ± 9.3	45.1 ± 9.5
Female	48	21	27
Male	78	34	44
Right position	55	40	15
Left position	61	46	15
Pain duration (months)	16.4 ± 16.2	15.3 ± 13.8	17.3 ± 18.9

Table 1. Demographic data.

Patients from the sham group were excluded in placebo analysis as soon as they crossed over to verum treatment. They were analyzed as "changers" (Table 4). Seven patients left the study for different reasons (2 operative treatments, 5 due to different systemic diseases). Four patients were lost during follow-up. We are able to re-examine 96.5% of patients during the follow-up period.

After one week, 73% of the verum patients and 28% of patients from the control group noticed an improvement. At the 4-week follow-up, the evaluation of subjective improvement was significantly better in the verum group compared to placebo. In the active group 63% indicated improvement (47% reported improvement of at least 40%), while in the control group 48% indicated an improvement of at least 40%. Twelve weeks after rESWT, most of the control patients could no longer be followed up as control patients because of persistent pain.

	Verum	Control
Awakening due to pain	26	24
Limitation during ADL	48	59
Limitation during sports	36	40
Limitation during work	45	43
Disturbance in finger extension	39	42
Disturbance in finger flexion	8	16

Table 2. Clinical evidence (%).

Postoperative Results	All	Verum	Control
Local skin irritation	51	45	6
Petechial bleedings	21	19	2
Hematoma	3	3	0
Swelling	35	30	5
Pain	39	34	5

Table 3. Adverse events (%).

In accordance with directives from the ethics commission, randomization was terminated after 4 weeks for patients without successful treatment (improvement less than 50%). These patients were offered verum treatment. At this point, 83% of verum patients indicated an improvement. Control patients without significant improvement had left the control group and experienced a verum treatment as changers. All of them were analyzed as changers after cross over. Only few control patients who noticed an improvement and whose randomization was not terminated remained in the control group. Even though they represent a positive selection from the control group, their results do not reach the primary or secondary verum and changer groups. After 52 weeks, only 11% of all patients reported no improvement, 70% of patients with primary or secondary verum treatment noticed improvements of at least 80% (Figure 1).

In terms of the criteria pressure pain, night pain, pain at rest and pain during exercise (Figures 2-5), the verum treatment proved clearly superior as shown in the specific tests as well (Figures 6-8).

	1 week	4 week	12 week	52 week
Verum	27	34	42	48
Control	44	50	17	16
Changer	-	-	37	41
All	71	84	96	105

Table 4. Number of patients in follow-up examinations.

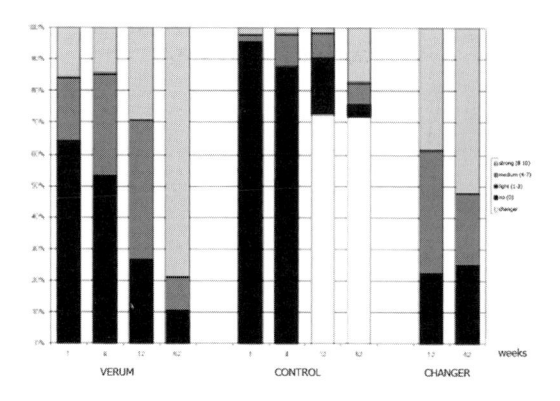

Figure 1. Subjective improvement (Visual Analog Scale).

The subjective evaluation shows a slight advantage of the verum group after 1 week. After 12 weeks only 5% of verum patients and 20% of changers obtained poor results. Among the patients who remained in the control group (improvement of a least 50%), 29% reported poor results. After 52 weeks, only 4% of patients within the verum group scored as poor. In contrast, the changer group was less successful (22% poor results) (Figure 9).

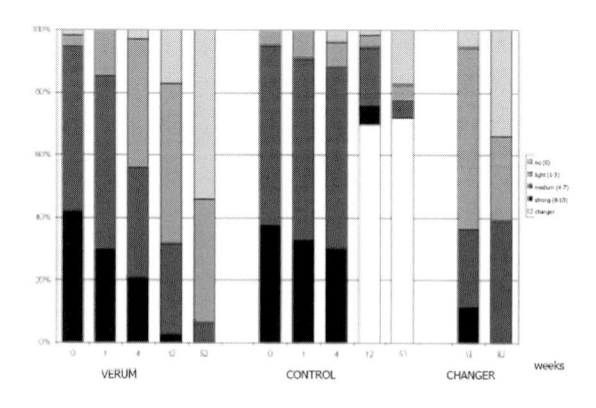

Figure 2. Local pain (Visual analog Scale).

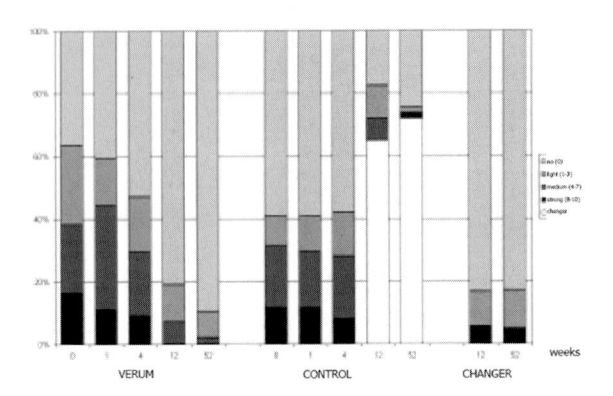

Figure 3. Night pain (Visual analog Scale).

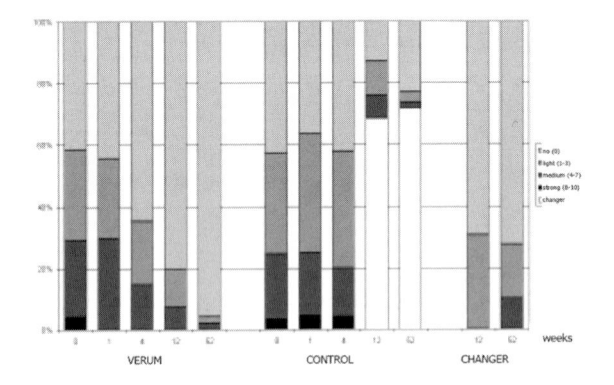

Figure 4. Pain at rest (Visual analog Scale).

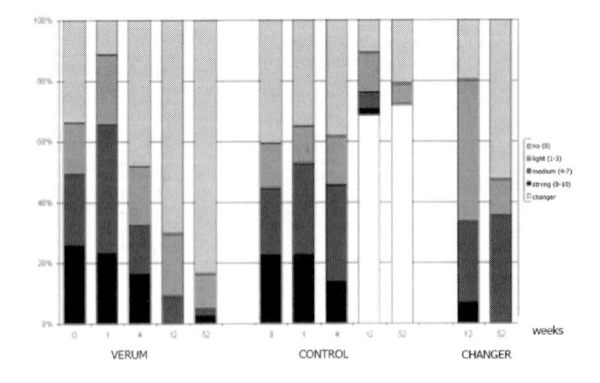

Figure 5. Pain during exercise (Visual analog Scale).

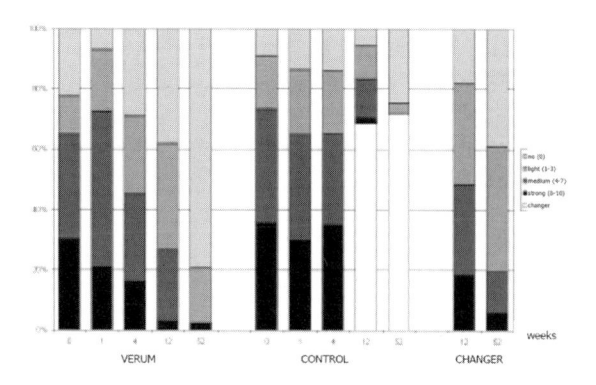

Figure 6. Thomsen-Test (Visual analog Scale).

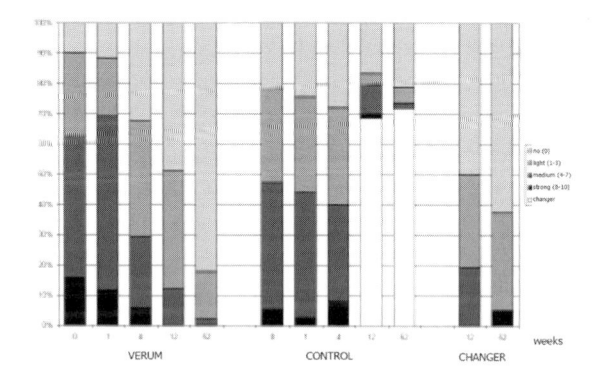

Figure 7. Midfinger-Test (Visual analog Scale).

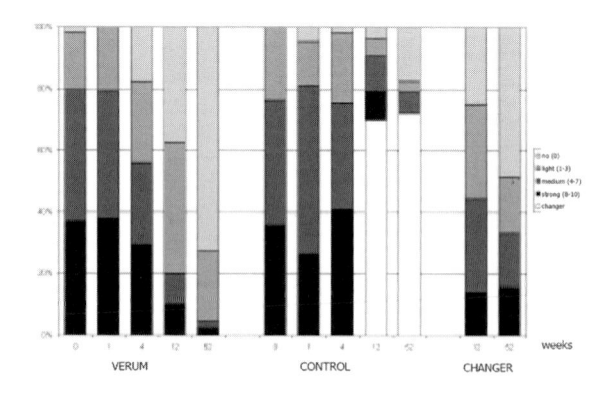

Figure 8. Chair-Test (Visual analog Scale).

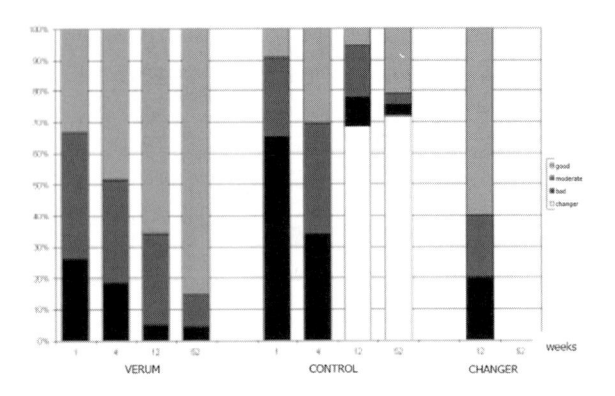

Figure 9. Subjective outcome.

Figure 10 shows the percentage of treatment recommendation by patients. 81% of all verum patients (primary verum and changers) would like to repeat the treatment after 52 weeks if the same pain would occur. Significant symptoms were reported to limit a variety of activities (Figures 11-13). The limitations decreased over time.

Only patients with these symptoms were included in the following evaluation. The analysis showed the percentage of patients who still suffered

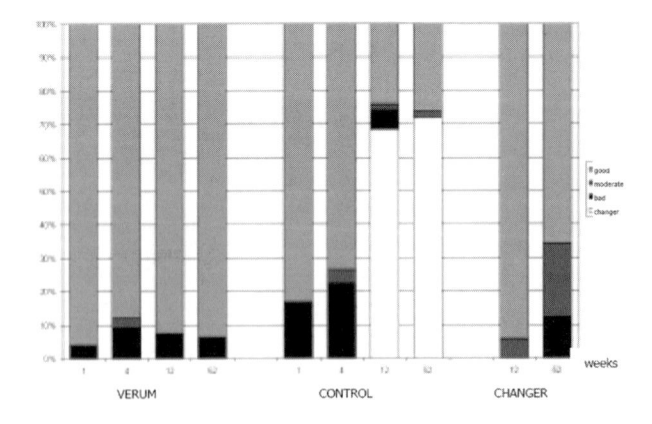

Figure 10. Patients recommendation for ESWT.

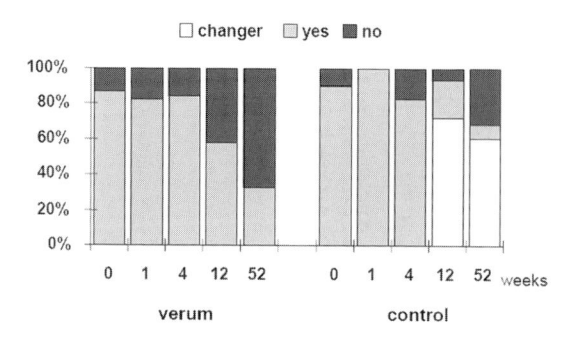

Figure 11. Limitation during sports (Percentage value of the original patients with this symptom).

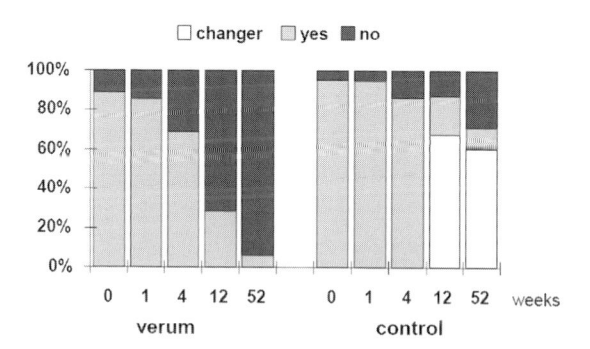

Figure 12. Limitation in daily life (Percentage value of the original patients with this symptom).

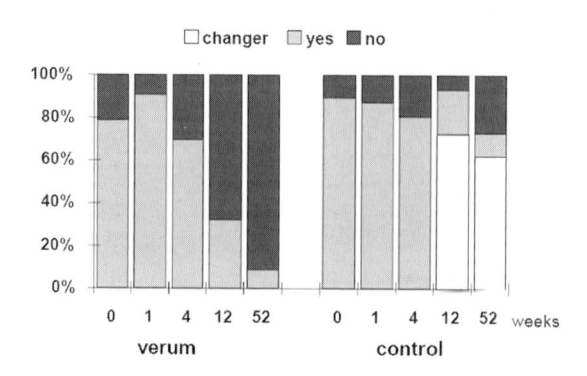

Figure 13. Restriction in occupation (Percentage of patients with this symptom).

from symptoms. After 12 weeks 64% of control patients had switched to verum treatment and 70% within 52 weeks because of persistent symptoms. That indicates a significant selection of control patients at this point in time, which resulted in biasing the overall study results.

Discussion

Dahmen was the first to treat soft tissue pain near bones with extracorporeal shockwaves[1]. Until December 1994 he treated 512 patients who received a total of 4892 shockwave treatments. Two hundred and eighty-nine of these patients had a minimum follow-up period of 6 months (average 12.1 months). Overall, a large variety of patients with 30 different syndromes were enrolled in this uncontrolled study. Of the patients, 52% had good results and 28% found an improvement. Only 3% of patients had surgery[2].

Haist reported 812 patients with enthesiopathies who received an average of 2.2 shockwave treatments with a Siemens Lithostar Overhead Module. Five hundred and twenty-five patients suffered from radial epicondylitis, 87 from ulnar epicondylitis and 113 patients were enrolled suffereing from periarthopathy humeroscalpularis. Of these patients, 76.5% had a follow-up of at least 3 months. Of patients with epicondylitis, 76.1% reported very good or good results whereas only 7.1% did not obtain a satisfactory condition[12].

In another study, Rompe treated 150 patients with epicondylitis after unsuccessful conservative therapy of at least 3 months, although the average conservative therapy was 15 months. On average, 5 conservative therapy attempts were conducted. As an example, 92% of patients had received steroid injections. A 3-week treatment period preceded shockwave therapy. Patients were enrolled only if surgery was indicated. An Osteostar was used to apply 1000 shockwaves 3 times at weekly intervals with an energy density of 0.06 mJ/mm^2. All 5 selected parameters (e.g. night pain, pain with or without activity) showed significant improvements. Forty-eight patients showed very good and 51% good results. Only 24 patients achieved no improvement. Fifteen of them were operated. In summary, a success rate of 84% was achieved in a patient group where, without shockwave therapy, operative therapy would have been performed[13].

With higher energies, the Ossatron achieved success in 8 of 10 patients with epicondylitis (n=10). Here the average conservative treatment rate was significantly lower at 1.3; no more than 3 treatments were performed[14]. Diesch obtained similar results in 80 patients with epicondylitis (success rate 68%)[3]. Using the same equipment, Richter, however, considered 6-month results as disappointing[4]. Schleberger, however, preferred the ultrasound-controlled MPL 9000 for shoulder treatments while he used the MFL 5000 for epicondylitis[5].

In summary, the studies mentioned above report success rates like those in this study. However, the generation of shockwaves is different: all studies mentioned above have used shockwave units emitting focused shockwaves. Radial shockwaves as used for this study obtained identical success rates but required fewer equipment resources.

Literature

1. Dahmen, G.P., et al., Extrakorporale Stosswellentherapie (ESWT) im knochennahen Weichteilbereich an der Schulter. Extracta Orthopaedica, 1992. 11: p. 25-27.
2. Dahmen, G.P., et al., Die Behandlung knochennaher Weichteilschmerzen mit Extrakorporaler Stosswellentherapie (ESWT), Indikation, Technik und bisherige Ergebnisse, in Die Stosswelle - Forschung und Klinik, C. Chaussy, et al., Editors. 1995, Attempto Verlag: Tübingen. p. 175-186.
3. Diesch, R., Persönliche Mitteilung. 1996.
4. Richter, D., A. Ekkernkamp, and G. Muhr, Die extrakorporale Stosswellentherapie - ein alternatives Konzept zur Behandlung der Epicondylitis humeri radialis. Orthopäde, 1995. 24: p. 303-306.
5. Schleberger, R., Anwendung der extrakorporalen Stosswelle am Stütz- und Bewegungsapparat im mittelenergetischen Bereich, in Die Stosswelle - Forschung und Klinik, C. Chaussy, et al., Editors. 1995, Attempto Verlag: Tübingen. p. 166-174.
6. Runge F: Zur Genese und Behandlung des Schreibkrampfes. Berliner Klinische Wschr. 1873: 10: 245
7. Morris H.: Riders sprain. Lancet 1882 2, 557
8. Allander E.: Prevalence, incidence, and remission rates of some common rheumatic diseases or syndromes. Scand. J Rheumatol. 1974 3:145
9. Verhaar J.A.: Tennis elbow. Anatomical, epidemiological and therapeutic aspects. Int. Othopaedics 1994 18:263
10. O'Dwyer K.J., Howie C.R.: Medial epicondylitis of the elbow. Int. Orthop. 1995 19:69
11. Haupt G., Menne A., Schulze M.: Medizinisches Instrument zur Behandlung von biologischem Gewebe. Patent Nr. 197 25 477 angemeldet am 17.06.1997 (1999)
12. Haist, J.: Die Osteorestauration via Stosswellenanwendung. Eine neue Möglichkeit zur Therapie der gestörten knöchernen Konsolidierung. In: Chaussy, C., F. Eisenberger, D. JochamD. Wilbert (Hrsg.): Die Stosswelle - Forschung und Klinik, Attempto Verlag, Tübingen (1995) 157-161.

13. *Rompe, J.D., C. Hopf, P. Eysel, J. Heine, U. Witzsch, B. Nafe*: Extrakorporale Stosswellentherapie des therapieresistenten Tennisellenbogens - Erste Ergebnisse von 150 Patienten. In: Die Stosswelle - Forschung und Klinik. (2. Konsensus Workshop der deutschen Gesellschaft für Stoßwellenlithotripsie vom 26. – 28.01.95). Ed. Christian Chaussy et al. Attempto-Verlag, Tübingen (1995) 147 – 152.

14. Haupt, G., P. Katzmeier: Anwendung der hochenergetischen extrakorporalen Stosswellentherapie bei Pseudarthrosen, Calcific tendinitis der Schulter und Ansatztendinosen (Fersensporn, Epicondylitis). In: Chaussy, C., F. Eisenberger, D. JochamD. Wilbert (Hrsg.): Die Stoßwelle - Forschung und Klinik, Attempto Verlag, Tübingen (1995) 143-146.

Efficiency of rESWT for Calcifying Shoulder Tendinitis

G. Gremion, A. Farron, P.F. Leyvraz

Introduction

The calcium hydroxyapatite crystal deposit disease, better known as calcific tendonitis of the shoulder, is characterized by the periarticular presence of basic calcium phosphate crystals. A variety of names were used in the same manner: peritendonitis calcarea, calcific periarthritis, periarticular calcification, Duplay's disease. In this report, the term calcifying tendonitis will be used when referring to calcium hydroxyapatite crystal deposit disease.

According to Wefling, the radiological incidence of calcium hydroxyapatite crystal deposit disease varies from 2.7% to 20% of asymptomatic shoulders. With regard to the shoulder rotator cuff muscles, several authors agree that the incidence of calcifying tendonitis is greatest in the supraspinatus tendon although there are some cases of several concomitant tendon injuries[2, 3, 4]. The deposits occur most frequently in the fourth and fifth decades. In most reports, women and those in sedentary professions seem to be more inclined[1, 3, 5].

Pathogenic aspect

The etiology of calcifying tendonitis is unclear. Some authors have attributed the etiology of calcifying tendonitis to a degenerative sickness associated with age and repeated tendon trauma leading to degeneration and collagen fiber necrosis, followed by calcification[6,7]. Several pathogenic explanations have been put forward depending on the progress phase of the affection[5].

As described by Gerdesmeyer and Magosch previously the natural course of the desease is divided into different phases: Pre-calcification phase, calcification phase, resorption phase and post-calcification phase[9].

Less than one person out of two suffering from radiologically visible rotator cuff calcification will present a symptomatic shoulder. If calcific tendonitis runs its course, chronic pain is variable in intensity and the patient is able to refer to the maximum pain spot which is usually located in front of the humeral head. The pain often radiates to the insertion of the muscle deltoid but also towards the arm and neck. It is often found to increase at night especially when the patient likes to sleep on the effected side. Clinically, a painful arch is found located between 70 and 110° of abduction. The pain symptomatology lasts for several months.

The acute pain within the resorption phase is characterized by severe pain, disability and, frequently, nocturnal discomfort. These symptoms normally disappear within a short time[10]. The therapy at this point has to be pain management only. Neither ESWT nor surgery is indicated anymore.

However in some cases, the natural cyclic course stops at the calcific stage for a year or more and chronic pain, slight or moderate, can remain during the phase. If pain becomes clinicically relevant, ESWT and surgery are indicated.

Therapeutic aspect

It is the progress of the disease that will dictate the treatment. During the formation phase, anti-inflammatory treatment is often combined with physiotherapy. A steroid/anesthesic injection is indicted if pain becomes severe as well as if pain occurs during the acute phase. Radio-guided percutaneous needle aspiration combined with lavage is used[11]. Arthroscopy is offered exceptionally, when pain resists conservative treatment option[12]. Extracorporal shockwave therapy (ESWT) should be indicated if pain becomes chronic and non-surgical options fail[13,14,15]. High-energy shockwaves are expected to exert a direct mechanically disintegrating effect on acoustic borderlines found around the calcific deposit. Low-energy extracorporal shockwave therapy is considered as a form of hyperstimulation analsegia. In this trial we have studied both energy alternatives in patients with chronic shoulder calcifying tendonitis.

Material and Methods

120 patients suffering from chronic shoulder calcifying tendonitis of the supraspinatus for at least 6 months were enrolled prospectively. Written informed consent was done prior to treatment. Conservative therapeutical options must have failed if patients were enrolled (cold, proprioception stretching, ultrasound and cortisone deposit infiltration, physiotherapy). Calcifying tendonitis was proven by standardized radiographs of the shoulder in anterioposterior (AP) view and AP internal-external rotation. The calcaneous deposits had to be at least 5 mm in diameter.

Patients suffereing from chronic/subacute pain as described by De Palma [16] were selected. The patients were assigned to two groups.

Group 1 consisted of 48 patients (33 women, 15 men), with a mean age of 42.2 years (+/- 8), and with duration of the pain at 6.4 months (+/- 5).

Group 2 comprised 72 patients (45 women, 27 men) with a mean age of 47.3 years (+/- 12), and with duration of the pain at 8.2 months (+/- 4).

The primary criteria chosen were: pain during rest quantified on the visual analogic scale (0-10), pain at night, pain during activities of daily living (ADL) and overall satisfaction expressed on a 0-10 scale. The assessment was done at baseline prior intervention and directly after the treatment and 6 months after last ESWT.

In group 1 the treatment was conducted using a the Sonocur® system. This machine provides high-energetic shockwaves adjustable in 8 levels from 0.04 mJ/mm^2 to 0.05 mJ/mm^2. In group 2 patients were treated by the Swiss Dolor-Clast® mashine which provides low energetic shockwaves between 0.02 mJ/mm^2 and 0.16 mJ/mm^2 energy flux density and a penetration depth of up to 30 mm.

Based on the manufacturer's instructions, we applied one 500 impulse session at a frequency of 2 Hz and weekly intervals in group 1.

The patients treated with the Swiss DolorClast® received 2000 impulses with a 4 Hz frequency at weekly intervals. In both cases the shockwave intensity was adjusted to the patient's tolerance.

High energy ESWT	Low energy ESWT
• Patients: 48 • Age: 42.2 +/- 8 • Duration: 6.4 +/-5 • 15 Male • 33 Female • Treatments: 4	• Patients: 72 • Age: 47.3 +/- 12 • Duration: 8.25 +/- 4 • 27 Male • 45 Female • Treatments: 4.8 +/-

Table 1. Clinical data for patients.

The statistical assessment was made in the form of an average and typical difference by analyzing the parametric data following the intra-group trend by variance analysis. The significance level was defined at 0.05.

Results

The clinical data of our patients are summarised in Table 1. At the beginning of the study, all 120 patients rated the condition of their shoulder as poor. Twenty-four weeks after ESWT application, 39% of the patients in group 1 and 34% in group 2 were documented as pain free and 35% in each group related an improvement of more than 75%. The results were found slightly better in group 1 compared to group 2 (Table 2).

The intensity of pain at baseline was 5.8 +/- 1.7 in group 1 and 5.5 +/- 1.4 in group 2 before treatment. Twenty-four weeks after treatment, the pain score was 1.9 +/- 0.6 in group 1 and 2.1 +/- 0.5 in group 2 (Table 3).

	Failure	< 50% better	< 75% better	100% pain free	Good results
Group 1 (48)	14.5%	11.3%	34.8%	39.4%	74.2%
Group 2 (72)	15.2%	20.1%	29.9%	34.8%	64.7%

Table 2. Subjective assessment of treatment success at 24 weeks after ESWT.

VAS Scale (1-10)

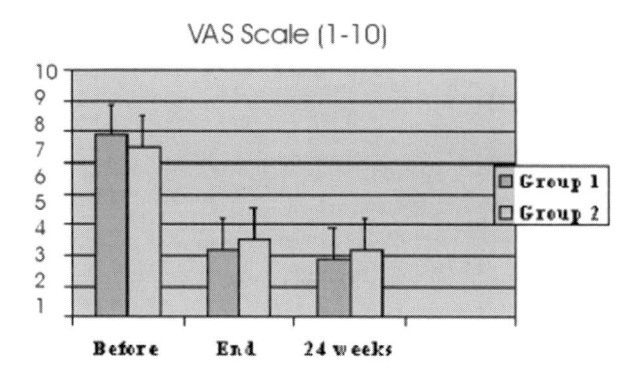

Table 3. Pain results measured on the visual analog scale at the end and 24 weeks after ESWT. Compared to baseline the table shows a significant pain reduction but non significant difference was found between both groups.

Seven patients in group 1 and 11 patients in group 2 did not respond to the treatment. Later on they underwent either a percutaneous needling or an arthroscopic surgery.

The score for discomfort in ADL at baseline was 3.5 +/- 1.3 for group 1 and 3.6 +/- 1.2 for group 2. After 6 months the scores were 1.1 +/- 0.4 and 1.0 +/- 0.5 respectively. (Table 4).

Function ability dissatisfaction

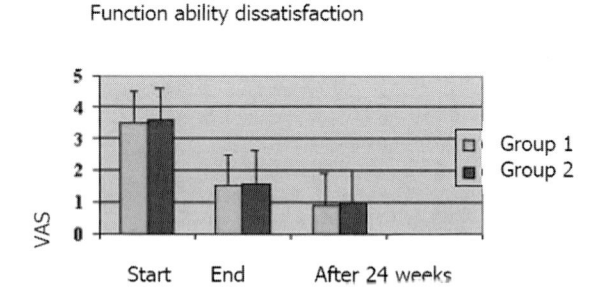

Table 4. Dissatisfaction with functional ability in daily life on VAS-scale before treatment, after treatment and 24 weeks after treatment with ESWT. The table is showing a significant improvement of activity in daily life and life quality.

Discussion

Chronic calcifying shoulder tendonitis treatments have not been standardized today and the correlation between pain and calcific deposit is not defined. Conservative treatment options are mostly polypragmatic. The intralesional cortisone injections are efficient within a short treatment interval but evidence is still lacking on long term observations. Reported success rates vary between 30% and 85% depending on author as well as treatment modality. A review of conservative treatment methods is not published but a few single excellent studies have shown some evidence regarding ESWT as well as short time effects after cortisone and physiotherapy.

The application of extracorporeal shockwaves is used in urology to treat kidney, urinary and biliary tract concrements. The technique used by orthopedists was introduced by Valchanou and Michailov in 1991 to treat non-union or delay-of-union in fractures[17]. In two separate studies, Loew et al. [13] reported satisfactory results after using high-energetic shockwaves in calcific tendonitis of the shoulder. After 12 weeks of follow-up, 75% of the patients showed a significant reduction in symptoms and pain. The functional outcome was scored by using the Constant Score and 30% improvement was found. Rompe et al. [14] reported a series of 40 patients with calcific tendonitis of the shoulder. They found increasing values on the Constant Scores up to 77 points compared to the baseline of 48 points. Their study had a 62% rate of partial or complete disintegration of calcareous deposits. Brunner et al. reported on 67 patients after ESWT. Again an improvement of 80% was found[18].

The current study has compared the effects of low-energy ESWT with high-energy shockwaves. Patients treated with high-energy shockwaves (group 1) had better results than patients treated with low-energy shockwaves (group 2). However, low-energy ESWT was successful in about 65% of the patients and no anesthesics were used. The application of low-energy extracorporeal shockwaves was easy to perfom and pain was reduced significantly after the 3rd intervention.

We found no clinically relevant side effects but we did find some minor petechial bleedings or bruising after high-energetic ESWT. These data corroborate published data[19].

One reason to explain the better results of high-energetic ESWT was that the application is ultrasound controlled. In contrast to the DolorClast® system, whose guidance is based on patient feedback, ultrasound guidance was used.

Additionally, focused high-energetic shockwaves are known for better penetration as necessary in calcific tendonitis of the shoulder.

Literature

1. Welfing I, Kahn MF, Desroy M, Paolaggi JP, De Sèze S: La maladie des calcifications tendineuses multiples. Rev Rhum, 32 : 325 – 334, 1965.
2. Ark JW, Flock TJ, Flatow EL, Bigliani LU: Arthroscopic treatment of calcific tendonitis of the shoulder. Arthroscopy 8 (2): 183 – 188, 1992.
3. De Palma AF, Kruper JS: Long-term study of shoulder joints afflicted with and treated calcific tendonitis. Clin Orthop 20: 61 – 72, 1972.
4. Hayes CW, Conway WF: Calcium hydroxyapatite deposition disease. Radiographics 10 (6): 1031 – 1048, 1990.
5. Uthoff HK, Sarkar K: Calcifying tendonitis. Baillières Clinical Rheumatology 3: 567 – 581, 1989.
6. Herherts P, Kadefors R, Hoyfors C, Sigholm G : Shoulder Pain and manual labor. Clin Orthop 191: 166 – 178, 1984.
7. Olsson O: Degenerative changes of the shoulder and their connection with shoulder pain. Acta Chirurgica Scandinavia, suppl 181 : 1 – 110, 1953.
8. Sengar DPS, Mc Kendry RJ, Uthoff HK : Increased frequency of HLAA A1 in calcifying tendinitis. Tissues antigens, 29: 173 – 174, 1987.
9. Gärtner J, Simons B: Analysis of calcific deposits in calcifying tendonitis. Clin Orthop. 254: 111 – 120, 1990.
10. Mc Laughlin HL: The selection of calcium deposit for operation: The technique and results of operation. Surg Clinic North Am 43 (6): 1501 – 1504, 1963.
11. Pfister J, Gerber H: Chronic calcifyinf tendonitis of the shoulder-therapy by percutaneous needle aspiration and lavage: A prospective open study of 62 shoulders. Clinical Rheumatology, 16 (3): 269 – 274, 1997
12. Jerosch J, Strauss JM, Schmiel S: Arthroscopic treatment of calcufic tendonitis of the shoulder. J Shoulder Elbow Surg. 7 (1): 30 – 37, 1998.
13. Loew M, Jugorwski W; Mau HC, Thomsen M: Treatment of calcifying tendonitis of rotator cuff by extracorporeal shockwaves: a preliminary report. J Shoulder Elbow Surg. 4: 101 – 106, 1995
14. Rompe JD, Rumler F, Hopf C, Nafe B, Heine J: Extracorporeal shockwaves therapy for calcifying tendonitis of the shoulder. Clin Orthop. 321: 196 – 201, 1995.
15. Rompe JD, , Hopf C, Küllmer K, Heine J, Bürger R: Analgesic effects of extracorporeal shockwaves therapy on chronic tennis elbow. J Bone Joint Surg br. 78-b: 233 – 237, 1996.
16. De Palma AF : Calcareous tendinitis In : De Palma, editor. Surgery of the shoulder. Philadelphia: JB Lippincott; 277 – 285, 1985.
17. Valchanou VD, Michailov P High-energy shockwaves in the treatment of delayed and non union of fractures. Int orthop. 15: 181-184, 1991.
18. Brunner W et al : Die extrakorporelle Stosswellentherapie im Rahmen der orthopädischen Schmerztherapie: 2-Jahres-Ergebnisse in 899 Fällen. Orthopädische Praxis 35: 12, 777-780, 1990.

19. Rompe JD, Bürger R, Hopf C, Eysel P: Shoulder function after extracorporal shockwave therapy for calcific tendonitis. J Shoulder Elbow Surg. 7 (5): 505-509, 1998.
20. Gerdesmeyer L, Wagenpfeil S, Haake M, Maier M, Loew M, Wörtler K, Lampe R, Seil R, Handle G, Gassel S, Rompe JD: Extracorporeal shockwave therapy for the treatment of chronic calcifying tendonitis of the rotator cuff – a randomized controlled trial. JAMA (2003);290:2573-2580

ESWT for the Treatment of Chronic Calcifying Tendonitis of the Rotator Cuff – a Randomized Placebo Controlled Multi-Center Trial

Ludger Gerdesmeyer, MD, PhD,[1] Stefan Wagenpfeil, MD, PhD,[2] Martin Russlies, MD, PhD,[3] Markus Maier, MD, PhD,[6] Markus Loew, MD, PhD,[7] Klaus Wörtler, MD,[5] Romain Sail, MD, PhD,[5] Gerhard Handle, MD,[9] Jan D. Rompe, MD, PhD[4]

Introduction

Calcific tendonitis of the rotator cuff is a common condition presenting in a general or orthopedic practice and is a known source of shoulder pain[1]. It initially was described more than 100 years ago as Maladie de Duplay. Reports on the overall incidence vary tremendously, ranging between 2.5% and 20% [1,2,3] depending not only on the clinical criteria used but also on the radiographic technique. The disease is usually self-limiting and the natural course varies[1-5]. Gärtner followed the natural evolution over 3 years. Deposits with sharp margins and homogenous or inhomogeneous structure disappeared in 33% of the cases in contrast with 85% of the

---

[1] Dept of Orthopedic Surgery and Sportstraumatology, Technical University Munich
[2] Institute of Medical Statistics and Epidemiology, Technical University Munich
[3] Dept of Orthopedic Surgery, University of Regensburg
[4] Dept of Orthopedic Surgery, Johannes Gutenberg University School of Medicine
[5] Dept of Radiology, Technical University Munich
[6] Dept of Orthopedic Surgery, Ludwig Maximilian University Munich
[7] Dept of Orthopedic Surgery, Ruprecht-Karls-University Heidelberg
[8] Dept of Orthopedic Surgery, University of Homburg
[9] Dept of Orthopedic Surgery, University of Innsbruck
[10] Dept of Orthopedic Surgery, University of Bonn

fluffy accumulations[6]. Annually 6.4% of calcific lesions showed spontaneous resorption[1]. It is very important to distinguish whether the shoulder pain is caused only by calcific tendonitis or from a rotator cuff tear[7]. Several authors have found that there was no correlation observed between a tendon tear and calcific tendonitis[4,7-10]. The treatment of patients with calcific tendonitis typically is conservative, including subacromial cortisone injections, physical therapy and systemic NSAIDs with limited evidence of efficacy[11,12]. Ultrasonic energy has been reported to accelerate functional improvement in acute cases with calcific tendonitis, while showing no better efficacy than placebo in a long term follow-up[13].

No evaluation was done in chronic cases. If pain becomes chronic, surgical removal of the deposits has been recommended[4,14]. Open or arthroscopic surgery is regarded as a dependable and quick method to remove the deposit [15-19] and is indicated in nearly 10% of the patients with clinically relevant calcific tendonitis[20,2].

Recently, extracorporeal shockwave therapy (ESWT) has shown encouraging results in the treatment of calcified deposits[21-25]. However, all of these trials showed numerous methodical deficiencies[12].

The goal of the current study was to compare the effectiveness of high-energy and low-energy ESWT versus placebo treatment in patients with chronic, symptomatic calcific tendonitis of the supraspinatus tendon.

Patients and Methods

The study is a subject and observer-blinded, placebo-controlled, randomized, multicentric, binational trial with parallel group design consisting of three groups: high-energy ESWT, low-energy ESWT and placebo ESWT. The trial was performed between February 1997 and March 2001 and was designed according to standardized guidelines of "Good Clinical Practice" from the International Conference on Harmonization[26,27]. A total of 164 patients were screened for eligibility. One hundred forty-four subjects gave signed, informed consent to participate in the study and were treated according to the study protocol in 7 centers in Germany and Austria (Figure 1). The trial was approved by an independent institutional review board and ethical committee. Subjects were assigned to one of three groups with use of concealed randomization.

Inclusion Criteria	Exclusion Criteria
• Symptomatic calcifying tendinopathy	• Glenohumeral or acromioclavicular joint arthritis
• At least a 6-month duration of symptoms	• Previous surgery of the painful shoulder
• Must have completed to conservative treatments with at least: Physiotherapy (n:20) *and* Subacromial injections (n:2) *and* Physical therapy (n:10) *and* Systemic NSAID´s	• Rheumatic diseases/ connective tissue disease / diabetes
	• Bursitis/ infection/ tumor of the shoulder
	• Instability/ rotator cuff lesion of the shoulder
• Treatment washout period of 4 weeks	• Deposit type III (Gärtner classifcation)*
• Deposit size at least 5mm	• Abnormal peripheral neurological findings
• Deposit type I or II (Gärtner classification)*	• Pregnancy
• Signed informed consent	• Coagulation disturbance
• Age greater than 18 years	• Previous unsuccocoful ESWT

* The radiological classification of calcified tendonitis according to Gärtner [6]

Type : I   Homogeneous structure, sharp margins
        II Inhomogeneous structure, sharp margins, or homogeneous structure, no defined margins
        III Inhomogeneous structure, no defined margins

Table 1. List of the inclusion and exclusion criteria.

Subjects were made aware of the trial by reports in the press, by health insurance companies, or by orthopedic practitioners or hospitals. They were referred to one of the participating centers in Germany and Austria.

To be eligible for the trial, subjects had to have a history of at least 6 months of pain or tenderness from idiopathic calcific tendonitis, type I or II according to Gärtner [6], that was resistant to conservative treatment.

Inclusion and exclusion criteria for selecting patients are shown in Table 1.

Rotator cuff lesions and subacromial bursitis were ruled out in all patients by sonographical examination, and in doubtful cases by magnetic resonance imaging prior to randomization and at all follow ups. Gärtner type III deposits were excluded because of the well known high probability for spontaneous resolution[6]. All patients had to have completed conservative treatments with physiotherapy, including active and passive exercise, mobilization, manual therapy and massage, muscle strengthening together with pendulum exercises, subacromial local anesthetic and cortisone injections, and ultrasound or iontophoresis with an anti-inflammatory drug. For systemic anti-inflammatory therapy, all patients had to have taken NSAIDS such as acetaminophen, ibuprofen or diclophenac.

Patients with acute subacromial bursitis were excluded by clinical examination and diagnostic ultrasound which was compared to the contralateral, unaffected side.

In doubtful cases, the diagnosis was confirmed by MRI.

Randomization

Using concealed randomization, subjects were assigned to receive high energetic extracorporeal shockwave (group I), low energetic shockwave (group II) or placebo (group III) treatment. Randomization was accomplished using a computer generated fixed block scheme with permutated blocks of 48 patients each.

Treatment allocation was determined immediately before the first treatment and was provided centrally by telephone and kept in sealed opaque envelopes. Thus, the subject, the physician applying the shockwaves and the follow up evaluator were unaware of the treatment assignments.

Method of Treatment

All subjects had at least a one-month therapy-free period before the first ESWT. The ESWT was applied by a mobile therapy unit especially designed for orthopedic use (Epos Fluoro®, Dornier MedTech®, Wessling, Germany), and licensed by the European Commission. The same unit was used in all patients. Shockwave focus guidance was established by out-line fluoroscopy. Before each intervention focus, position and fluoroscopy function were verified by an engineer. The total energy flux density (ED) output was 0.32 mJ/mm² per shockwave in Group I, 0.08 mJ/mm² in Group II, and 0 mJ/mm² in Group III, based on measurements with glass-fiber hydrophones in accordance with IEC (International Electrotechnical Commission) 61846 procedures. A total of two treatments were performed with an interval of 2 weeks between each ESWT. All patients were treated on an outpatient basis by orthopedic surgeons who have significant experience using ESWT. The first treatments were done under instruction by the monitor. All treatment and device set ups were also controlled and monitored to be sure that the application performance was consistent and according to the study protocol in all centers.

Intervention

Active treatment. Immediately after randomization, the subject was placed in the prone position. Using fluoroscopy, in an anterior-posterior view, the shoulder was rotated until the calcific deposit was identified in a free position. Then the shockwave head was coupled to the shoulder and a coupling gel was applied to the head only in the active group. A thin polyethylene (PE) foil was placed between the shockwave head and the shoulder. Coupling gel was used at the patient and the shockwave head site.

The exact focus position was fluoroscopy controlled during the ESWT and adjusted if necessary. After the energy level was increased up to the assigned treatment level (0.32 mJ/mm^2 in Group I and 0.08 mJ/mm^2 in group II), 1,500 high-energy shockwaves were applied in Group I, and 6,000 low-energy shockwaves in Group II to reach a total energy of 0.960 J/mm^2 in both groups. One hundred twenty impulses were applied per minute. If the treatment was too painful, an adequate combination of analgesics and sedation, administered intravenously, was performed. Local anesthetics were prohibited. ESWT was repeated with an interval between treatments of 14 ± 2 days. Due to the fluoroscopy controlled technique, the varied deposit locations, the need to refocus the shockwaves and the individual pain tolerance with the necessity to give sufficient analgesics, the procedure could take up to 1 hour per treatment. Measurements with glass-fiber hydrophones in accordance with IEC 61846 procedures showed that shockwaves were unaffected by the PE-foil with ultrasound coupling gel on both sides of the foil.

Sham treatment. Subjects were blinded as to which treatment they were assigned. The set-up in all groups was identical except for an air-chambered PE-foil with coupling gel on the patient site and no coupling-gel on the shockwave head site. The air-chambered PE-foil in the placebo group (Group III) was placed between the subject and the water cushion of the ESWT device in the same technique as in the treatment groups (Groups I and II). Measurements with glass-fiber hydrophones in accordance with IEC 61846 procedures showed that no shockwave could pass through the foil. The placebo subjects received 1500 shockwaves per treatment with one hundred twenty impulses applied per minute after the energy level reached the assigned treatment level (0.32 mJ/mm²). A total energy of 0.960 J/mm² was emitted from the ESWT device but no energy could pass through the air chambered PE foil. The prone position of the subjects prevented the subjects from seeing anything from the device, but they could hear the impressive, typical sound of shockwaves being generated.

The subjects of all groups were informed that sometimes the procedure could be painful and could take up to 1 hour each due to the necessity to control and refocus the shockwaves exactly.

Concomitant therapies. Subjects of all groups underwent physiotherapy 10 times after the intervention. Physiotherapy includes active and passive exercise mobilization techniques, massage, and manual therapy to prevent worsening in range-of-motion, muscular deficit or imbalance.

Rescue medication was allowed if pain became "unbearable" throughout the entire study: Up to 14 days following the last treatment, 2g Paracetamol/day (Ben-u-ron®) or 2g Acetaminophen/day (Tylenol®) and up to 2g Paracetamol/week or 2g Acetaminophen/week later than 2 weeks after ESWT. No other therapies (e.g. chiropractic, laser, acupuncture, ultrasound, other NSAIDs or corticosteroids) were allowed until the 6-month follow-up.

Primary outcome measure. The primary endpoint was defined as the increase from baseline to six months post-treatment in the Constant-Murley Score (CMS), a widely used shoulder score[28]. The 6 month analysis were pre-specified in the study protocol. The other results were pre-specified as secondary outcome measures to provide further information.

The CMS is a standardized simple clinical method of shoulder functional assessment and has a maximum score of 100 points with both subjective (35 points) and objective (65 points) components. The score has a low systematic inter– and intraobserver error in patients suffering from shoulder pain. The subjective parameters assess the degree of pain perception (15 points) and the ability to perform the normal tasks of daily living in both activity and position-related terms (20 points). The objective parameters include testing of active range of motion (40 points) and shoulder power (25 points). All blinded observers who assessed the CMS were experienced and used a goniometer to evaluate the active forward and lateral elevation and body land marks, reached by the patient, to assess the internal/external rotation. The power in abduction was measured using a spring balance.

The 6-month interval was selected because it was expected that the healing process would likely be evident (although not necessarily complete) at this point. Clinically relevant improvement was defined as a 30% increase from baseline. Patients who needed additional therapies, except the allowed amount of rescue medication and physiotherapy, were defined as failing treatment.

Secondary outcome measure. Secondary endpoints were defined as a reduction from baseline at all points of evaluation post-treatment on a visual analog scale (VAS, 0 points = no pain; 10 points = unbearable pain) for daily pain.

The presence of the calcified deposit was assessed by conventional x-rays. The technique used was standardized in terms of position of the shoulder and arm, distance from the x-ray film and exposure. The localization of calcifications within a specific tendon was determined by anteriorposterior radiographs of the shoulder obtained in 45° external and 45° internal rotation[30]. These two standard anterior-posterior (AP) views were obtained within 14 days before intervention (to exclude spontaneous healing before treatment), at three months, six months and 12 months post treatment and analyzed by an independent skeletal radiologist without knowledge of the type of treatment. Success was defined as complete dissolution of the deposit.

Side effects and adverse reactions were recorded on standardized written forms.

Statistics

Changes in CMS, VAS and deposit size were defined as the difference between the 3-month, 6-month and 12-month measurement and respective baseline values. These absolute changes were the variables of primary interest and analysis.

All analysis was performed with SPSS for Windows statistical software[31]. Computed p-values are two-sided and subject to a 5% significance level. For group comparisons of changes we used the t-test for independent samples or Welch-test, where appropriate. Quantitative values are given as a mean with 95% confidence intervals (CI). Qualitative values are presented as percentages. To adjust for multiplicity, the Bonferroni-Holm procedure was performed. Study examination was carried out according to the principle of intention-to-treat. Missing values in the analysis were replaced by the technique of 'Last Observation Carried Forward' (LOCF). Leaving missing values and analyzing the reduced data set only marginally changed the results. Significance, however, was unaffected.

For the secondary end-points and explorative analysis, descriptive statistics with a 95% confidence interval were calculated, without adjusting for multiplicity.

The success rate was determined as an improvement of >15% better than placebo. The sample size calculation was performed with nQuery Version 2.0, $\alpha=$ 0.025 two sided significance level, $\beta=$ 10% (power = 90%). To prove the efficacy of ESWT it was necessary to enroll 144 patients in the study, including an expected drop-out rate of 10%. To detect selection bias we used the method according to Berger and Exner[32].

Results

A total of 144 patients (48 per group) were treated as randomized according to the study protocol. The required number of pulses per treatment was achieved in all cases. Only 11 patients were lost to follow-up (7.6%) prior to the six months endpoint. (Figure 1).

The mean age of patients at time of randomization was 49.7 ± 11.0 years. The average clinically relevant pain history was 42.2 ± 25.8 months. Relative to the main criteria, the mean CMS was 62.3 ± 12.8, pain sensation on the VAS was 6.0 ± 1.6 and the size of the deposit at baseline was 168.7 ± 144.6 mm2. The epidemiological baseline data are displayed in Table 3. No statistical differences in baseline data of primary or secondary efficacy data or epidemiological data were found in the three analyzed study groups by using the 0.49 from the Kruskal-Wallis test (p =0.49) (Table 4). No selection bias could be detected according to the method of Berger and Exner[32]. Alternative evaluation with the permutation test yielded comparable results. Significance did not change.

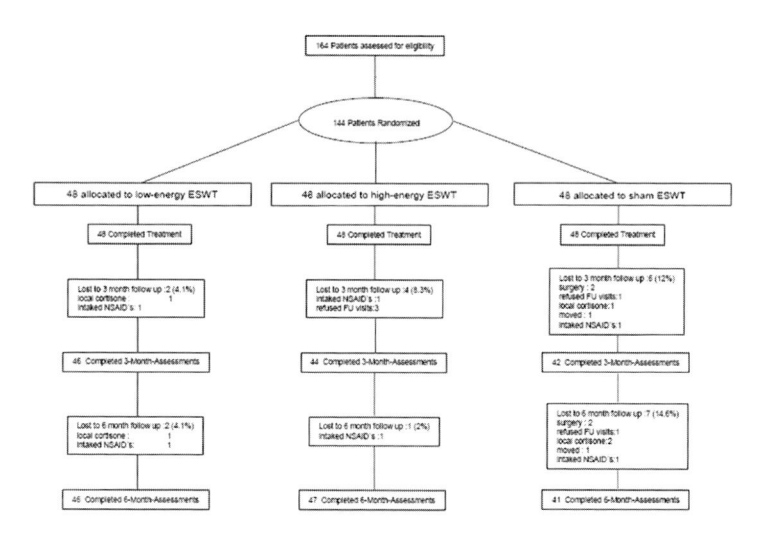

Figure 1. Flow of participants through the trial.

Primary outcome measure. The mean Constant-Murley Score of patients in Group I (35 female/13 male, mean age 42.6 ± 8.5 years, 28 right-handed, 20 left-handed, mean duration 42.6 ± 23.2 months) was 60.2 ± 11.4 points at baseline, 91.4 ± 9.4 points at six months and 91.8 ± 10.0 points at 12 months (Table 2a). The improvement was significant and rated clinically relevant as defined above (> 30%).

The mean score of patients in Group II (32 female/16 male, mean age 47.3 ± 8.5 years, 28 right-handed, 20 left-handed, mean duration 42.8 ± 25.2 months) was 62.7 ± 14.0 points at baseline, 77.4 ± 16.5 points at six months and 80.1 ± 16.1 points at 12 months, but improvement did not reach clinical relevance. (Table 2b).

The average score in Group III (28 female/20 male, mean age 52.3 ± 9.8 years, 27 right-handed, 21 left-handed, mean duration 41.3 ± 28.6 months) was 64.2 ± 12.8 points at baseline, 70.8 ± 14.4 points at six months and 77.9 ±14.9 points at 12 months (Tables 2a, 2b).

The different parts of the score (pain, activity of daily living, range of motion and power) showed the same changes after shockwave therapy in all groups. Detailed results of the subjective and objective parts of the score are given in Tables 2a and 2b.

	3 Months			
	Mean [95% CI] Change			
Outcome measure	Group I High energy n:44	Group III Placebo n:42	Between-Group Difference (95% CI)	P Value
Constant-Murley Score [0-100]	26.2 [22.3 to 30.2]	9.8 [5.1 to 14.5]	-16.4 (-22.5 to -10.3)	<.001
30% improvement	0.77 [0.62 to 0.89]	0.21 [0.10 to 0.37]		<.001
Pain	7.2 [6.0 to 8.4]	2.4 [1.1 to 3.7]	4.8 [3 to 6.6]	<.001
ADL	6.5 [5.1 to 7.8]	1.9 [0.7 to 3.2]	4.5 [2.7 to 6.3]	<.001
ROM	7.5 [5.7 to 9.3]	3.3 [1.1 to 5.4]	4.3 [1.5 to 7]	.004
Power	5.1 [3.8 to 6.3]	1.9 [0.7 to 3.1]	3.2 [1.5 to 4.9]	<.001
Pain (VAS) [0-10]	-5.0 [-5.7 to -4.2]	-1.8 [-2.5 to -1.1]	3.2 (2.2 to 4.2)	<.001
Size (mm²)	-128.9 [-170 to -87.7]	-30.3 [-53.7 to -7.0]	98.6 (51.8 to 145.4)	<.001

	6 Months			
	Mean [95% CI] Change			
Outcome measure	Group I High energy n:46	Group III Placebo n:41	Between-Group Difference (95% CI)	P Value
Constant-Murley Score [0-100]	31.0 [26.7 to 35.3]	6.6 [1.4 to 11.8]	-24.4 (-31.0 to -17.8)	<.001
30% improvement	0.89 [0.77 to 0.96]	0.17 [0.07 to 0.32]		<.001
Pain	8.7 [7.6 to 9.8]	1.1 [-0.2 to 2.5]	7.6 [5.9 to 9.3]	<.001
ADL	7.5 [6.5 to 8.5]	0.3 [-1.0 to 1.6]	7.2 [5.6 to 8.8]	<.001
ROM	10.2 [8.6 to 11.9]	1.4 [-0.9 to 3.7]	8.8 [6 to 11.6]	<.001

	6 Months			
	Mean [95% CI] Change			
Power	5.9 [4.7 to 7.1]	1.1 [-0.2 to 2.4]	4.8 [3.1 to 6.6]	<.001
Pain (VAS) [0-10]	-5.5 [-6.2 to -4.8]	-1.1 [-1.8 to -0.5]	3.7 (2.7 to 4.7)	<.001
Size (mm^2)	-152.8 [-195 to -110]	-41.0 [-66.0 to -16.1]	111.8 (63.2 to 160.5)	<.001

	12 Months			
	Mean [95% CI] Change			
Outcome measure	Group I High energy n:35	Group III Placebo n:32	Between-Group Difference (95% CI)	P Value
Constant-Murley Score [0-100]	31.6 [27.3 to 36.0]	13.7 [8.4 to 19.0]	-17.9 (-24.7 to -11.1)	<.001
30% improvement	0.94 [0.81 to 0.99]	0.22 [0.09 to 0.40]		<.001
Pain	10.0 [9.4 to 10.6]	4.4 [2.9 to 5.9]	5.6 [4 to 7.2]	<.001
ADL	7.9 [7.1 to 8.7]	3.1 [1.8 to 4.4]	4.8 [3.3 to 6.4]	<.001
ROM	11.7 [9.9 to 13.5]	4.3 [2.3 to 6.2]	7.4 [4.8 to 10.1]	<.001
Power	6.3 [5 to 7.6]	2.8 [1.1 to 4.4]	3.5 [1.5 to 5.6]	0.001
Pain (VAS) [0-10]	-5.6 [-6.3 to -4.9]	-1.9 [-2.7 to -1.2]	3.7 (2.7 to 4.7)	<.001
Size (mm^2)	-162.2 [-204 to -120]	-46.8 [-74.3 to -19.3]	115.4 (65.4 to 165.4)	<.001

Table 2a. Mean changes in outcome measures after high-energetic shockwave therapy from baseline at three, six and 12 months. ESWT indicates extracorporeal shockwave therapy; SD, standard deviation; CI, confidence interval.

3 Months

Outcome measure	Group II Low energy n:46	Group III Placebo n:42	Between-Group Difference (95% CI)	P Value
Mean [95% CI] Change				
Constant-Murley Score [0-100]	16.6 [11.8 to 21.0]	9.8 [5.1 to 14.5]	-6.6 (-13.1 to -0.1)	.047
30% improvement	0.40 [0.26 to 0.55]	0.21 [0.10 to 0.37]		0.07
Pain	3.7 [2.5 to 5.0]	2.4 [1.1 to 3.8]	1.3 [-0.5 to 3.2]	0.148
ADL	3.9 [2.7 to 5.1]	1.9 [0.7 to 3.2]	2 [0.2 to 3.7]	0.028
ROM	5.5 [3.7 to 7.4]	3.3 [1.1 to 5.4]	2.3 [-0.6 to 5.1]	0.119
Power	3.2 [2.1 to 4.3]	1.9 [0.7 to 3.1]	1.4 [-0.3 to 3]	0.106
Pain (VAS) [0-10]	-2.7 [-3.3 to -2.1]	-1.8 [-2.5 to -1.1]	0.9 (0.0 to 1.8)	.060
Size (mm²)	-56.3 [-106.7 to -5.8]	-30.3 [-53.7 to -7.0]	26.0 (-29.1 to 81.1)	.350

6 Months

Outcome measure	Group II Low energy n:46	Group III Placebo n:41	Between-Group Difference (95% CI)	P Value
Mean [95% CI] Change				
Constant-Murley Score [0-100]	15.0 [10.2 to 19.8]	6.6 [1.4 to 11.8]	-8.4 (-15.4 to -1.4)	<.001
30% improvement	0.41 [0.27 to 0.57]	0.17 [0.07 to 0.32]		0.02
Pain	3.7 [2.5 to 4.9]	1.1 [-0.2 to 2.5]	2.6 [0.8 to 4.4]	0.006
ADL	3.0 [1.8 to 4.3]	0.3 [-1.0 to 1.6]	2.8 [1 to 4.6]	0.003
ROM	5.3 [3.4 to 7.1]	1.4 [-0.9 to 3.7]	3.9 [0.9 to 6.8]	0.012

6 Months

Outcome measure	Group II Low energy n:46	Group III Placebo n:41	Between-Group Difference (95% CI)	P Value
Power	3.2 [2.0 to 4.5]	1.1 [-0.2 to 2.4]	2.2 [0.4 to 4]	0.021
Pain (VAS) [0-10]	-2.4 [-3.1 to -1.7]	-1.1 [-1.8 to -0.5]	1.3 (0.4 to 2.2)	.008
Size (mm²)	-77.7 [-130 to -24.9]	-41.0 [-66.0 to -16.1]	36.7 (-21.2 to 94.6)	.210

12 Months

Mean [95% CI] Change

Outcome measure	Group II Low energy n:44	Group III Placebo n:32	Between-Group Difference (95% CI)	P Value
Constant-Murley Score [0-100]	17.7 [13.2 to 22.3]	13.7 [8.4 to 19.0]	-4.1 (-11.0 to 2.8)	.241
30% improvement	0.45 [0.30 to 0.61]	0.22 [0.09 to 0.40]		0.05
Pain	4.2 [3.1 to 5.3]	4.4 [2.9 to 5.9]	-0.2 [-2 to 1.7]	0.859
ADL	3.5 [2.2 to 4.7]	3.1 [1.8 to 4.4]	0.4 [-1.4 to 2.2]	0.681
ROM	6.6 [4.7 to 8.6]	4.3 [2.3 to 6.2]	2.4 [-0.4 to 5.1]	0.093
Power	3.6 [2.3 to 4.8]	2.8 [1.1 to 4.4]	0.8 [-1.2 to 2.9]	0.422
Pain (VAS) [0-10]	-2.6 [-3.2 to -1.9]	-1.9 [-2.7 to -1.2]	0.7 (-0.3 to 1.7)	.179
Size (mm²)	-91.5 [-148 to -35.1]	46.0 [-74.3 to -19.3]	44.7 (-17.6 to 107.0)	.157

Table 2b. Mean changes in outcome measures after low-energetic shockwave therapy from baseline at three, six and 12 months. ESWT indicates extracorporeal shockwave therapy; SD, standard deviation; CI, confidence interval.

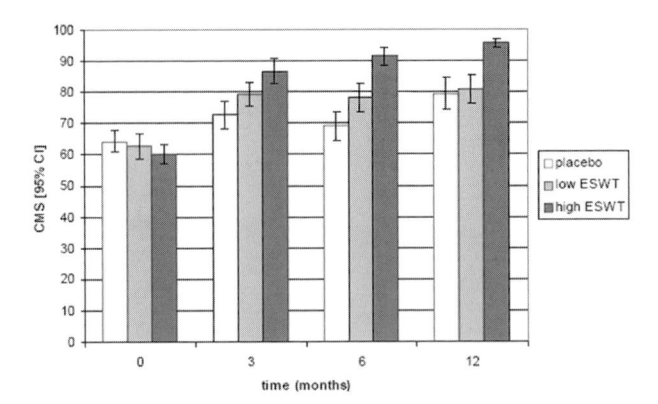

Figure 2. Absolute mean change of CMS measurements from baseline stratified according to treatment groups and time in weeks.

The outcome after high-energetic shockwave therapy was better, compared to low-energetic shockwave therapy. Significantly more patients showed more than 30% improvement ($p<0.01$) in all follow-ups (Figure 2).

<u>Secondary outcome measure.</u> Improvement of pain on the VAS developed parallel results with the CMS.

Concerning the size of the deposit, complete disappearance was observed in Group I in 60% of the patients after six months and in 86% after 12 months. In Group II complete disappearance was found in 21% and 37%, respectively. In the placebo group (Group III), spontaneous complete disappearance was observed in 11% after six months and in 25% after one year (Figure 3).

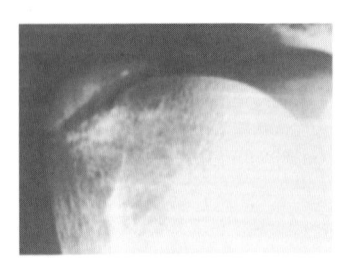

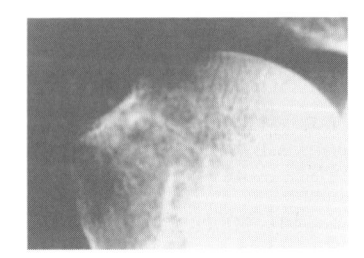

Figure 3. X-ray control of the deposit at baseline (left) and at six months post treatment (right).

	High-energy ESWT	Low-energy ESWT	Placebo ESWT
Location: SSP	42	41	43
Location: ISP	6	7	4
Location: TM	0	0	0
Location: SSC	0	0	1
Deposit classification type I	34	30	32
Deposit classification type II	14	18	16
Deposit classification type III	0	0	0
Afflicted site right	28	28	27
Afflicted site left	20	20	21
Male	13	16	28
Female	35	32	20
Age	51.6 ± 8.5	47.3 ± 8.5	52.3 ± 9.8
Pain duration (month)	42.6 ± 23.2	42.8 ± 25.2	41.3 ± 28.6
Previous surgery	0	0	0
Experience with ESWT	0	0	0
Constant Score total	60 ± 11	62.7 ± 14.0	64.2 ± 12.8
- Constant score pain	4.8 ± 2.7	5.9 ± 3.3	5.1 ± 2.8
- Constant score ADL	10.9 ± 2.9	11.9 ± 3.3	12.0 ± 3.0
- Constant score ROM	26.7 ± 5.5	26.22 ± 6.7	28.0 ± 6.1
- Constant score power	17.8 ± 3.9	18.6 ± 3.7	18.9 ± 4.4
VAS	6.5 ± 1.3	5.7 ± 1.9	5.6 ± 1.6
Deposit size (mm^2)	182 ± 135	195 ± 166	128 ± 112

* ESWT indicates extracorporeal shockwave therapy, ADL activity of daily living, ROM range of motion, SSP supraspinatus, ISP infraspinatus, SSC subscapularis, TM teres minor, value given as mean ± standard deviation

Table 3. Epidemiological data and baseline values.

Differences of change between the groups are given in Tables 2a and 2b.

Up to the one year follow-up, more of the additional therapies were used in the control group (Figure 1). Five patients (10%) in the control group needed surgery compared to none in the low-energy ESWT group and one in the high-energy ESWT group.

After 12 months, local cortisone injections, needed for shoulder pain, were used in 8% of the control group, 4% of the low-energy ESWT group and 2% of the high-energy ESWT group.

Side effects

Side effects were recorded on standardized forms by clinical examination, ultrasound and by subject questionnaire directly after the ESWT and after every follow-up visit. It was explicitly asked whether reddening of the skin, swelling, petechia, reaction to the anesthetic used, bleeding, acute bursitis or syncope occurred after the therapy. In addition, subjects were also asked whether they had suffered any other side effects. Unexpected adverse or severe adverse events had to be reported separately, but did not occur. Pain, caused by the shockwaves during the treatment, was analyzed separately. Clinically relevant side effects (e.g. nerval disorders, tendon ruptures, infections) or severe adverse events or effects were observed neither at the one month nor at the 6 or 12 month follow-up.

In the high-energy shockwave group, 20 patients reported moderate and 16 severe pain. Eight of those patients needed intravenous analgesics during intervention. Ten patients had insignificant or no pain during the ESWT. In the low-energy shockwave group, moderate pain was found in 22 cases and severe pain in five cases, with two of them needing intravenous pain medication. Twenty-one patients reported slight or no pain.

In the placebo group, shockwave induced pain sensation could be found in 25 cases. Four of them had severe pain and one of them required additional intravenous pain medication. Insignificant or no pain sensation was observed in 23 cases.

Petechia, bleeding and hematoma have been put into one category and were found, directly after the treatment, in 36 cases for Group I, in 32 cases for Group II and in eight cases in the placebo group (Group III).

Rotator cuff lesion, transient bone edema, aseptic humerus head necrosis, infection, neural disturbance or deep hematoma were absent during clinical examination, ultrasound or x-ray evaluation.

Discussion

Shoulder pain due to calcific tendonitis of the shoulder is a common problem observed in daily clinical practice and conservative therapy is sometimes frustrating[1,5]. In these cases, ESWT has been proposed as an alternative to operative procedures[21,24,33]. Unfortunately, there was a lack of evidence for this hypothesis due to methodological flaws in all published studies[12].

We could confirm positive findings of smaller, uncontrolled or non-placebo controlled studies [23,24,34] in a randomized trial that was conducted according to ICH/GCP standards[26,27]. These previous trials either had no placebo [24,34] or only a wait list control [23,35], a small sample size [21-25,34] or subjects who were not randomly assigned to the intervention groups. Also, recent studies published in other peer reviewed journals showed significant methodical or biometrical flaws with unblinded control groups, unbalanced treatment and control groups, no randomization, different treatment parameters and protocols or the additional application of local anesthetics[36,37]. In contrast to previous studies, ESWT is compared for the first time in this study to a placebo therapy and the sample size is based on power calculations. In the study, subjects were randomly assigned to three groups to receive either fluoroscopy-guided ESWT given twice within two weeks (Group I: high-energy shockwaves; Group II: low-energy shockwaves) for a total energy flux density of 0.96 J/mm² or identical placebo (Group III). Clinical assessment at six months after treatment showed a significant and clinically relevant improvement in shoulder function in Group I and a significant improvement in Group II without clinical relevance, but no significant improvement in the control group. Patients in the control group showed the well-known spontaneous progress[4]. They needed more pain medication and there were more cases of surgery during follow-up than in the ESWT groups.

ESWT-induced deposit elimination and clinical improvement has been known to last up to 4 years after high energy ESWT[35].

Similar to the importance of stone removal in the therapy of nephrolithiasis, most of the authors stress the necessity of complete disintegration of the calcified deposit in orthopedics[38].

Radiologically, a complete disappearance of the deposit was observed in 60% of the patients in Group I after six months and in 86% after 12 months. In contrast, the x-rays of 21% of patients in Group II and 11% of patients in the placebo group showed complete deposit resorption after 6 months. Other authors discussed the potential disintegrating capability of extracorporeal shockwaves regarding calcified deposits of the rotator cuff, but the working mechanisms still remain unclear[39-41].

Several reports indicate that there is a correlation between the applied energy of each shockwave, and of the rate of disintegration [23,25] as long as exact focusing was provided[42].

For the moment, it is unclear by which parameter of shockwaves a higher rate of complete resorption of the deposit can be achieved. The parameter "energy flux density" (ED) is generally assumed to be the primary parameter for physical and biological effects[43]. Obviously, by simply doubling the number of applied shockwaves compared with a previous study, neither an increase of the elimination rate nor an improvement of the clinical outcomes were possible[24,25]. We suppose that the energy level seems to be a more important parameter. The high-energy and low-energy group received the same total acoustic energy but showed different clinical and radiological outcome. Besides the number of shockwaves and energy level, the frequency of incoming shocks may have an influence. Recent studies in kidney stones found that fragmentation efficiency, due to cavitation effects, was significantly enhanced, if the interval between two shocks is about 250 and 400 microseconds[44]. These findings support the theory that the appearances of cavitation effects may be one reason for the disintegrating effect of ESWT[45,41].

It is important for a possible future clinical application of shockwaves in cases of tendinopathies of the shoulder that an effect of ESWT was only found for calcifying tendinopathy but not for the non-calcifying impingement syndrome[46,47].

In contrast to other authors, three months after intervention, no side effects were observed in our study. We found neither petechial bleeding nor skin lesions as described previously[22,23]. Different shockwave generators used in the trials with different physical parameters may be the reason for this.

Short term morphological pathologies in tendons of rabbits were reported if ESWT was applied with an energy level of at least 0.6 mJ/mm^2[48]. Neither the biomechanical properties of tendons or the cartilage of joints were affected by shockwaves below this energy level[49,50]. In this study, no evaluation of the shoulder by means of magnetic resonance tomography was performed after the intervention to detect these side effects, but neither tendon ruptures nor aseptic necrosis of the humeral head [51] were documented. Long term observations four years after high energetic shockwave therapy showed no tendon lesions or other side effects due to shockwaves in patients who underwent surgery[52]. Cost analysis showed that ESWT has a better cost efficacy compared to surgery[53].

The findings of this study may be limited by the different amounts of intravenous sedation used in the treatment groups (8 patients, 16%, in Group I; 2 patients, 4%, in Group II; and 1 patient, 2%, in the placebo group) which was confounded with the effects of the active therapy and the amount of shockwave energy. It is unlikely that intravenous sedation alone may have influenced the chronic pain condition.

There is a need to confirm our findings in high quality clinical trials with different treatment protocols with changed treatment parameters (frequency, number of shockwaves and energy levels) to optimize the efficacy and dose. Up to now, the threshold energy level that provides good clinical and radiological outcome is still unknown. The intravenous sedation used is a limitation to apply our regimen on an outpatient basis. It has to be proven whether similar results can be achieved with other forms of anesthesia, like scalenus block or local anesthesia, applied outside a hospital setting.

Conclusion

Evidence was found for a beneficial effect of high-energy ESWT with two treatments of 1,500 impulses with an energy density of 0.32 mJ/mm² over placebo on shoulder function and disintegration of the calcified deposit six months after treatment for chronic calcific tendonitis. High-energy ESWT was found more effective than low-energy ESWT, but threshold energy still has to be defined. No clinically relevant side effects were observed.

Literature

1. Bosworth B. Calcium deposits in the shoulder and subacromial bursitis: a survey of 12122 shoulders. JAMA 1941;116:2477-2489
2. Rupp S, Seil R, Kohn D. Tendinosis calcarea der Rotatorenmanschette. Orthopäde 2000;29:852-867
3. Welfling J, Kahn MF, Desroy M. Les calcifications de l épaule. II. La maladie des calcifications tendineuses multiples. Rev Rheum 1965 ;32:325–334
4. Uhthoff HK, Loehr JF Calcifying tendinitis. In: Rockwood CA, Matsen FA (eds): The shoulder. Saunders, Philadelphia (1998),989-1008
5. Harmon PH. Methods and results in the treatment of 2580 painful shoulders with special reference to calcific tendinitis and the frozen shoulder. Am J Surg 1958;95:527-544
6. Gärtner J. Tendinosis calcarea- Behandlungsergebnisse mit dem needling. Z Orthop Ihre Grenzgeb 1993;131:461-469
7. Jim YF, Hsu HC, Chang CY, Wu JJ, Chang T. Coexistence of calcific tendonitis and rotator cuff tear: an arthrographic study. Skeletal Radiol 1993;22:183–185.
8. Chiou HJ, Chou YH, Wu JJ, Hsu CC, Huang DY, Chang CY. Evaluation of Calcific Tendonitis of the Rotator Cuff Role of Color Doppler Ultrasonography. J Ultrasound Med 2002;21:289–295
9. Loew M, Sabo D, Mau H, Perlick L, Wehrle M. Proton spin tomography imaging of the rotator cuff in calcific tendinitis of the shoulder. Z Orthop Ihre Grenzgeb. 1996;134(4):354–9
10. Maier M, Stabler A, Schmitz C, Lienemann A, Kohler S, Durr HR, Pfahler M, Refior HJ. On the impact of calcified deposits within the rotator cuff tendons in shoulders of patients with shoulder pain and dysfunction. Arch Orthop Trauma Surg. 2001;121:371–8
11. Rompe JD, Buch M, Gerdesmeyer L, Haake M, Loew M, Maier M, Heine J. Muskuloskeletale Stosswellenapplikation - Aktueller Stand der klinischen Forschung zu den Standardindikationen. Z Orthop Ihre Grenzgeb 2002;140:267–274
12. Green S, Buchbinder R, Glazier R, Forbes A. Systematic review of randomised controlled trials of interventions for painful shoulder: selection criteria, outcome assessment, and efficacy. BMJ 1998;316:354–360
13. Ebenbichler GR, Erdogmus CB, Resch KL et al. Ultrasound therapy for calcific tendinitis of the shoulder. N Engl J Med 1999;340:533–8
14. Maier M, Krauter T, Pellengahr C, et al. Operationsverfahren bei Tendinosis calcareader Schulter - Begleitpathologien beeinflussen das Operationsergebnis. Z Orthop Ihre Grenzgeb 2002;140:656–661
15. Rubenthaler F, Wittenberg RH. Mittelfristige Nachuntersuchungsergebnisse der operativ versorgten Tendinosis calcarea des Schultergelenkes. Z Orthop Ihre Grenzgeb 1997;135:354–359
16. Rochwerger A, Franceschi JP, Viton JM. Surgical management of calcific tendinitis of the shoulder: an analysis of 26 cases. Clin Rheumatol 1999;18:313–316
17. Gazielly DF, Bruyère G, Gleyze P, Thomas T. Open acromioplasty with excision of calcium deposits and tendon suture. In: Gazielly DF, Gleyze P, Thomas T (eds) The cuff. Elsevier, Paris,1997,181–184
18. Ark JW, Flock TJ, Flatow EL, Bigliani LU. Arthroscopic treatment of calcific tendinitis of the shoulder. Arthroscopy 1992;8:183–188

19. Molé D, Kempf JF, Gleyze P, Rio B, Bonnomet F, Walch G. Résultat du traitement arthroscopique des tendopathies non rumpues, II: les calcifications. Rev Chir Orthop 1993;79:532-541
20. Maier M, Krauter T, Pellengahr C, Schulz CU, Trouillier H, Anetzberger H, Refior HJ.Open surgical procedures in calcifying tendinitis of the shoulder - concomitant pathologies affect clinical outcome. Z Orthop Ihre Grenzgeb. 2002;140:656-61.
21. Loew M, Jurgowski W. Erste Erfahrungen mit der extrakorporalen Stoßwellen-Lithotrypsie (ESWL) in der Behandlung der Tendinosis calcarea der Schulter. Z Orthop Ihre Grenzgeb 1993; 131: 470-473
22. Loew M, Jurgowski W, Thomsen M. Die Wirkung extrakorporaler Stoßwellen auf die Tendinosis calcarea der Schulter. Urologe 1995; 34:49-53
23. Loew M, Daecke W, Kusnierczak D, Rahmanzadeh M, Ewerbeck V. Extracorporal shockwave application – an effective treatment for patients with chronic and therapy-resistant calcifying tendinitis? J Bone Joint Surg 1999;81-B:863-867
24. Rompe JD, Rumler F, Hopf C, Nafe B, Heine J. Extracorporal shockwave therapy for calcifying tendinitis of the shoulder. Clin Orthop 1995;321:196-201
25. Rompe JD, Burger R, Hopf C, Eysel P. Shoulder function after extracorporeal shockwave therapy for calcific tendinitis. J Shoulder Elbow Surg 1998;7:505-509
26. The European Agency for the Evaluation of Medicinal Products – Human Medicines Evaluation Unit. ICH Topic E 9, Guideline for Statistical Principles in Clinical Trials, CPMP/ICH/363/96E9. Document III/3630/92-EN 1998. www.emea.eu.int/pdfs/human/ich/036396en.pdf.
27. The European Agency for the Evaluation of Medicinal Products – Human Medicines Evaluation Unit. ICH Topic E 6, Guideline for Good Clinical Practice, CPMP/ICH/135/95. 1996. www.emea.eu.int/pdfs/human/ich/ 013595en.pdf
28. Constant CR, Murley AHG. A clinical method of functional assessment of the shoulder. Clin Orthop 1987;214:160-164
29. Conboy VB, Morris RW, Kiss J, Carr AJ. An evaluation of the Constant-Murley shoulder assessment. J Bone Joint Surg 1996;78-B:229-32
30. Kilcoyne RF, Reddy PK, Lyons F. Optimal plain film imaging of the shoulder impingement syndrome. Am J Roentgenol 1989;53:795-797. SPSS for Windows, release 11.5. Chicago: SPSS, 2002
31. Berger VW, Exner DV. Detecting selection bias in randomized clinical trials. Controlled Clinical Trials 1999;20:319-327
32. Rompe JD, Zöllner J, Nafe B. Shockwave therapy versus conventional surgery in the treatment of calcifying tendinitis of the shoulder. Clin Orthop 2001;387:72-82
33. Seil R, Rupp S, Hammer DS, Ensslin S, Gebhardt T, Kohn D. Extracorporeal shockwave therapy in tendionosis calcarea of the rotator cuff: comparison of different treatment protocols. Z Orthop Ihre Grenzgeb. 1999;137:310-5
34. Daecke W, Kusnierczak D, Loew M. Long-term effects of extracorporeal shockwave therapy in chronic calcific tendinitis of the shoulder. J Shoulder Elbow Surg 2002;11:476-480
35. Wang CJ, Yang KD, Wang FS, Chen HH, Wang JW. Shockwave therapy for calcific tendinitis of the shoulder: a prospective clinical study with two-year follow-up. Am J Sports Med. 2003;1:425-30.
36. Cosentino R, De Stefano R, Selvi E, Frati E, Manca S, Frediani B, Marcolongo R. Extracorporeal shockwave therapy for chronic calcific tendinitis of the shoulder: single blind study. Ann Rheum Dis. 2003;62:248-50
37. Rompe JD, Zoellner J, Nafe, B. Bedeutung der Kalkdepotelimination bei Tendinosis calcarea der Schulter. Z Orthop Ihre Grenzgeb 2000;138:335-339

38. Perlick L, Korth O, Wallny T. Die Desintegrationswirkung der Stoßwellen bei der extrakorporalen Stoßwellenbehandlung der Tendinosis calcarea – ein in vitro Modell. Z Orthop Ihre Grenzgeb 1999;137:10-16
39. Maier M, Lienemann A, Refior HJ. Are there magnetic resonance tomographic changes following shockwave treatment of tendinitis calcarea? Z Orthop Ihre Grenzgeb 1997;135:Oa20-1.
40. Delacretaz G, Rink K, Pittomvils G, Lafaut JP, Vandeursen H, Boving R.: Importance of the implosion of ESWL-induced cavitation bubbles. Ultrasound Med Biol 1995;21:97-103
41. Haake M, Deike B, Thon A, Schmitt J. Exact focusing of extracorporeal shockwave therapy for calcifying tendinopathy. Clin Orthop 2002;397:323-31
42. Granz B, Kohler G. What makes a shockwave efficient in lithotripsy? J Stone Dis 1992;4:123-128
43. Loske AM, Prieto FE, Fernandez F, van Cauwelaert J.: Tandem shockwave cavitation enhancement for extracorporeal lithotripsy. Phys Med Biol 2002;47:3945-57
44. Sapozhnikov OA, Khokhlova VA, Bailey MR, Williams JC Jr, McAteer JA, Cleveland RO, Crum LA: Effect of overpressure and pulse repetition frequency on cavitation in shockwave lithotripsy. J Acoust Soc Am 2002;112:1183-95
45. Schmitt J, Haake M, Tosch A, Hildebrand R, Deike B, Griss P: Low energy extracorporeal shockwave therapy (ESWT) of supraspinatus tendinitis - A prospective randomised study. J Bone Joint Surg (Br) 2001;83:873-876
46. Speed CA, Richards C, Nichols D, Burnet S, Wies JT, Humphreys H, Hazleman BL. Extracorporeal shockwave therapy for tendonitis of the rotator cuff. A double-blind, randomised, controlled trial. J Bone Joint Surg 2002;84-B:509-12
47. Rompe JD, Kirkpatrick CJ, Kullmer K, Schwitalle M, Krischek O: Dose-related effects of shockwaves on rabbit tendo Achillis. A sonographic and histological study. J Bone Joint Surg 1998;80-B:546-52
48. Maier M, Tischer T, Milz S, Weiler C, Nerlich A, Pellengahr C, Schmitz C, Refior HJ. Dose-related effects of extracorporeal shockwaves on rabbit quadriceps tendon integrity. Arch Orthop Trauma Surg. 2002;122:436–41
49. Vaterlein N, Lussenhop S, Hahn M, Delling G, Meiss AL. The effect of extracorporeal shockwaves on joint cartilage-an in vivo study in rabbits. Arch Orthop Trauma Surg. 2000;120:403–6
50. Durst HB, Blatter G, Kuster MS: Osteonecrosis of the humeral head after extracorporeal shockwave lithotripsy. J Bone Joint Surg 2002;84-B:744-746
51. Daecke W, Kusnierczak D, Loew M : Importance of extracorporeal shockwave therapy (ESWT) in chronic calcific tendinitis of the shoulder. Orthopade 2002;·31:645–651
52. Haake M, Rautmann M, Wirth T. Assessment of treatment costs of Extracorporeal Shockwave Therapy (ESWT) - Comparison of ESWT and surgical treatment in shoulder diseases. Int J Tech Ass Health Care 2001;17: 612–617

22

Painful Heel - Anatomy, Clinical Study and Therapy Result after Radial Extracorporeal Shockwave Therapy (rESWT)

L. Gerdesmeyer,[1] M. Henne,[1] H. Gollwiitzer,[1] P. Diehl,[1] M. Russlies[2]

Introduction

Plantar heel pain is one of the most common disorders in the foot region and has been studied for more than one hundred years without doctors reaching a precise uniform diagnosis. As early as 1922, Stiell observed that "due to its inexact diagnosis, the painful heel did not allow any specific intervention[1]." Lapidus and Guidooti found that the term "painful heel" is to be preferred because the exact pathophysiological pathways remain unclear[2]. Today the term "painful heel" is mostly used in literature as well as "heel spur" even though it is not always documented in x-rays.

The term "fasciitis plantaris" refers to an inflammatory condition of the plantar fascia close to the calcaneal insertion area and/or of the short muscles affecting the fascia. Like epicondylitis humeri radialis, plantar fasciitis is generally viewed as a primary insertion enthesiopathy[3]. Woolnough also referred to "tennis heel[4]." Out of 323 patients analyzed by Lapidus and Guidotti, 76% were aged between 40 and 70 years[2]. Sex distribution varied[2, 5, 6]. Very often patients were found to be obese. Obesity significantly impacts the symptoms and has to be defined as predictive factor[7, 8].

---

[1] Dept. of Orthopedic Surgery and Sportstraumatology, Technical University Munich
[2] Dept. of Orthopedic Surgery, University of Lübeck

ESWT is used to provide an increase in blood supply by inducing neovascularisation which affects local inflammatory processes in order to favor regional metabolism. Studies by Wang demonstrated that low-energy ESWT leads to increased perfusion if applied to the tendon insert area. In addition, a positive vasculogenetic effect was observed[43, 44].

Clinical Study and Diagnosis

The pain threshold decreases by walking barefoot especially within the first steps in the morning. Various pathologies such as foot deformities or ligament insufficiencies with hypermobility of the hind foot were known as predictive factors regarding plantar heel pain[3]. Typically, pain could be generated by palpation of the Tuberculum mediale calcanei[11]. Typically, patients complain about morning pain as well as pain after rest which may occur at different times. Symptoms might worsen as a result of professional or sports activities[12]. Just a few patients also suffered from night pain. When the inflammation becomes chronic, a thickening of the fascia was found by ultrasound exploration.

The heel spur itself was found as an ossification of the tendon insertion zone close to the tuberculum mediale of the calcaneus where plantaraponeurosis, M. abductor hallucis and M. abductor digiti quinti originate. The length of the spur varies between 2 mm and 15 mm but no correlation was found between the spur itself and clinical symptoms[9, 10, 13, 14].

Spontaneous resorption of the spur does not exist[5]. Epidemiological x-ray analysis reported heel spur to be present in about 50% of all patients suffering from heel pain[15-17]. In 1963, Tanz found 16 heel spurs in 100 x-rays taken of patients with acute injuries without plantar heel pain. In another study, Shmokler et al. described an incidence of 13.2% by analyzing 1000 cases, but only 5.2% were found to be clinically significant[18].

Tomographic MR images and ultrasound exams may also reveal a fasciitis plantaris. Most commonly, the thickening of the fascia was associated with soft-tissue edema[19]. In 1995, Lin et al. reported a diagnostic sensitivity of 94% if technetium methyl diphosphonate was used in bone scintigraphy[20].

Inclusion Criteria	Exclusion Criteria
• Patient's history over 6 months • Unsuccessful conservative therapy • Clinically relevant heel spur pain	• < 18 years old • Dysfunctions in the ankle joint and foot region • Local arthrosis/arthritis; rheumatoid arthritis • Pathological neurological and/or vascular findings • Tarsal tunnel syndrome • Pregnancy • Disturbance of coagulation • Infections • Tumors

Table 1. Inclusion and exclusion criteria.

Patients and Method

A total of 79 patients (95 heels) were enrolled in the study. All of them had to fulfill specific inclusion and exclusion criteria as listed in Table 1.

The treatment was performed by using the DolorClast® device from July 2001 to March 2002. The mean age was 56.4 years (24 to 81 years), sex distribution women:men was 52:27. Prior to the first treatment, weight and size were measured in all patients. The mean calculated Body Mass Index (BMI) at baseline was 27.1 kg/m^2 (20.3 to 48.8 kg/m^2) which corresponds to obesity stage 1 according to the WHO classification.

The study population involved 46 right and 49 left heels. Mean pain history was reported as 21 months (2 weeks to 15 years). All heels were examined by x-rays. A plantar spur was found in 65 of 95 heels; the mean length was about 3.7 mm (1 to 11 mm).

Treatment Method

Radial extracorporeal shockwave therapy (rESWT) was performed with the EMS Swiss DolorClast®. After localization by patient biofeedback, the region

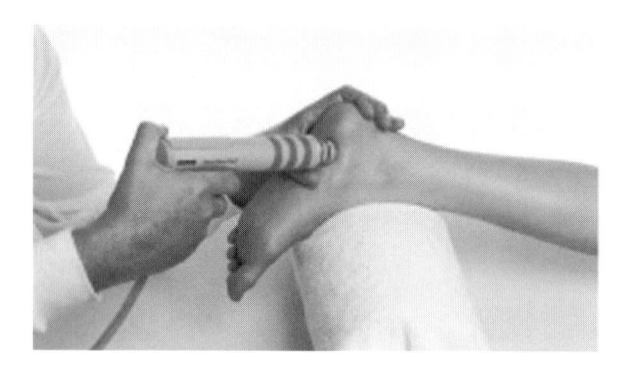

Figure 1. Treatment of heel spur.

was marked and coupling gel was applied to the skin. Then the applicator was placed on the marked area to start the treatment (Figure 1). Two thousand impulses with an energy density of 0.08 mJ/mm^2 at a frequency of 8 Hz and application pressure of 4 bar were delivered three times within 6-week intervals. Even though the treatment was reported as painful, no local anesthesics were used in order to exclude any additive effects.

Evaluation

The primary criterion was defined as change regarding pain during first steps in the morning. The values were scored on the Visual Analog Scale (VAS). Secondary criteria were subjective pain at activities of daily living (ADL). The primary end point was defined at 12 months after the last treatment. Additional follow-up exams were conducted 6 weeks, 3 and 6 months after the last rESWT. Pain indications by the patients were entered on a 10-point VAS scale whereby 0 correlates to no pain. Another secondary criterion was outcome scored by the Roles and Maudsley score (Table 2).

An independent blinded observer as used to perform re-examination and evaluation and data management.

The statistical evaluation was also carried out independently from the physicians. The t-test for 2 dependent variables was carried out to test the primary

Roles and Maudsley Score	
Very good	No pain, no limitation in occupational or leisure activities
Good	Low remaining pain, no limitation in occupational or leisure activities
Satisfactory	Tolerable remaining pain, limitations in occupational and leisure activities
Poor	Activity-limiting pain

Table 2. Roles and Maudsley Score.

hypothesis in terms of the primary criteron based on group differences. The statistical significance level was defined as $p<0.05$. A statistical analysis of the secondary criterion, outcome measured by Roles and Maudsley score, was described by using the Wilcoxon rank sum test.

Results

All but one patient followed the recall for re-examination (78 out of 79). One patient dropped out because of an additional cortisone injection within the treatment period. Seventy-eight patients (94 heels) were included in the analysis 6 weeks, 3, 6 and 12 months after intervention. Five out of 78 patients received specific heel pain related interventions. They were ruled out and data were replaced by the last value prior to the additional intervention. This data management technique is called the "last value carried forward" technique. Intention-to-treat analysis was performed.

At the baseline examination, patients reported an average VAS value of 6.0 +/- 3.0. After the last rESWT, pain dropped down to 1.67 +/- 2.46 at the 6-week follow-up, down to 1.43 +/- 2.37 at the 3-month follow-up, down to 1.31 +/- 2.27 at the 6-month follow-up and down to 1.11 +/- 2.12 at the 12-month follow-up (Figure 3). These differences were analyzed and found to be statistically significant ($p< 0.01$) as well as clinically relevant.

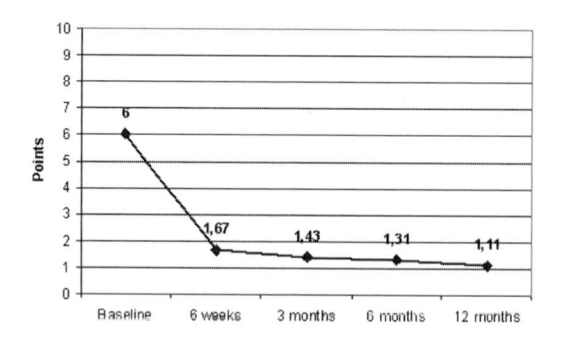

Figure 3. VAS (first steps in the morning). Primary criterion: Pain during first steps in the morning

Secondary Target Criterion

Pain during ADL decreased as well. Comparable to pain in the morning, pain dropped down from 7.0 +/- 2.0 at baseline to 1.73 +/- 2.42 after 6 weeks, to 1.68 +/- 2.45 after 3 months, to 1.67 +/- 2.54 after 6 months and finally down to 1.39 +/- 2.35 after 12 months (Figure 4). These changes as well were statistically significant ($p<0.01$) and clinically relevant.

Roles and Maudsley Score

The same outcome was found regarding the Roles and Maudsley Score. At baseline, 72 heels were rated as poor (76.6%) and 22 as satisfactory (23.4%). A significant improvement was found after shockwave intervention. Six weeks after the last treatment, 32 heels were rated as good (34.0%) and 43 as very good (45.7%). Another 6 weeks later, 24 patients (25.5%) reported good results and 49 (52.1%) very good results. After 6 months, 24 patients (25.5%) were scored as good and 51 (54.3%) as very good. At the primary end point (12 months after the last rESWT), 57 heels could be documented as very good (60.6%), 18 good (19.1%), 9 satisfactory (9.6%) and 10 poor (10.6%). Overall 4 out of 5 obtained good or very good results (Figure 5).

Discussion

Heel pain in the sense of a plantar fasciitis is one of the most common diseases of the foot and occurs primarily at an older age. The prevalence is reported as 12.5 to 15%[25].

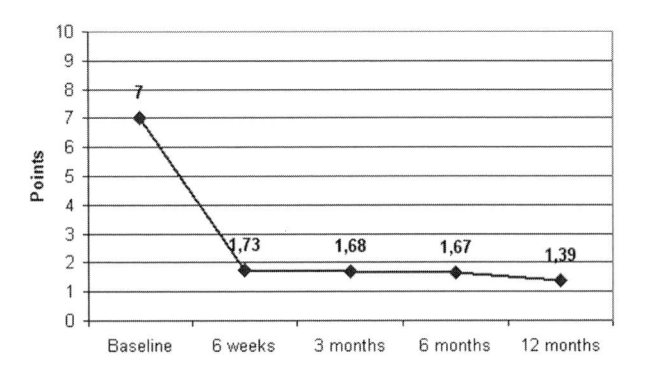

Figure 4. Pain during ADL.

A uniform etiology for plantar heel pain cannot be shown. Factors that may contribute to plantar fasciitis are deformities such as differences in leg length, tarsal coalition, shortening of the Achilles tendon, obesity or sudden weight gain and training errors in athletes such as rapid increase in running distance, running speed and duration[26]. Riddle found in a study that factors such as reduced dorsal extension in the ankle joint, obesity with a body mass index >30 kg/m2 and job-related weight exertion of the heel lead to problems[27].

Whether in terms of conservative or operative treatments, few or no multi-centered, controlled studies have been done on plantar fasciitis. Therefore,

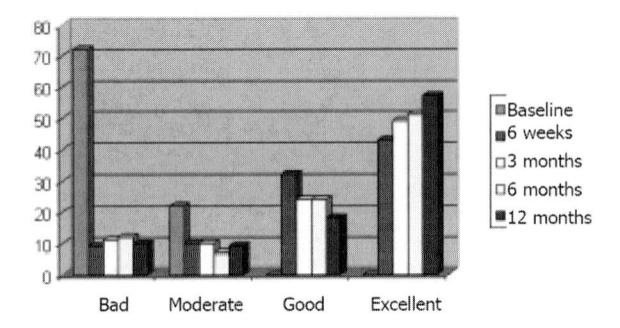

Figure 5. Roles and Maudsley Score.

an evaluation of their validity is difficult[28]. Crawford compared eleven randomized studies with 465 patients and came to the conclusion that the quality of the setup was so unsatisfactory that a pooling of the results was not possible. Only seven studies compared treatment with placebo or no treatment. They showed a low evidence of the effectiveness of local cortisone injections, night splints or low energy shockwaves[29]. Only six studies involved a randomized and controlled analysis (night splints, shoe inlays, tape, laser, iontophoresis with Dexamethason). Only one study, in which the laser was found to be ineffective for the treatment of plantar fasciitis, involved a placebo-controlled examination[26].

No randomized studies were available on radiation therapy or surgery[29]. Boyle reported on the results of endoscopic release of plantar fasciitis on 17 feet. All patients were satisfied with the procedure and reported improved walking distance, and 82.4% reported no or minimum pain[30]. Brekke as well obtained very good and good results in 54 Fascectomy treatments (endoscopic, minimal incision and open)[31]. Nevertheless, a conservative therapy is to be preferred over operative treatment.

In the past 30 years, studies have been performed on the different effects of physical factors on the healing processes of bone and soft tissues. A new physical medium was introduced with extracorporeal shockwave therapy for kidney stone fragmentation[32, 33]. This made it possible to achieve effects in the body without surgery. It became logical to use the therapy for the treatment of other intracorporeal concrements such as gallstones, pancreatic and salivary duct stones[34, 35, 36].

In orthopedics, shockwaves were used for the first time in 1986 to stimulate healing processes. High-energy shockwaves are found to have a marked physical effect on Model stones and bone tissue while low energy shockwaves have a neurophysiological effect on human connective tissue[37].

In 2001 Ogden et al. conducted a double-blinded, placebo-controlled multicentered study on 302 patients with heel spur, 260 randomized and 42 non-randomized. He used an electrohydraulically operated shockwave unit (Ossa Tron). Inclusion criteria were a history of pain over 6 months, failure of at least three conservative therapy options, the clinical evidence of plantar fasciitis and an evaluation of pain during first steps in the morning on the Visual Analog Scale of > 5. The mean age was 49.6 years and 65.9% of patients were women. Pain history was reported as 19 months on average. After randomization all patients were treated with 1500 impulses at a frequency of 18 kV. In the placebo group, foam material was placed between the coupling membrane and heel for the purpose of absorption. The four main criteria were indication of pain with pressure applied to the heel (as measured with the Dolormeter) (1), morning pain (2), activity pain during the day (3), as well as reduction in consumption of pain killers (4) after 12 weeks. An improvement of 50% or more was entered as successful. The following results were obtained:

Group	Dolormeter	Pain first steps	Pain during ADL		Pain Average	
Randomized, verum	7.68→3.13	62.2%	8.02→3.48	59.7%	3.49→1.72	69.74%
Randomized, placebo	7.87→4.37	43%	8.14→4.2	48.2%	3.53→1.88	34.65%
Non-randomized, verum	8.05→2.01	80%	6.86→2.1	70.7%	2.63→0.85	80.5%

Of the patients in the verum group, 47.06% met all four criteria versus 30.17% in the placebo group. Statistic significance was found by p = 0.008. Of the non-randomized patients, 58.54% met all four target criteria[38].

Buchbinder et al. questioned the efficacy of extracorporeal shockwaves in a placebo-controlled study. One hundred sixty-six patients were randomly assigned to receive ESWT three times at weekly intervals by an ultrasound-controlled Dornier MedTech EPOS unit. This device delivered focused shockwaves. Patients assigned to active treatment received 2000-2500 impulses with a frequency of 3 Hertz and an energy flux density between 0.02 and 0.33 mJ/mm^2 depending on pain tolerance. The placebo intervention as performed by applying 100 impulses at 1 Hertz and 0.02 mJ/mm^2. The primary criteria were also defined as pain during first steps in the morning and during ADL, walking time, Maryland Foot Score, the Problem Elicitation Technique, the SF-36 Health Survey, side effects and self-evaluation. The primary endpoints were 6 and 12 weeks after last ESWT. A significant improvement was not found in either group with 20% after 6 weeks and 25% after 12 weeks. Similar results were obtained for the other criteria. No statistically significant difference was found between the two groups[39]. The study was significantly limited by the fact that no chronic but rather acute heel spur patients were enrolled and a real sham treatment was not performed as well.

Similar results were reported by Haake et al. who performed another randomized placebo-controlled multicentered trial in 2003. They were also unable to show clinically relevant evidence to support shockwave application. They enrolled a total of 272 patients suffering from chronic plantar fasciitis. All patients got shockwaves by a Dornier Epos Ultra Lithotripter. Similar to the Buchbinder study, it must be noted that all treatments were carried out with low-energy focused shockwaves combined with local anesthetics, which is known to compromise shockwave efficacy as described later on by Rompe et al. In the Haake trial, patients received 3 x 4000 impulses at two-week intervals with an energy flux density of 0.22 mJ/mm^2. Primary criteria were defined as success rates analyzed 12 weeks after the last ESWT and the Roles and Maudsley Score 6 weeks, 12 weeks and 1 year after the last intervention. Secondary criteria were described as night pain, pressure pain as well as improved walking distance. The success rate after 12 weeks was 34% for ESWT and 30% for the sham treatment. Six weeks after ESWT, the Roles and Maudsley Score improved in the same way. A better outcome was found after active ESWT but without clinical relevance[40].

Significantly better results were published by Rompe et al. Rompe studied 45 runners with chronic fasciitis plantaris and a pain history of at least 12 months. He reported a significant improvement after ESWT compared to placebo. He stated a clearly positive impact of ESWT[45].

Our clinical study as well showed an excellent outcome 6 weeks and later on after rESWT. Particularly, it was noticed that no recurrence of pain occurs.

In conclusion, low energy radial shockwave therapy (rESWT) is suitable as an effective procedure in chronic plantar fasciitis of the heel. After rESWT clinical side effects occurred.

Literature

1. Stiell WF: Painful heel. Practitioner 108:169, 1922
2. Lapidus PW., Guidotti FP. Painful heel: report of 323 patients with 364 painful heels, Clin Orthop 39: 178, 1965
3. Loew H., Rompe J.D.: Stosswellenbehandlungen bei orthopädischen Erkrankungen. Enke Verlag Stuttgart: 34, 1998
4. Woolnough, J. Tennis heel. Med. J. Aus. 1954; 2:857-861
5. Greer Richardson, E. Painful heel. In Campbells's Operative Orthopaedics (Ed. Crenshaw, A.H.). Mosby St. Louis 1992; Vol.4, 2787-2792

6. Barrett, S.L.; Day, S.V.; Pignetti, T.T.; Egly, B.R. Endoscopic heel Anatomy: analysis of 200 fresh frozen specimens. J. Foot Ankle Surg. 1995; 34:51-56
7. Hill JJ, Cutting PJ: Heel pain and body weight. Foot Ankle 9:254-256, 1989
8. Furey JG: Plantar fasciitis: the painful heel syndrome. J Bone Joint Surg 57A:672-673, 1975
9. Haglund, P.: Beitrag zur Klinik der Achillessehne. Z. orthop. 49. 49.52, 1928
10. Hohmann, G.: Fuß und Bein. Bergmann München, 1951
11. Rompe JD: Extrakorporale Stosswellentherapie; Grundlagen, Indikation, Anwendung. Chapman & Hall: 110, 1997
12. Ogden, J.A. et al: Shockwave therapy for chronic proximal plantar fasciitis. Clinical Orthopaedics and Related Research 387: 47, 2001
13. Haglund, P.: Beitrag zur Klinik der Achillessehne. Z. orthop. 49: 49-52, 1928
14. Hohmann, G.: Fuß und Bein. Bergmann München, 1951
15. Snook, G.A., Chrisman O.D.: The management of subcalcaneal pain. Clin Orthop 82_ 163-168, 1972
16. Tanz S.S.: Heel pain. Clin Orthop 28: 169-178, 1963
17. Baxter D.E., Pfeffer G.B., Thigpen C.M.: Chronic heel pain: treatment rationale, Orthop Clin North Am 20: 563-569, 1989
18. Shmokler R.L., Bravo A.A., Lynch F.R. et al.: A new use of instrumentation in fluoroscopy controlled heel spur surgery. J Am Podiatr Med Assoc 78. 194-197, 1988
19. Berkowitz J.F., Kjer R., Rudieel S.: Plantar fasciitis: MR imaging. Radiology 179: 665-667,1991
20. Lin W.Y., Wang S.J., Lang J.L. et al.: Bone scintygraphy in evaluation of heel pain in Reiter´s disease: compared with radiography and clinical examination. Scand J Rheumatology 24: 18-21, 1995
21. Rompe JD: Extrakorporale Stosswellentherapie; Grundlagen, Indikation, Anwendung. Chapman & Hall: 112, 1997
22. Rompe JD: Extrakorporale Stosswellentherapie; Grundlagen, Indikation, Anwendung. Chapman & Hall: 113, 1997
23. Schepsis AA, Leach RE, Gorzyca J: Plantar fasciitis. Etiology, treatment, surgical results and review of the literature. Clin Orthop 266: 185-196, 1991
24. Rompe JD: Extrakorporale Stosswellentherapie; Grundlagen, Indikation, Anwendung. Chapman & Hall: 114, 1997
25. Krischek O., Rompe JD, Herbsthofer B., Nafe B.: Symptomatische niedrigenergetische Stosswellentherapie bei Fersenschmerzen und radiologisch nachweisbarem plantaren Fersensporn. Z. Orthop 136: 169-174, 1998
26. Buch M, Knorr U, Fleming L, Theodore G, Amendola A, Bachmann C, Zingas C, Siebert WE: Extrakorporale Stosswellentherapie beim symptomatischen Fersensporn. Orthopäde 31: 637-644, 2002
27. Riddle DL, Pulisic M, Pidcoe P, Johnson RE: Risk factors for plantar fasciitis: a matched case-control study. J Bone Joint Surg Am 85-A(5): 872-877, 2003
28. Atkins D, Crawford F, Edwards J, Lambert M:a systematic review of treatments for the painful heel. Rheumatology (Oxford) 38(10):968-973, 1999
29. Crawford F, Atkins D, Edwards J: Interventions for treating plantar heel pain. Cochrane Database Syst Rev CD000416, 2000
30. Boyle RA, Slater GL: Endoscopic plantar fascia release: a case series. Foot Ankle Int 24(2): 176-179, 2003

31. Brekke MK, Green DR: Retrospective analysis of minimal-incision, endoscopic and open procedures for heel spur syndrome. J Am Podiatr Med Assoc 88(2): 64-72, 1998
32. Chaussy C: Extracorporeal shockwave lithotripsy. Basel: Karger, 1982
33. Chaussy C, Eisenberger F, Wanner K, Forssmann F, Hepp W, Schmiedt E, Brendel W: The use of shockwaves for the destruction of renal calculi without direct contact. Urol. Res. 4: 175, 1976
34. Iro H, Schneider H, Födra C, Waitz G, Nitsche N, Heinritz HH, Benninger J, Ell C: Shockwave lithotripsy of salivary duct stones. Lancet 339: 1333-1336, 1992
35. Sauerbruch T, Delius M., Paumgartner G., Holl J., Wess O., Weber W., Hepp W., Brendel W: Fragmentation of gallstones by extracorporeal shockwaves. New England J. Med. 314: 818-822, 1986
36. Sauerbruch T, Holl J, Sackmann M, Werner R, Wotzka R, Paumgartner G: Disintegration of a pancreatic duct stone with extracorporeal shockwaves in a patient with chronic pancreatitis. Endoscopy 19: 207-208, 1987
37. Loew H, Rompe JD: Stosswellenbehandlungen bei orthopädischen Erkrankungen. Enke Verlag Stuttgart: 9, 1998
38. Ogden, JA, Alvarez R, Levitt R, Cross GL Marlow M: Shockwave therapy for chronic proximal plantar fasciitis. Clinical Orthopaedics and Related Research 387: 47-59, 2001
39. Buchbinder R, Ptasznik R, Gordon J, Buchanan J, Prabaharan V, Forbes A: Ultrasound-guided extracorporeal shockwave therapy for plantar fasciitis. A randomized controlled trial. JAMA 288: 1364-1372, 2002
40. Haake M, Buch M, Schoellner C, Goebel F: Extracorporeal shockwave therapy for plantar fasciitis: randomised controlled multicentre trial. British Medical Journal 327: 1-5, 2003
41. Gerdesmeyer L., Maier M., Haake M.: Physikalisch-technische Grundlagen der extrakorporalen Stosswellentherapie. TechnGrundlageOrthopädie2002-V4.doc
42. Haupt G, Menne A, Schulz M: Medizinisches Instrument zum Erzeugen und Weiterleiten von extrakorporalen nicht fokussierten Druckwellen auf biologisches Gewebe. Patentanmeldung, 1997
43. Wang CJ, Huang HY, Pai CH. Shockwave-enhanced neovascularization at the tendon-bone junction: an experiment in dogs. J Foot Ankle Surg 2002; 41: 16-22.
44. Wang CJ, Wang FS, Yang KD, Weng LH, Hsu CC, Huang CS, Yang LC. Shockwave therapy induces neovascularization at the tendon-bone junction. A study in rabbits. J Orthop Res 2003; 21: 984-989
45. Rompe JD, et al. Shockwave application for chronic plantar fasciitis in running athletes – a prospective, randomized, placebo- controlled trial. Am J Sports Med 2003; 31:268-275

Short and Medium-Term Results in the Treatment of Epicondylitis Humeri Radialis with rESWT

L. Gerdesmeyer,[1] M. Henne,[1] H. Gollwiitzer,[1] P. Diehl,[1] M. Russlies[2]

Introduction

Epicondylitis humeri radialis, well known as tennis elbow, was firstly described as "writer's cramp" by Runge in 1873[1]. It is rather a perostium inflammation which causes microtrauma of the insertion zone of the extensor muscles[2]. In this regard, the extensor carpi radialis seems to be the key point[3]. Wilhelm and Gieseler discussed a local neuritis of local nerves innervating the lateral epicondyle[4]. Trigger factors were also discussed such as a microtrauma [12] or just a muscular insufficiency[13]. Peripheral and cervical nerve compression syndromes have to be ruled out as well as para-articular and intra-articular disorders corresponding to lateral epicondyle pain[14].

In addition to local tendon pathologies, there was also evidence of collagen tissue degeneration followed by vessel ingrowth, degeneration of fibrocytes and fibrilles, necrosis, calcifications and cartilage changes known as local metaplasia[5].

The lateral epicondyle is afflicted up to 5 times more often than the medial epicondyle. The incidence is described as 1 to 9% and a prevalence was found near 10%. The lateral epicondylitis has an important impact in middle-aged patients within the fourth decade[6].

---

[1] *Dept. of Orthopedic Surgery and Sportstraumatology, Technical University Munich*
[2] *Dept. of Orthopedic Surgery, University of Lübeck*

Clinically, radial epicondylitis is characterized by local pain around the extensor muscle insertion zone. Pain could be generated by increased extension load or palpation of the epicondyle. However, neither active nor passive mobility within the elbow joint is limited. Pain may be also triggered by performing the Chair Test or Thomson Test.

In terms of predictive factors, data are limited to define any[15].

Imaging in lateral epicondylitis is less frequently used because clinical examinations could simply be used to determine the exact diagnosis. MRI as well as x-ray exams are used to exclude some differential diagnosis. MRI and sonography imaging show local edema[16].

The suppinator syndrome is also known to generate elbow pain if nerve entrapment was found. Regarding the lateral epicondylitis, an entrapment of the R. profundus of the N. radialis exists. This has to be excluded by electromyography[4].

Material and Methods

Sixty-four patients were enrolled into this prospective study. All of them suffered from chronic lateral epicondylitis. They were indicated to receive radial extracorporeal shockwaves. The study was performed at the Orthopedic Department of the Technical University Munich.

Inclusion criteria were defined as pain history of at least 6 months and failed conservative treatment with at least two different methods. Exclusion criteria were defined as: rheumatoid diseases, disturbance of coagulation, tumors, osteoarthritis of the elbow joint, nerve entrapment, symptomatic HWS disorders, pregnancy and age below 18.

The mean age at baseline was 43.5 years (21 to 68 years), gender distribution was almost equal (women:men 34:30). In 56 patients (87.5%) the dominant arm was affected. Only 6 patients (9.4%) were evaluated as active tennis players.

Patients were seated with elbow flexion at 90° during the treatment. All patients received a total of 2000 impulses with a frequency of 8 Hz and an application pressure of 4 bar. The treatment was performed three times at 4-week

Very good	No pain, no limitation in occupational or leisure activities
Good	Low remaining pain, no limitation in occupational or leisure activities
Satisfactory	Tolerable remaining pain, limitations in occupational and leisure activities
Poor	Activity-limiting pain

Table 1. Roles and Maudsley Score.

intervals. Only a few patients needed a slow increasement of application pressure due to pain but no local anesthesia was required.

The primary criterion was defined as pain during daily activities (ADL) measured by the Visual Analog Scale (VAS). Secondary criteria were the local pressure threshold scored using the DolorMeter and pressure measurement scored on the Visual Analog Scale (VAS). Furthermore, the Thomson Test and Chair Test as the well as the Roles and Maudsley Score (Table 1) were used to determine the outcome after rESWT. The primary endpoints were defined as 6 and 12 weeks after the last rESWT.

An independent blinded observer was used to perform re-examination and evaluation and data management.

The statistical evaluation was also carried out independently from the physicians. The t-test for 2 dependent variables was carried out to test the primary hypothesis in terms of the primary criterion based on group differences. The statistical significance level was defined as $p<0.05$. A statistical analysis of the secondary criterion, the outcome measured by the Roles and Maudsley score, was described using the Wilcoxon rank sum test.

Results

Sixty-four out of 64 patients could be re-examined within the complete follow up period.

In terms of the defined primary criteron measured on the VAS, a significant improvement was observed in all patients. Six weeks after rESWT, the VAS value representing pain during daily activities decreased down to 3.4 points compared

Pain with	Baseline	6 weeks	12 weeks
General activity	7.6	3.4	2.8
Pressure (DolorMeter)	9.4	6.9	6.5
Thomson test	7.1	5.0	3.0
Chair test	8.4	4.9	3.7

Table 2. Pain sensation on the Visual Analog Scale (VAS).

to 7.6 at baseline. The same reduction was measured 12 weeks after the last rESWT, indicating statistically as well as clinically significant improvement. At the end of the 12th week, the VAS score had to be determined at 2.8 points, which corresponds to an improvement of at least 4.8 points. These findings were below the predefined level of significance ($p<0.05$).

Regarding the outcome scored for the secondary criteria, we found the same effects after rESWT as described above. The Thomson and Chair Tests were found to improve significantly with further improvement 12 weeks after rESWT. To determine pressure pain, a DolorMeter and an exact application pressure were used in a standardized fashion. Tests were conducted 6 and 12 weeks after intervention. The applied pressure was the same as applied at baseline. A moderate improvement of 2.9 points was observed after 12 weeks. Table 2 and Figure 1 summarize the outcome.

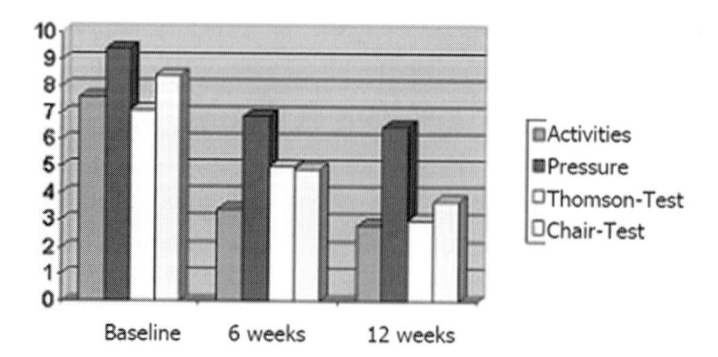

Figure 1. Pain sensation on the Visual Analog Scale (VAS).

	Baseline	6 Weeks	12 Weeks
Very good	0	5	12
Good	0	41	43
Satisfactory	16	11	4
Poor	48	7	5

Table 3. Change in Roles and Maudsley Score.

A similar outcome was found if scored by the Roles and Maudsley score. At baseline patients were qualified as poor (75%) or satisfactory (25%) but changed significantly 6 weeks after intervention (71% were scored as very good or good). Twelve weeks after rESWT, further improvement was found (85.9% were scored as very good or good). Results are shown in Table 3 and Figure 2.

No clinically relevant side effects occurred. Fifty-one patients (79.7%) reported pain following treatment but the pain disappeared soon. A few minor side effects including petechial bleeding (70.3%) or transient swelling (65.6%) and small hematoma (6 patients) were documented but disappeared completely within 2 weeks without any specific treatment.

Discussion

The epicondylitis humeri radialis is caused by many factors. Vessel ingrowth and hyaline changes in histological cross-sections of chronic epicondylitis point to a degenerative rather than an inflammatory process. The spontaneous healing process without further intervention is unknown. Nevertheless, epicondylitis humeri radialis is considered by many authors as a self-limiting disease thus implying that this disorder eventually leads to healing independently of other supportive interventions. Today hundreds of different treatments are available and published for chronic lateral epicondylitis, but evidence is still lacking. Local steroids and shockwave therapy have shown little evidence. Neither corticoid injections nor non-steroidal antirheumatics significantly affect the disease in the long term.

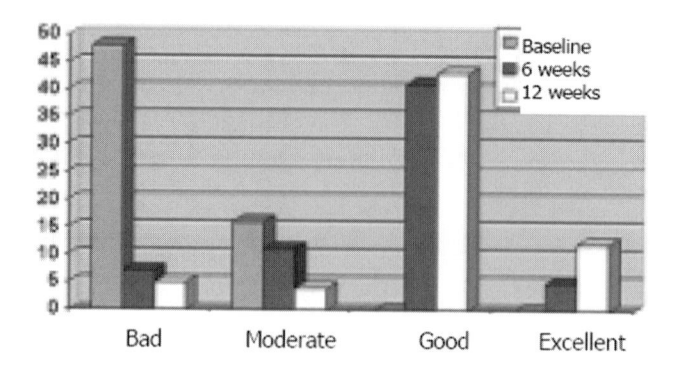

Figure 2. Change in Roles and Maudsley Score.

Nirschl et al. analyzed cortisone injections in 199 patients enrolled in a randomized double-blinded placebo-controlled trial. Two days after injection, patients improved 2.3 points on the VAS compared to 1.4 points in the placebo group. One month after intervention, improvement was found down 2.4 points compared to 1.9 points after sham injection. Finally, 52% improved after 2 days versus 33% in the placebo group, and 54% one month after injection compared to 49% after placebo[8].

Another randomized trial was performed by Smidt et al. The authors compared corticoid injections to physiotherapy and a wait-and-see policy. One hundred eighty-five patients were randomly assigned to one of the treatments. Six weeks after intervention, the success rate was 92% for injection versus 47% for physiotherapy and 32% for the wait-and-see period. Injections proved significantly better than the other treatments. However, the relapse rate was also correspondingly high. Fifty-two weeks after treatment only 69% reported to be pain free for injection versus 91% for physiotherapy and 83% for the wait-and-see period. No significance could be detected between the different options[9].

A large variety of surgical approaches are known as well, but evidence is much less compared to non-invasive techniques. Most studies were conducted retrospectively with heterogeneous patient groups. Finally all studies published 80% improvement overall but without any evidence[10].

Ko et al. conducted a prospective study. They enrolled a total of 56 tennis elbow patients. Shockwave therapy was performed with 1000 impulses at a voltage of 14 kV. The therapy was administered using the OssaTron machine from HMT. Twelve weeks after treatment, 13.2% reported their condition as very good, 44.7% as good, 36.8% as satisfactory and 5.3% remained unchanged or poor. At the follow-up examination 24 weeks after ESWT, 30.8% were scored as very good, 42.3% as good and 26.9% as satisfactory. None of the patients deteriorated[7].

In a prospective study, Decker et al. treated 85 patients with chronic therapy-resistant epicondylitis humeri radialis three times at one-week intervals. After local anesthesia with 3 ml Mepivacain 1%, treatment was performed with an energy flux density of 0.05 to 0.18 mJ/mm^2. The mean follow-up time was 30.7 months. Outcome measurement was performed using the VAS rating system and the Roles and Maudsley score. In the post-exam VAS improvement totaled 4.5 points and 30.8% of patients scored themselves as very good, 42.3% as good, 11.5% as satisfactory and 15.4% as poor[11].

With a total of 71.9% very good and good results after 6 weeks and 85.9% after 12 weeks, our findings correspond with the studies already published. No deterioration was found in any of the patients. Even though local pressure pain improved less in VAS versus the other criteria, this did not affect activity.

With regard to the treatment of epicondylitis with focused low-energy shockwave therapy, excellent clinical prospective randomized placebo-controlled studies now exist. However, neither the work group of Haake [17] nor that of Speed [18] were able to produce evidence of efficacy while other groups found a difference in favor of ESWT[7, 19, 20].

Until now, no high quality studies were available on the use of radial ESWT for the treatment of chronic radial epicondylitis. The efficacy of rESWT is still considered controversial. However, studies published so far allow us to entertain the justified assumption that rESWT can be used as a non-operative treatment option prior to any interventional technique.

In summary, radial extracorporeal shockwave therapy (rESWT) can be recommended for epicondylitis humeri radialis. Results published so far stated efficacy as well as safety

Literature

1. Runge F: Zur Genese und Behandlung des Schreibkrampfes. Berliner Klinische Wschr. 1873: 10: 245
2. Hohmann G: Das Wesen und die Behandlung des sogenannten Tennisellenbogens. Münch. Med. Wschr. 1933: 80: 250-252
3. Rompe J-D: Extrakorporale Stosswellentherapie. Grundlagen, Indikation, Anwendung. Chapman & Hall 1997: 83
4. Hipp EG, Plötz W, Thiemel G: Orthopädie und Traumatologie. Thieme 2003: 532
5. Putz R, Müller-Gerbl M: Anatomie und Pathologie der Sehnen. Orthopäde 1995: 24: 180-186
6. Loew H, Rompe J-D: Stosswellenbehandlungen bei orthopädischen Erkrankungen. Enke Verlag Stuttgart 1998: 30
7. Ko J-H, Chen H-S, Chen L-M: Treatment of lateral epicondylitis of the elbow with shockwaves. Clin Orthop 2001: 60-67
8. Nirschl RP, Rodin DM, Ochiai DH, Maartmann-Moe C: Iontophoretic administration of dexamethasone sodium phosphate for acute epicondylitis. AJSM 2003: 31: 189-195
9. Smidt N, van der Windt DA, Assendelft WJ, Deville WL, Korthals-de-Bos IB. Bouter LM: Corticosteroid injecions, physiotherapy, or a wait-and-see policy for lateral epicondylitis: a randomsed controlled trial. Lancet 2002: 23: 657-62
10. Rompe J-D: Extrakorporale Stosswellentherapie. Grundlagen, Indikation, Anwendung. Chapman & Hall 1997: 87-88
11. Decker T, Kuhne B, Göbel F: Extrakorporale Stosswellentherapie (ESWT) bei Epicondylitis humeri radialis. Kurz- und mittelfristige Ergebnisse. Orthopäde 2002: 31: 633-636
12. Chard MD, Hazleman B (1989) Tennis elbow- a reappraisal. Br J Rheum 28:186-190
13. Koydl P, Voigt K, Kochte E (1983) Diagnostische und therapeutische Probleme der Epicondylitis humeri. Orthopädische Praxis 1:26-28
14. Totkas D, Noack W (1995) Bedeutung des Radialiskompressionssyndrom (RKS) für die Diagnostik und operative Therapie der sogenannten Epikondylitis humeri radialis and (Epic. hum. rad.). Z Orthop Ihre Grenzgeb 133:317-22
15. Assendelft W, Hay E, Adshead R, Bouter L (1996) Corticosteroid injections for lateral epicondylitis: a systematic overview. Br J Gen Pract 46:209-216
16. Maier M, Steinborn M, Schmitz C, Stabler A, Kohler S, Veihelmann A, Pfahler M, Refior HJ. Extracorporeal shockwave therapy for chronic lateral tennis elbow—prediction of outcome by imaging. Arch Orthop Trauma Surg. 2001 Jul;121(7):379-84.
17. Haake M, Konig IR, Decker T, Riedel C, Buch M, Muller HH; Extracorporeal Shockwave Therapy Clinical Trial Group.:Extracorporeal shockwave therapy in the treatment of lateral epicondylitis : a randomized multicenter trial. J Bone Joint Surg Am. 2002 Nov;84-A(11):1982-91.
18. Speed CA, Richards C, Nichols D, Burnet S, Wies JT, Humphreys H, Hazleman BL. Extracorporeal shockwave therapy for tendonitis of the rotator cuff. A double-blind, randomised, controlled trial. J Bone Joint Surg Br. 2002;84:509-12
19. Rompe, J.D., C. Hopf, K. Küllmer, et al.:Analgesic effect of corporal shockwave therapy on chronic tennis elbow. JBJS Vol. 78 B (2) March (1996) 233 ff
20. Hammer DS, Rupp S, Ensslin S, Kohn D, Seil R. Extracorporal shockwave therapy in patients with tennis elbow and painful heel. Arch Orthop Trauma Surg 2000;120(5-6):304-7

rESWT – Benefit in the Treatment of Tendinopathies

H. de Labareyre, G. Saillant

It is becoming difficult to talk about the treatment of tendinopathies without raising the possibility of treatment with shockwaves (SW). This technique which has developed recently is still relatively unknown. A few concepts need to be explained about the presumed mechanisms of action to at least partially explain the therapeutic effects which are seen. We describe the results obtained from a series of 467 patients treated with radial SW during 4 years.

Presumed mechanism of action

We did not have the advantage of radial SW experimentation on animals prior to its use in human beings. Use in a veterinary environment was started in parallel to use in human beings (horse-racing) and there are still only few histological data (8-10) in the setting of so-called extra-corporeal SW. Our understanding about the mechanisms of action is therefore in the hypothetical stage.

The role of SW is probably related to that of certain "rough" physiotherapy techniques which are recognised to be effective (Cyriax deep transverse massages, de-fibrosing massages, etc.) and combine both a mechanical action and a biochemical analgesic and/or local anti-inflammatory action. It has been shown by echo-Doppler that local hypervascularization is produced after an extra-corporeal SW session on the rotator cuff[9]. This is liable to increase local metabolism. Events occur as if the SW create fresh micro-injuries which are liable to heal in a second stage, conversely to a chronic non-progressive desperately painful injury (this principle is used in the treatment of some pseudarthroses).

Methods

We have used the Swiss DolorClast® in the setting of a sports traumatology consultation service since July 1999, very cautiously initially and then far more readily because of the scarcity of side effects and the complete absence of clinical worsening in patients suffering from lower limb tendinopathies. Poor initial experience in the treatment of lateral epicondylitis led us to stop our study in this indication for 2 years before re-starting it using less aggressive parameters.

Teatment protocol

There are three device parameters: the number of shocks applied, their frequency and their energy level. As we wished to keep within the most reproducible protocol setting as possible we made our initial choices guided by previous Swiss and German studies. These choices represented a "gamble" as the parameters chosen were not necessarily those which were liable to produce the best results. Some were slightly modified during our evaluation and other studies are currently ongoing.

Device parameters used

Calcaneal tendon, plantar aponeurosis and high enthesopathy of the hamstrings muscles: 2000 shocks, 9 Hz, 2.5 bar

Calcaneal enthesopathy, patellar tendonitis, lateral and medial epicondylitis: 2000 shocks, 15 Hz, 1.5 bar (an attempt using 4 Hz on the patellar tendon was not satisfactory) (if tolerance is good we gradually increase the pressure to 2 or even 2.5 bar)

Frequency of sessions – number of sessions

The protocol chosen involved 1 session per week most frequently and twice per week for high level sportsmen/women, with a total number of sessions up to 6 or less.

We reduced the recommended time between two sessions, which was two weeks, as we wished to offer a relatively short term treatment which is invariably better appreciated by populations of sporting patients. We therefore obtained a maximum treatment time of 18 days for high level sportsmen/women and 36 days for others. We did not observe any intolerance reactions as a result of shortening the period between two sessions.

Objective

Our objective was to demonstrate that if radial shockwaves were effective in the treatment of tendinopathies, they could also be effective by using a smaller number of sessions. For this reason we limited our protocol to a maximum of 6 sessions. The patient could decide to stop his treatment sooner when he felt a sufficient improvement.

After the treatment and the 6 weeks following, it is clear that in cases of partial improvement, which were considered to be inadequate by the patient, a few additional sessions were able to improve the result. We have conducted this experiment on many occasions although previously results were always defined as poor.

Application force on the applicator tip

We always exerted the maximum pressure tolerated by the patient on the treatment head (feed-back control using the pain), on the most painful area without sweeping. We did not use contact gel initially although we subsequently used it systematically (following technical demonstrations by the physicists from the EMS company), and gained a favorable outcome from its use. On the other hand, we never used local anesthesia. The wide head (20 mm) must be used as the 5mm applicator may cause skin lesions.

Concomitant treatment

The patient was requested not to follow any concomitant treatment except for wearing heel supports, which were recommended in all cases for calcaneal tendinopathies, and wearing an inextensible bracelet at the top of the forearm for elbow tendinopathies.

No indication	Contraindications
• Bursitis • Tenosynovitis • Painful syndromes without validated tendinopathies	• Circulatory disorders • Anti-coagulant therapies • Pregnancy • Children – growth disorders • Local tumors • Local neurological disorders

Table 1. Contraindications.

Sporting activities

Rest was not requested. Quite in contrast, patients were required to try to continue sporting activities provided that their pain did not return during exercise. We did however allow warming up and cooling down pains. This choice was logical with respect to the presumed mechanism of action of SW: if micro-injuries are created, reasonable continuation of activities guides healing towards improved functional quality which would not be achieved by rest alone.

This choice is debatable and may in part be responsible for the very average (i.e. modest) results which we obtained for certain locations. We shall return to this further on.

Indications and contraindications

Apart from contraindications on principle (pregnancy, children, local tumor disease) we felt it was more important to place the emphasis on local neurological or circulatory disorders, coagulation disorders and anti-coagulant therapies, and algodystrophies. We did not have an upper age limit (Table 1).

Our series included mostly tendinopathies of the lower limb (84%): calcaneal tendinopathies, plantar aponeurositis (and probably also incorrectly labelled talalgia, liable to reduce the performance of the treatment), high enthesopathies of the hamstrings muscles (all proven by MRI) and patellar tendinopathies. Elbow tendinopathies were not as prevelant (16%) because we started our study later.

The length of follow-up is still too short for the shoulder tendinopathies and a large study is currently ongoing in a rheumatological setting. The possibility of destroying rotator cuff calcifications which is envisaged by the promoters of the technique by extrapolation from the destruction of urinary calculi is a reality, although it is not obtained in all cases[7]. The purely analgesic effect of the treatment is clearly not to be ignored.

Evaluation of the results

Our evaluation is based on 467 patients with figures updated in September 2003. All performed without any accompanying therapy. See Table 2.

Indication	VS + S	I + D
Corporeal calcaneal Tendon. (nodular or fusiform) n = 205	74.6 %	25.4 %
mean number of sessions	4	4.5
Calcaneal tendon insertion. n = 35	68.6 %	31.4 %
mean number of sessions	4.1	5.1
Plantar aponeurositis. n = 73	67.1 %	32.9 %
mean number of sessions	4	4.5
Hamstring enthesopathy. n = 25	76 %	24 %
mean number of sessions	4.4	4.5
Patellar tendon. n = 51	52.,9 %	47.1 %
mean number of sessions	3.3	3.9
Epicondylitis humeri radialis. n = 50	58 %	42 %
mean number of sessions	4.3	5.3
Epicondylitis humeri ulnaris. n = 12	61.5 %	38.5 %
mean number of sessions	4.7	5.1

VS + S = Very Satisfactory + Satisfactory; I + D = Inadequate + Disappointing
Table 2. Results.

Discussion

The results obtained should be compared to those which we have published previously[3-6]. The 24 patients (5%) who could not be re-contacted were considered as lost to follow-up. All evaluations were performed a minimum of 6 weeks after the final session. This waiting time is the necessary time for the healing of the micro-lesions we have created with SW.

The rESWT was well tolerated by all patients in our protocol. Only a few patients with lateral epicondylitis or experienced severe pain from use of the small 5mm applicator, which was then modified to the large one. None of the patients with lower limb tendinopathies got worse after rESWT using the described parameters. We should highlight that the satisfactory results were obtained with a limited number of sessions. The mean number of sessions was between 4 and 5, representing treatment for 22 to 29 days if sessions are separated by one week. This is less constraining for the patient, both in terms of time and cost.

The sessions are undoubtedly painful, although this is not an obstacle to treatment. We did not observe immediate side-effects (wounds, bruising) using the large head and the parameters chosen. The delayed side effects (hyperalgic reaction, oedema, ecchymoses) were minor and occurred in approximately 10% of cases.

It is clear from our results that all the tendons do not respond in the same way to the SW, although it is possible that these figures may be modified using different protocols. The table shows results for calcaneal enthesopathies and even for the patellar tendon after changing the force and frequency of shocks. The initial results were considerably poorer. Other authors have obtained different, better results using different parameters[1]. Many older German publications have reported very satisfactory results.

We have looked for predictive factors affecting the results from our 120 initial cases of calcaneal tendinopathy[6]. Neither patient age, length of history of symptoms, type of tendinopathy, or sporting level showed any impact. Results were better in women than in men although the female population was considerably smaller.

It is currently not possible to provide a definitive assessment for some of our groups of diseases because of their small size.

A few comments are needed about our choice to permit the continuation of sporting activities provided that pain was respected.

Although it is easy for a long distance runner to stop his/her activities as soon as pain develops, this is a highly theoretical concept when the sport involves a more "explosive" activity. In the former situation the patient does not inflict any true additional suffering on his/her tendon and we consider that this is a help to radial SW treatment, although in the latter situation (in a football or tennis player for example) it is possible that the sportsman/woman can greatly exceed the resistance threshold of their tendon with a specific action and maintain the damage process, which will adversely affect treatment. We are in the process of changing our approach to limit "explosive" activities.

Conclusion

A new arrival in the range of treatments available for use in tendinopathies, radial extracorporeal shockwave therapy is a non-invasive technique and provides not insignificant results. The efficacy of relatively short term treatments and the ability to continue physical activities in a controlled manner are significant arguments towards offering this technique to the population of sportsmen/women, although this is not the only indication.

Although we have tested this technique in isolation, it is possible that results may be improved by associating it with conventional treatments.

Literature

1. Brunet-Guedj E, Brunet B, Girardier J, Renaud E: Traitement des tendinopathies chroniques par ondes de choc radiales J Traumatol Sport, 2002, 19, 239-243
2. Gremion G, Augros R, Gobelet Ch, Leyvraz PF : Efficacité de la thérapie par ondes de choc extra-corporelle dans les tendinopathies rebelles. J Traumatol Sport, 1999, 16, 117-121
3. Labareyre H (de), Saillant G : Evaluation de l'efficacité des traitements par ondes de choc radiales sur les tendinopathies du membre inférieur chez le sportif. Le spécialiste de Médecine du Sport, 2000, 28, 34-40
4. Labareyre H (de), Saillant G : Tendinopathies calcanéennes ; formes cliniques et évaluation de l'efficacité des ondes de choc radiales. J Traumatol Sport, 2001, 18, 59-69

5. Labareyre H (de), Saillant G : Tendinopathies du membre inférieur chez le sportif ; intérêt du traitement par ondes de choc radiales. Reflexions Rhumatologiques, 2002, 47, 40-42
6. Labareyre H (de), Saillant G : A propos du traitement des ondes de choc radiales ; actualisation des résultats. J Traumatol Sport, 2002, 19, 244-246
7. Noel E : Prise en charge des calcifications de la coiffe des rotateurs. 4ème Symposium de Rhumatologie, « Tête, Cou, Epaule », Paris, May 2002
8. Orhan Z, Alper M, Akman Y et al: an experimental study of extracorporeal shockwaves in treatment of tendon injuries; preliminary report. J Orthop Sci, 2001, 6, 566-570
9. Peers K, Brys P, Lysens R: Power Doppler sonography measurement of tendon vascularity after ESWT. Muskuloskeletale Stosswellentherapie, Mainz, March 2001
10. Wang CJ, Ko JY, Chen HS: Shockwave-enhanced neovascularization at the tendon-bone junction; an experiment in dogs. J Foot Ankle Surg, 2002, 41, 16-22
11. Wang CJ, Wang FS, Yang KD, Weng LH, Hsu CC, Huang CS, Yang LC: Shockwave therapy induces neovascularization at the tendon-bone junction. A study in rabbits. J Orthop Res, 2003, 21, 984-989

25

Different Results in Repetitive Low Energy ESWT for Chronic Plantar Fasciitis - The Effect of Local Anesthesia?

Jan-Dirk Rompe,* Vinzenz Auersperg,** Gerold Labek**
and Ludger Gerdesmeyer***

The term "plantar fasciitis" refers to inflammatory conditions of the plantar fascia (fasciitis) on the calcaneus and/or tendons of the planta pedis (tendinitis).

Pain achieves clinical relevance when it passes the pain threshold while walking barefoot, while taking first steps in the morning or while walking after rest. Typically pressure pain may be triggered by palpation above the tuberculum tibiale of the calcaneum. This pressure point on the insertion area of the plantaraponeurosis prompted Woolnough to speak of "tennis heel" in reference to the term "tennis elbow."

Like patients with tennis elbow, patients with "tennis heel" and persistent subcalcanear pain only rarely require surgery. Cryotherapy, shoe inlays and shoe modifications, night splints, soft pads, stretching exercises, oral NSAR and/or local steroid injections are effective in acute cases. An interruption in training is advised for the athlete. A polypragmatic therapy regimen includes NSAR, ultrasound, phonophoresis, iontophoresis and steroid injections but cast immobilization is not advised. The course of the disease itself is often protracted. Radiation therapy is controversial. Risks, especially linked to steroid injections, are soft tis-

---

* *Orthopedic Dept. University of Mainz*
** *Orthopedic Dept. University of Linz*
****Orthopedic and Traumatology Dept. Technical University of Munich*

sue calcification, rupture of the plantar fascia and local infections such as osteomyelitis. Success rates between 75% and 100% have to be assessed carefully because prospective studies including control groups are not available. In many studies the sample size is insuffcient, follow-up often does not exceed 24 weeks and uniform evaluation criteria are not available. However, it is well accepted to prefer non invasive procedures to the surgical option.

More than ten years ago, German teams directed by Dahmen [1] and Schleberger [2] were the first to use extracorporeal shockwaves (known since the pioneering work of Chaussy) in pilot studies for musculoskeletal disorders. The impact of low energy ESWT in plantar fasciitis is controversial.

In a placebo-controlled pilot study on 30 patients, Rompe et al. [4] reported a drop in local pain from 80 points on the Visual Analog Scale (with a range from 0-100 points) to 21 points 6 months after ESWT. They performed 3 session of low energetic ESWT but no local anesthetics were used. Compared to active treatment, the placebo patient group reported a drop from 75 points at baseline down to 60 points.

Rompe et al. [5] included 112 patients in a prospective randomized controlled pilot study. Patients in Group I (therapy group) got three treatments of 1000 impulses of low energy flux density shockwaves without any local anesthesia. Patients enrolled in Group II (control group) received 10 impulses.

Six months after ESWT, 58% of the therapy group and 11% of the control group reported an excellent or good result. Local pain in Group I went down from 77 to 19 points, in Group II from 79 to 77 points. In Group I, 50% of the patients were completely free from pain but none were found in the control group (Group II). The results were significantly different. After 5 years, significance was no longer measurable between both groups. By this time 13% of the 38 follow-up patients in the therapy group required surgery compared to 58% of 40 follow-up patients in the control group.

The results of this study were contradicted by Buchbinder et al. [6] They enrolled 166 patients in a multicentered double-blinded placebo-controlled study. Patients received low energy ESWT three times at weekly intervals up to a total dose of at least 1.0 mJ/mm^2 or an identical placebo treatment. After 3 months both groups had improved similarly; a difference between the groups was not found.

Rompe et al. [7] conducted a randomized placebo-controlled study on 45 runners. After three applications of 2100 impulses of low energy flux density shockwaves without local anesthesia, the primary criterion defined as pain during first steps in the morning dropped down from 6.9 to 2.1 points in the verum group and from 7.0 to 4.7 points in the placebo group within 6 months after ESWT. Even after 12 months, the group difference of 1.5 and 4.4 points respectively remains highly significant. After 6 months the pain value was reduced by more than half in 63% and 30% respectively of patients (secondary criterion). After one year the pain value was reduced by more than half in 81% and 37% of patients respectively.

Haake et al. [8] reported on a prospective randomized multicentered study to analyze evidence of ESWT in plantar faciitis. A total of 271 patients were randomly assigned to verum therapy (three applications of 4000 impulses of 0.08 mJ/mm^2 at two-week intervals under local anesthesia) or identical placebo (insertion of a PE foil between the shockwave unit and heel with an otherwise identical treatment protocol). In a non-validated Roles and Maudsley score, 33.6% of the verum group and 30.5% of the placebo group obtained an excellent or good result after 12 weeks but the difference did not pass the level of significance. The use of local anesthesia as a systematic bias effect was considered partly responsible for the negative result of the Haake study.

Labek et al. [9] therefore studied, in a three-part prospective randomized single-blinded pilot study on 20 patients with chronic fasciitis, the results of three sessions of low-energy ESWT with 1500 impulses at 0.09 mJ/mm^2 at daily intervals without local anesthesia (Group I), three applications of low energy ESWT with 1500 impulses at 0.09 mJ/mm^2 at daily intervals with local anesthesia (Group II) and three sessions of low energy ESWT with 1500 impulses of 0.18 mJ/mm^2 at daily intervals with local anesthesia (Group III). A six-week interval without any therapy was advised. The primary criterion was defined as pain symptoms in the morning as rated on a 10-point Visual Analog Scale. Furthermore, efficacy was analyzed by evaluating the number of patients with a subjective improvement of at least 50% without any concomitant therapy in accordance with the classification in stages 6 or 7 of the 7-stage Auersperg score. All groups reported an improvement in pain symptoms. Statistically significant differences between Group I and Groups II and III were found in terms of the primary criterion (VAS of first steps in the morning). A success rate of at least 60% improvement indicated the excellent outcome from Group I. These patients showed significant superiority compared to Group II (29.6%) as well as Group III (36.3%) even in terms of the Auersperg score.

Criteria	3 month (95% CI) Group I ESWT without LA	Goup II ESWT with LA	Group difference (95% CI) Group I vs Group II	P-value
Pain during stand-up-load [0-10]	0.67 (0.52 - 0.81)	0.29 (0.15 - 0.44)	0.37 (0.17 - 0.58)	<.001
No of patients with ≥50% improvement	0.60 (0.44 - 0.74)	0.29 (0.16 - 0.46)	0.31 (0.10 - 0.52)	.005
No of patients with ≥50% improvement	0.67 (0.51 - 0.80)	0.24 (0.12 - 0.40)	0.43 (0.21 - 0.63)	.001

LA=Local anesthesia; CI=Confidence interval
Table 1. Number of patients showing at least 50 % improvement compared to baseline.

On the basis of the data of the Austrian pilot study, Rompe et al. [10] conducted a confirmatory randomized placebo-controlled study after an adequate sample size calculation was performed. Eighty-six patients were enrolled who suffered from chronic plantar fasciitis. They received repetitive low energy ESWT without local anesthesia (Group I, n=45; 3 treatments of 2000 impulses with 0.09 mJ/mm^2 at weekly intervals) or an identical ESWT with local anesthesia (Group II, n=41). The primary criterion was defined as pain during first steps in the morning 3 months after ESWT. Outcome was measured on the numeric analog scale in terms of morning pain. No differences were found at baseline in terms of efficacy criteria. After 3 months, the mean pain value was 2.2 ± 2.0 points for Group I and 4.1 ± 1.5 points for patients assigned to Group II. This difference was statistically significant as well as the overall successrate defined as improvement of at least a 50% pain reduction. For Group I 67% reported such a reduction and for Group II 29%. (Table 1)

Animal experiments conducted by Ohtori [11], Takahashi [12, 13] and Maier [14, 15] found that ESWT is able to destroy selectively unmyelinized sensory afferences but only in the shockwave focus. The use of local anesthesia inhibits correct focusing at least in the case of low-energy application and may therefore lead to a limitation of the changes described above. It is also known that local anesthesia is capable of significantly reducing hyperfusion induced by (mechanical) pain irritation. This may have impact in terms of blood supply at the tendon-bone interface following low-energy ESWT as described by Wang. Furthermore, local anesthesics have a negative impact on the activation of central pain-inhibiting neuromodulatory mechanisms. Once again, they can only be activated on the point of pain when focusing is precise.

In summary, the use of of local anesthesia is recently discussed to compromise the positive effects of ESWT for musculoskeletal indications. Local anesthesics should no longer be used to blind patients in shockwave trials. When applying low energy shockwaves, local anesthesia should not be used until further animal experiments and clinical studies have been conducted.

Literature

1. Dahmen GP, Meiss L, Nam VC, Skruodies B. Extrakorporale Stoßwellentherapie (ESWT) im knochennahen Weichteilbereich an der Schulter. Extracta Orthopaedica 1992; 15:25-28.
2. Schleberger R, Senge T. Non-invasive treatment of long bone pseudarthrosis by shockwaves (ESWL). Arch Orthop Trauma Surg 1992; 111:224-227
3. Chaussy C, Eisenberger F, Wanner K, Forssmann F, Hepp W, Schmiedt E, Brendel W. The use of shockwaves for the destruction of renal calculi without direct contact. Urol Res 1976; 4:181-188.
4. Rompe JD, et al. Low-energy extracorporeal shockwave therapy for painful heel. Arch Orthop Trauma Surg 1996; 115:75-79.
5. Rompe JD, Schoellner C, Nafe B. Evaluation of low energy extracorporeal shockwave application and treatment in chronic plantar fasciitis. J Bone Joint Surg 2002; 84-A: 335-341.
6. Buchbinder R, et al. Ultrasound-guided extracorporeal shockwave therapy for plantar fasciitis. JAMA 2002; 288: 1364-1372.
7. Rompe JD, et al. Shockwave application for chronic plantar fasciitis in running athletes – a prospective, randomized, placebo- controlled trial. Am J Sports Med 2003; 31:268-275.
8. Haake M, et al. Extracorporeal shockwave therapy for plantar fasciitis: randomised controlled multicentre trial. BMJ 2003 ; 327:75-79.
9. Labek G, et al. Einfluß von Energie und Lokalinfiltration auf klinisches Outcome nach ESWT bei plantarem Fersensporn. Vortrag, 2. Dreiländertreffen der Österreichischen, Schweizer und Deutschen Gesellschaften für Orthopädische ESWT, Linz, 2002.
10. Rompe JD, et al. Low-energy shockwave application without local anesthesia is more efficient than low-energy extracorporeal shockwave application with local anesthesia in the treatment of chronic plantar fasciitis. Persönliche Mitteilung.
11. Ohtori S. et al. Shockwave application to rat skin induces degeneration and reinnervation of sensory nerve fibres. Neurosci Lett 2001; 315:57-60.
12. Takahashi N, et al. Application of shockwaves to rat skin decreases calcitonin gene-related peptide immunoreactivity in dorsal root ganglion neurons. Auton Neurosci 2003; 107:81-84.

13. Takahashi N, et al. The mechanism of pain relief in extracorporeal shockwave therapy. Poster # 448, AAOS Annual Meeting San Francisco, 2004. http://www.aaos.org/wordhtml/anmt2004/poster/p448.htm.
14. Maier M, et al. Substance P and prostaglandin E2 release after shockwave application to the rabbit femur. Clin Orthop 2003; 406:237-245.
15. Maier M, et al. Selective loss of unmyelinated and small myelinated fibers within the femoral nerve and reduction in substance P production in dorsal root ganglia L5 to L7 following high-energy extracorporela shockwave application to the ventral side of the distal femur of rabbits. Pain 2004, in press.
16. Wang CJ, et al. Shockwave therapy induces neovascularization at the tendon-bone junction. A study in rabbits. J Orthop Res 2003; 21:984-989.
17. Petrovic P, Ingvar M. Imaging cognitive modulation of pain processing. Pain 2002; 95:1-5.

26

Morton's Interdigital Neuroma: Indications, ESWT Technique, and Clinical Experience

Lowell Scott Weil, Jr., D.P.M., M.B.A., F.A.C.F.A.S.[1]
and Thomas S. Roukis, D.P.M., A.A.C.F.A.S.[2]

Introduction

Morton's interdigital neuroma (a.k.a., anterior metatarsalgia, interdigital neuritis, Morton's toe, and Morton's disease) is one of the most common nerve problems afflicting the foot, being documented as the cause of forefoot symptomatology in 9.3% of patients presenting to one foot and ankle surgeon practice[1]. This condition was originally described by Durlacher [2] in 1845 and later by Morton [3] in 1876. Historically, a myriad of etiologies have been proposed; however, they can essentially be divided into anatomical and mechanical factors (Table 1).

The most common clinical presentation is a that of a middle-aged female patient complaining of pain, described as a burning, tingling, throbbing, cramping, fullness, within her forefoot which is aggravated in shoes with a narrow toe-box and high-heel[7, 17-19]. This type of shoe gear increases the plantar pressure in the forefoot under the metatarsal heads and tethers the interdigital nerve since the digits assume a more dorsiflexed/extended position[19]. Alternatively, the pain sensation may range from complete anesthesia to severe lancinating pain within a specific interdigital space and/or adjacent digits, which radiates proximally into the

---

[1] *Fellowship Director, Weil Foot and Ankle Institute, 1455 E. Golf Road, Des Plaines, Illinois 60016 U.S.A.*
[2] *Staff Member, Weil Foot & Ankle Institute*

medial arch or distally along the digital branches. The patient may describe the sensation of walking on a "pea-sized lump," often likened to a rolled or bunched-up sock. Usually, the symptoms are intermittent and somewhat relieved by rest and/or removing the shoe gear and massaging the forefoot[18, 19].

Physical examination typically reveals no actual sensory loss within the interdigital space or within the digits themselves. Additionally, there is typically no evidence of intrinsic muscle atrophy or cramping[18]. Reproduction of the patient's symptomatology can usually be induced through dorsal and plantar compression of the involved interdigital space (pinch test), medial and lateral compression of the forefoot (lateral squeeze test), medial and lateral compression of the forefoot with repeated dorsiflexion of the lesser digits (Gauthier test), and/or direct palpation of the web space with a pencil eraser sized instrument (Straub test)[18, 19]. These tests are considered positive if they reproduce the patient's symptomatology within the involved interdigital space. The most widely utilized and recognized clinical test involves simultaneously performing dorsal and plantar compression of the interdigital space (pinch test) with medial and lateral compression of the forefoot (lateral squeeze test). This has been coined "Mulder's test" and is considered positive when a palpable and/or audible "click" is present within the interdigital space which reproduces the patient's symptomatology[1, 3, 18, 19].

Classically, Morton's neuroma is found in the third interdigital space between 50% [7] and 91% [20] of the time, with the second interdigital space being the next most common location[7, 18]. The first and fourth interdigital spaces are rarely, if ever, involved[21]. Although no direct correlation between the development of a symptomatic interdigital neuroma and any particular foot type has been demonstrated [19], there seems to be a predominance of symptomatic interdigital neuroma formation in patients with a flexible forefoot and concomitant gastrocnemius equinus deformity.

Diagnostic tests include local anesthetic nerve block of the suspected interdigital space [17, 18], weightbearing radiographs [23], computed tomography [24], magnetic resonance imaging [25], ultrasonographic imaging [26], and sensory nerve conduction tests[27].

A local anesthetic nerve block is a widely utilized diagnostic method and involves infiltration of a few milliliters of short acting local anesthesia delivered through a dorsal approach just proximal and deep to the deep transverse intermetatarsal ligament. When properly placed, the injection usually results in immediate relief of symptoms, providing confirmation of the diagnosis. If the injection is placed too far distal, or superficial to the deep transverse metatarsal ligament, the injection may fail to provide pain relief, resulting in a false negative response. Although generally considered an essential component of the diagnosis of Morton's interdigital neuroma prior to surgical intervention, Younger and Claridge [22] found that diagnostic nerve blocks did not improve the end result of surgical excision of the neuroma and recommended against its routine use.

Weightbearing radiographs may confirm a space-occupying lesion, which, if large enough, may produce lateral splaying or deviation of the adjacent lesser toes (i.e., Sullivan's or Peace sign) or even a faintly radiopaque shadow at the level of the base of the proximal phalanx of the adjacent lesser digits[18, 23]. Additional radiographic findings include close approximation of the adjacent metatarsal heads, enlarged metatarsal heads, and/or metatarsal heads rotated within the frontal plane[18].

Computed tomography [24], magnetic resonance imaging [25], and ultrasonographic imaging [26] modalities have all been shown to be effective at determining the presence, location, and volume of an interdigital neuroma. However, routine utilization of these modalities to diagnose Morton's interdigital neuroma is not cost-effective (in the case of computerized tomography and magnetic resonance imaging) and is highly user-dependent (in the case of ultrasonographic imaging). The patient's description of symptomatology along with a clinical examination performed by an experienced clinician are still the most reliable means of diagnosing a Morton's interdigital neuroma.

Electrodiagnostic sensory nerve conduction tests for the diagnosis of Morton's interdigital neuromas are not popular due to the extreme difficulty in accurately isolating a single interdigital nerve and the pain involved in performing the study itself[17].

The histopathology characteristic of a Morton's neuroma is that of endoneural sclerosis, perineural fibrosis, edema, fibrinoid degeneration, vessel wall fibrosis, nerve fiber degeneration, amorphous eosinophilic deposition, and demyelination with fibroproliferative changes evident[28]. Therefore, a more accurate description would be a perineural fibroma to distinguish it from traumatic or amputation neuromas, which show signs of axonal sprouting in an attempt to regenerate[28]. Regardless, the term "Morton's interdigital neuroma" is in common use with foot and ankle surgeons throughout the world.

The differential diagnosis of Morton's interdigital neuroma includes: peripheral neuritis, neuropathy, tarsal tunnel syndrome, or lumbosacral disk disease; systemic diseases (rheumatoid arthritis); local soft-tissue space-occupying lesions (rheumatoid nodules, soft-tissue tumors, enlarged adventitial bursae); metatarsal (stress fracture, osseous tumors) or metatarsophalangeal joint pathology (Freiberg's infraction or degenerative joint disease, flexor tendonitis, plantar capsulitis, synovitis or rupture of the metatarsophalangeal plantar plate)[18, 19, 23]. Each of these entities can readily be differentiated from a true Morton's interdigital neuroma by taking an accurate patient history and performing careful physical and clinical examinations.

A myriad of conservative and surgical forms of treatment have been proposed for Morton's interdigital neuroma. Non-operative treatment is always attempted for a period of time prior to entertaining the thought of surgical intervention. Initial treatment is directed towards decreasing pressure on the ball of the foot and correcting any underlying mechanical faults through the use of shoe gear with a wider toe box and lower heel height, tape strapping, metatarsal padding, and functional foot orthosis to control excessive pronation[18, 29]. However, Kilmartin and Wallace [30] found that changing the position of the foot with either pronated or supinated orthoses did not significantly alter the pain associated with a Morton's interdigital neuroma.

Therapeutic injection therapies with vitamin B12 solutions [31], corticosteroid mixtures [32], and ethyl alcohol solutions [18] have all been advocated. Greenfield et al. [17] found that 30% of patients had complete relief and 50% had partial relief following infiltration of a mixture of local anesthetic and corticosteroid. Unfortunately, the recurrence rate is extremely high following a single corticosteroid injection[33]. Although multiple corticosteroid injections increase the improvement of symptoms [17], this practice has the distinct disadvantage of causing hyperpigmentation, thinning of the skin and subcutaneous tissue, and severe fat pad atrophy at the site of injection[34]. More recently, Dockery [18] found that 89% of patients had either complete or partial resolution of symptomatology following a series of between 3 and 7 injections of 0.5 ml of 4% sclerosing solution and 0.5% bupivicane with epinephrine repeated in 5 to 10-day intervals. While encouraging, Dockery's study was not performed as a double-blinded study using a placebo or compared with corticosteroid injections. Additionally, it has been shown that the addition of epinephrine to the bupivicane solution increases nerve axonal degeneration and may in itself be neurotoxic, perhaps responsible for the positive results in Dockery's study rather than the ethyl alcohol[35].

When non-operative interventions prove unsuccessful in alleviating the patient's symptomatology, then operative intervention can be entertained. There are essentially four options for operative intervention. First, the deep transverse intermetatarsal ligament can be transected through either an open or endoscopic approach with preservation of the nerve. Second, an external and/or internal neurolysis of the involved nerve can be performed. Third, transposition of the involved nerve dorsal to the level of the deep transverse intermetatarsal ligament can be performed. Fourth, the nerve can be transected and a neurectomy performed through either a dorsal longitudinal linear, plantar transverse, or plantar longitudinal linear incision with or without transposition of the remaining nerve stalk within adjacent muscle.

This is a preliminary study on the effectiveness of ESWT as a noninvasive alternative to the surgical technique for neurectomy of a primary Morton's interdigital neuroma. The procedure is indicated in the healthy, active patient with a symptomatic Morton's interdigital neuroma, which has failed non-operative treatments. This procedure can be utilized in the presence of severe atrophy of the interspace secondary to corticosteroid injection over-utilization. This procedure is contraindicated in the presence of active superficial or deep infection.

ESWT Technique

The procedure is performed on an outpatient basis with the patient under intravenous sedation. The patient is positioned on the operating table in the supine position. Local anesthesia is performed with 5 cc's of 0.5% Bupivicaine infiltrated in the appropriate interspace proximal to the actual neuroma. The bladder of the ESWT device is placed against the plantar aspect of the appropriate distal interspace with coupling gel. In order to perform exact targeting, the treating physician deeply palpates with dorsal to plantar pressure with one finger into the interspace overlying to region of neuroma. When the ESWT machine is started the physician will feel the "shockwaves" into their finger and know that precise application is occurring. Two thousand shocks at 21 Kv or 0.3 mJ/mm^2 are applied with the physician maintaining accurate targeting throughout.

Immediate weightbearing with normal shoegear is permitted, with return to full activities on the first post-operative day or to tolerance. Patients are prescribed NSAIDs for 2 weeks following the procedure to prevent any post treatment discomfort.

Methods and Materials

A pilot study of 29 patients and 30 feet showed excellent results. All patients had failed appropriate conservative and non-invasive care for their painful neuroma. All patients were candidates for open surgical resection of the neuroma. Patients were given an option of trying the ESWT to treat their painful neuroma. Twenty-nine patients and (30 feet) agreed to this option. Patients were evaluated pre-treatment and post-treatment by a physician and completed a pre-treatment and post-treatment questionnaire.

Results

Patients in the study had suffered with pain for 41 months (10 to 120 months) prior to treatment. Twenty-seven of the 30 feet (90%) were successfully treated by the ESWT. Overall, there was a reduction in patients' VAS from 7.5 to 2.1. In the 27 feet that were successfully treated, the VAS improved from 7.9 to 1.7 with patients stating there was an overall improvement of 92% (75% to 100%). In the 3 feet that failed, 2 patients noted no improvement and 1 patient noted 50% improvement.

Discussion

This preliminary report shows that ESWT may have an important place in the treatment of painful neuromas of the foot. Unlike other aspects of ESWT therapy, the goal of shockwave treatment for neuromas is not to create healing, but to create irreversible damage to the pathologic nerve while not damaging surrounding tissue. Patients are able to avoid the lengthy disability associated with open surgical techniques and eliminate the possible risks and complications which are well documented from surgery.

Further studies evaluating the mechanism of action and long term follow-up will be necessary to predict long term efficacy. Additionally, double-blinded placebo-controlled studies will be necessary to definitively assess the true value of ESWT for the treatment of painful foot neuromas.

Literature

1. Youngswick, F. D. Intermetatarsal neuroma. Clin. Podiatr. Med. Surg. 11(4):579-592, 1994.
2. Durlacher, L. Treatise on corns, bunions, the disease of nails and general management of feet, pp.52, London, 1845.
3. Morton, T.G. A peculiar and painful affection of the fourth metatarsophalangeal joint articulation. Am. J. Med. Sci. 71:35-45, 1876.
4. Betts, L. O. Morton's metatarsalgia: neuritis of the fourth digital nerve. Med. J. Aust. 1:514-515, 1940.
5. Nissen, K. I. Plantar digital neuritis: Morton's metatarsalgia. J. Bone Joint Surg. 31-A:84-94, 1948.
6. Bossley, C. J., Cairney, P. C. The intermetatarsophalangeal bursa: it's significance in Morton's metatarsalgia. J. Bone Joint Surg. 62-B:184-187, 1980.
7. Mann, R. A., Reynolds, J. C. Interdigital neuroma: a critical clinical analysis. Foot Ankle 3:238-243, 1983.
8. Graham, C. E., Graham, D. M. Morton's neuroma: a microscopic evaluation. Foot Ankle 5:150-153, 1984.
9. Jones, J. R., Klenerman, L. A study of the communicating branch between the medial and lateral plantar nerves. Foot Ankle 4(6):313-315, 1984.
10. Levitsky, K. A., Alman, B. A., Jevsevar, D. S. Digital nerves of the foot: anatomic variations and implications regarding the pathogenesis of interdigital neuromas. Foot Ankle 4:208-214, 1993.
11. Sgarlato, T. E. A Compendium of Podiatric Biomechanics, pp. 276, California College of Podiatric Medicine, San Francisco, 1971.
12. Root, M. L., Orien, W. P., Weed, J. H. Abnormal motion of the foot: neuromas, ch. 9. In Normal and Abnormal Function of the Foot, vol. 2, pp. 322-325, Clinical Biomechanics Corp., Los Angeles, 1977.
13. Tate, R. O., Rusin, J. J. Morton's neuroma: its ultrastructural anatomy and biomechanical etiology. J. Am. Podiatr. Assoc. 68:797-807, 1978.
14. Lassman, G. Morton's toe. Clin. Orthop. 142:73, 1979.
15. Gauthier, G. Thomas Morton's disease: a nerve entrapment syndrome. Clin. Orthop. 142:90-92, 1979.
16. Wachter, S. D., Nilson, R. Z., Thul, J. R. The relationship between foot structure and intermetatarsal neuromas. J. Foot Surg. 23:436-439, 1984.
17. Greenfield, J., Rea, J. Jr., Ilfeld, F. W. Morton's interdigital neuroma: indications for treatment by local injections versus surgery. Clin. Orthop. 185:142-144, 1984.
18. Dockery, G. L. The treatment of interdigital neuromas with 4% alcohol sclerosing injections. J. Foot Ankle Surg. 38(6):403-408, 1999.
19. Weinfeld, S. B., Myerson, M. S. Interdigital neuritis: diagnosis and treatment. J. Am. Acad. Orthop. Surg. 4(6):328-335, 1996.
20. Friscia, D. A., Strom, D. E., Parr, J. W. Surgical treatment for primary interdigital neuroma. Orthopedics 14:669-672, 1991.
21. Thompson, F. M., Deland, J. T. Occurrence of two interdigital neuromas in one foot. Foot Ankle 14:15-17, 1993.
22. Younger, A. S., Claridge, R. J. The role of diagnostic block in the management of Morton's neuroma. Can. J. Surg. 41:127-130, 1998.
23. Wu, K. K. Morton's interdigital neuroma: a clinical review of its etiology, treatment, and results. J. Foot Ankle Surg. 35:112-119, 1996.

24. Turan, I., Lindgren, U., Sahlstedt, T. Computed tomography for diagnosis of Morton's neuroma. J. Foot Surg. 30:244-245, 1991.
25. Hoskins, C. L., Sartoris, D. J., Resnick, D. Magnetic resonance imaging of foot neuromas. J. Foot Surg. 31:10-16, 1992.
26. Sobiesk, G. A., Wertheimer, S. J., Schulz, R., Dalfovo, M. Sonographic evaluation of interdigital neuromas. J. Foot Ankle Surg. 36:364-366, 1997.
27. Guiloff, R. J., Seadding, J. W., Klenerman, L. Morton's metatarsalgia: clinical, electrophysiological and histological observations. J. Bone Joint Surg. 66-B:586-591, 1984.
28. Rush, S. Interdigital neuroma: a histopathological perspective. Foot Ankle Review (Official Student Journal of the California College of Podiatric Medicine) 1(1):28-29, 1996.
29. Hirshberg, G. G. A simple cure for Morton's neuralgia. J. Am. Podiatr. Med. Assoc. 90(2):100, 2000.
30. Kilmartin, T. E., Wallace, W. A. Effect of pronation and supination orthosis on Morton's neuroma and lower extremity function. Foot Ankle Int. 15:256-262, 1994.
31. Steinberg, M. D., The use of vitamin B12 in Morton's neuralgia. J. Am. Podiatr. Assoc. 45:41-42, 1955
32. Bennett, G. L., Graham, C. E., Maudlin, D. M. Morton's interdigital neuroma: a comprehensive treatment protocol. Foot Ankle Int. 16:760-763, 1995.
33. Rasmussen, M. R., Kitaoka, H. B., Patzer, G. L. Nonoperative treatment of plantar interdigital neuroma with a single corticosteroid injection. Clin. Orthop. 326:188-193, 1996.
34. Reddy, P. D., Zelicof, S. B., Rutolo, C., Holder, J. Interdigital neuroma. Local cutaneous changes after corticosteroid injection. Clin. Orthop. 317:185-187, 1996.
35. Selander, D., Brattsand, R., Lundborg, G., Nordborg, C., Olsson, Y. Local anesthetics: importance of mode of application, concentration and adrenaline for the appearance of nerve lesions. An experimental study of axonal degeneration and barrier damage after intrafascicular injection or topical application of bupivicane (Marcain). Acta. Anaesthesiol. Scand. 23:127-136, 1979.

27

Extracorporeal Shockwave Therapy (ESWT) in Traumatology

Wolfgang Schaden, Andreas Fischer, Andreas Sailler

Summary

Since December 1998, more than 1,000 patients from 83 referring hospitals with non-unions or delayed healing fractures were treated with ESWT in the Trauma Center Meidling. After shockwave therapy the non-unions were immobilized like acute fractures. This kind of fixation is not appropriate for stable non-unions fixed by osteosynthetic material without clinical or radiological signs of loosening.

At this moment the results of 613 patients are available. Out of these 613 non-unions, 466 (76%) achieved bony healing. Atrophic or oligotrophic non-unions did not show any significant difference in the results in comparison to hyperthrophic or infected non-unions.

Beside the well known side effects of shockwave therapy, such as local swelling, petecheal bleedings and hematoma, no complications were observed. Although the working mechanism of shockwave therapy remains unclear, ESWT is considered as a first line option for non-unions and delayed healing fractures not needing surgical corrections due to its efficacy and the lack of complications. ESWT is less cost intensive and provides more comfort to the patient compared to the surgical procedures.

Introduction

Extracorporeal shockwaves have been used successfully in urology for several decades without major side effects. Despite the high energy flux density used in the process, no significant complications such as malignant degeneration of the treated tissue are known.

It is thanks to the German urologist Haupt [1–4] that this therapy is also used in orthopedics and trauma surgery. Urologists knew from empiric studies that higher energies or a larger number of impulses were required to fragment stones in the ureter and bladder than to disintegrate kidney stones. Neither physicists nor physicians initially had any reasonable explanation. In follow-up x-ray exams to exclude recurrent ureteral or bladder stones, Haupt noticed for the first time in 1986 a bony thickening of the iliac crest where shockwaves had traveled on their way to the calculi. This indicated absorption of shockwaves as well as shockwave induced bony effect at the iliac crest. It appears that shockwaves are suitable to trigger any biological reaction. Haupt demonstrated the osteoinductive effect of shockwaves in animal experiments as he wrote in previous chapters.

Mechanism

While physical properties of the shockwaves have a significant impact in urology in terms of their effect, these were also of primary interest to basic research in the area of orthopedics and trauma surgery.

Mechanical Model

The mechanism of shockwaves may be due to the microlesions which are found after high energetic ESWT in the focused tissue. The shockwaves do not destroy the surrounding soft tissue and therefore trigger repair processes for healing.

This model was also the reason why we [5] used high numbers of impulses (up to 12,000 for long bones in the first application period to treat pseudarthrosis). For technical reasons we were forced to terminate a few treatments at 3,000 to 4,000 impulses. Surprisingly we observed that pseudarthroses were nevertheless (or therefore) brought to heal compared to those treated with a complete high energetic shockwave therapy cycle. This finding coincided with the basic research of Maier [6, 7] who found an optimum osteoinductive effect of shockwaves on the femurs of rats. His analysis demonstrated that osteoinductive effects were already observed if no histological cell damage was found. This led to the fact that worldwide basic research focused increasingly on the biological effect of shockwaves.

Wang from Taiwan [8-19], Russo from Italy [20] and Takahashi from Japan [21, 22] showed that during and after the application of shockwaves, various biologically highly active substances are released in the tissue. The production of nitrogen monoxide (NO), vascular endothelial growth factor (VEGF), bone morphogenetic protein (BMP) and other growth factors were documented. In addition, Maier showed that the effect of shockwaves brings about a reduction in myelinisized nerve cells which may explain the analgesic effect of shockwaves.

As a result, the mechanical model was pushed aside more and more to be replaced by a bio-engineered tissue model.

This model attempts to explain the effect of ESWT as a result of ingrowth of blood vessels and the concomitant release of various growth factors. Improved metabolism in the presence of these growth factors may be responsible for the healing of the chronically inflamed tissue. The reduction in afferent nerve fiber is known to induce the analgesic effect.

ESWT appears to be a technology which may effect bioengineering (production of growth factors).

In trauma surgery these properties are used primarily for the treatment of delayed healing fractures or non-healing fractures (pseudarthrosis). But ESWT is also increasingly used for the treatment of early phases of osteochondritis dissecans [23, 24] and femur head necrosis[25-27].

Patients and Methods

Following a series of pilot studies, the treatment of non-unions and delayed healing fractures with ESWT started in December 1998 at AUVA's Meidling Trauma Center, Austria as part of a major prospective study. From the very beginning, more than 50 patient-specific data were entered in a specially developed database which also allows us to combine widely differing parameters not only for the purpose of quality assurance but also to make it possible to define optimum treatment parameters and other key criteria. This database for documenting the treatment of non-unions with ESWT is available at no charge to all users and can be obtained from the authors.

Since December 1998, more than 1,000 patients from 83 referring clinics and hospitals with non-unions and delayed healing fractures were treated. Today, the results from 613 patients are available, made up of 196 (32%) women and 417 (68%) men. The mean age of the patients was 43.7 (10 to 90 years); the mean age of non-unions was 16.1 months. In 556 cases (91%) non-unions resulted from fractures, in 57 cases (9%) they occurred after osteotomies. One hundred thirty-seven patients (22%) received conservative treatment before shockwave therapy; the other 476 (78%) received primary operative care. In this group, 266 underwent one operation, 120 two, 41 three and 49 four or more surgical interventions involving the bones prior to ESWT. In just 2/3 of the cases (392), the osteosynthesis material was in situ at the time of shockwave therapy. In 62 patients (10%), a deep infection with osteomyelitis was documented prior to ESWT. These patients were prevented from treatment to the acute inflammation, which was identified through clinical investigation and laboratory results.

Exclusion criteria are:

- Coagulopathies
- Epiphyseal plate in focus
- Nerve structures in focus
- Tumor tissue in focus
- Lung tissue in focus
- Pregnancy
- Acute infection

Shockwave therapy was performed with the OssaTron from HMT (High Medical Technologies, Lengwil, Switzerland) and is viewed in principle as a one-time treatment. Depending on the affected region, patients are treated under general, regional or local anesthesia.

The patient is positioned so that the x-ray clearly shows the bony gap in a.p. view. The focus is positioned onto this gap. Between 2,000 and 4,000 impulses are applied (1,000 impulses each per localization) depending on the size of the area to be treated. For all bone treatments we use a voltage of 26 kV, which corresponds to an energy flux density (ED) of 0.38 mJ/mm^2.

Following shockwave therapy, the non-union is immobilized like a fresh fracture. Customarily this is done with casts. In some cases where the non-union is particularly mobile especially in the lower limb, an external Fixater is also placed. This fixation is not necessary if the non-union is supplied with corresponding osteosynthesis material which has not been found to show signs of loosening. Since we can assume that initial healing begins with an ingrowth of the blood vessels, we attempt to avoid micromovements in the non-unions during the first 3 weeks in order to prevent a tearing of the capillaries. If in doubt, this may require a support for the affected extremity during that time. This makes it necessary to fully inform the patients; indeed, due to the analgesic effect of the shockwaves, they are often free from pain immediately following the treatment and therefore are willing to put a full load on the affected extremity. A pseudarthrosis non-union more than 5 mm wide in long bones is to be considered as subject to an unfavorable prognosis.

We commonly treat only those fractures which are older than 3 months (from the date of the accident or of the last operation involving the bone).

Results

Six hundred thirteen non-unions received ESWT, 466 (76%) achieved bony healing (see Table 1). To evaluate the results, x-rays were performed in two planes and the patient was clinically assessed. If in doubt, x-ray in oblique view or CT scans must be done. In small bones (metacarpal, metatarsal) the results can be determined mostly after 2 to 3 months. In long bones, one should wait up to 6 months before evaluating the final result (see Tables 2 and 3).

If symptoms such as bending or load bearing pain as well as swelling, reddening and overheating drop in the early phase (2 to 3 months after ESWT), one can remain confident even if x-ray findings are unclear. In this phase clinical findings take priority over x-rays.

Region	Number	Recovered	Not recovered
Humerus	51 (8%)	34 (67%)	11 (33%)
Radius	36 (6%)	32 (89%)	4 (11%)
Ulna	42 (7%)	29 (69%)	13 (31%)
Scaphoid	85 (14%)	55 (65%)	30 (35%)
Hand	40 (6%)	34 (85%)	6 (15%)
Becken	7 (1%)	6 (86%)	1 (14%)
Femoral neck	5 (1%)	4 (80%)	1 (20%)
Femur	85 (14%)	61 (72%)	24 (28%)
Tibia	181 (30%)	150 (83%)	31 (17%)
Arthrodesis	11 (2%)	5 (45%)	6 (55%)
Fibula	19 (3%)	17 (89%)	2 (11%)
Foot	51 (8%)	39 (76%)	12 (24%)
Total	613 (100%)	466 (76%)	147 (24%)

Table 1. Overall results.

Number	Unsure	Recovered	Not recovered
613 (100%)	81 (13%)	383 (63%)	149 (24%)

TAble 2. Results after 3 months.

Number	Unsure	Recovered	Not recovered
613 (100%)	0	466 (76%)	147 (24%)

Table 3. Results after 6 months.

Region	Number	Recovered	Not recovered
Humerus	1	1	0
Radius	3	3	0
Ulna	3	2	1
Scaphoid	2	0	2
Hand	4	3	1
Femur	9	7 (77%)	2
Tibia	34	25 (76%)	9
Fibula	1	1	0
Arthrodesis	4	4	0
Patella	1	1	0
Total	62	47 (76%)	15 (24%)

Table 4. Infected Non-union.

Of the 62 infected non-unions, 47 (76%) achieved bony healing (see Table 4). In principle, there was no prophylaxis with antibiotics but if the patient was already receiving antibiotic treatment, this was continued. Not a single case was found to bring about a floride infection following ESWT.

If within an appropriate time no bony healing was found, the patient was offered surgical treatment. This was rejected by many, mostly patients who had already undergone an operation, which brought about a relatively high number of second treatments (see Table 5). In exceptional cases, a third and in one case even a fourth treatment was performed (Tables 6 and 7). These patients also included those for whom major non-union surgery was impossible to perform for internal reasons or associated high risk factors.

As expected, the 152 delayed healing fractures (ESWT 3-6 months after the trauma or after the last surgery involving the bone) showed the best results. One hundred thirty-three (88%) achieved healing. Of the 445 non-unions older than six months, 320 (72%) achieved bony healing. Even in the subgroup of 185 non-unions who showed no spontaneous healing tendency more than one year after the last treatment, 132 (71%) achieved bony healing 3 to 6 months following ESWT (see Table 8). The result is relatively constant for non-unions which are 12

Region	Number	Recovered	Not recovered
Humerus	9	7	2
Radius	6	5	1
Ulna	7	3	4
Scaphoid	8	4	4
Hand	5	1	4
Ilium	1	1	0
Femur	14	7	7
Tibia	30	21 (70%)	9
Fibula	1	0	1
Artrodesis	4	0	4
Foot	4	1	3
Total	89	50 (56%)	39 (44%)

Table 5. Second Treatment.

Region	Number	Recovered	Not recovered
Ulna	1	1	0
Femur	2	1	1
Tibia	3	3	0
Arthrodesis	1	0	1
Total	7	5 (71%)	2 (29%)

Total 6. Third Treatment.

Region	Number	Recovered	Not recovered
Femur	1	1	0

Table 7. Fourth Treatment

Duration	Number	Recoverd	Not recovered
> 3 < 6 Months	152 (29%)	133 (88%)	19 (12%)
> 6 < 12 Months	191 (36%)	146 (76%)	45 (24%)
> 12 < 18 Months	85 (16%)	65 (76%)	20 (24%)
> 18 < 24 Months	40 (8%)	30 (75%)	10 (25%)
> 24 < 36 Months	29 (5%)	21 (72%)	8 (28%)
> 36 Months	31 (6%)	16 (52%)	15 (48%)
Total	528 (100%)	411 (78%)	117 (22%)

Table 8. Success rate dependence to duration of non-union (except scaphoid)

to 36 months old (76% to 72% healing rate). In fact, the success rate does not drop significantly (52%) until the non-union is 3 years old since the last operation. One exception is scaphoid since results become increasingly worse with increasing age of the non-union (see Table 9).

Atrophic or oligotrophic non-unions showed no significant difference in the results when compared to hypertrophic or infected non-unions (see Table 10). Of note is also the correlation between the number of impulses and healing success (see Table 11). It shows that the best results are obtained with 3,000 impulses or less. Once again, the scaphoid is an exception: 4,000 impulses proved to be best (see Table 12).

Duration	Number	Recovered	Not recovered
3 – 12 Months	37 (43%)	29 (78%)	8 (22%)
1 – 2 Years	26 (31%)	16 (62%)	10 (38%)
2 – 4 Years	12 (14%)	5 (42%)	7 (58%)
> 4 Years	10 (12%)	5 (50%)	5 (50%)
Total	85 (100%)	55 (65%)	30 (35%)

Table 9. Success rate dependence to duration (Scaphoid).

Discussion

The purpose of any bone fracture treatment is a fully restored functioning of the injured skeletal part and fracture healing in anatomic position in the shortest possible time. Despite highly developed technologies and good primary care, 1% of all bone fractures become non-unions. A "gold surgical standard" is the surgical treatment with resection of the pseudarthrotic tissue, autologeous spongiosa plasty and internal stabilization with osteosynthesis material. These procedures, especially on long bones, are very demanding for the patient, require substantial resources and time, and are very complicated. In the past decades less complicated and less costly alternatives have been sought.

The often required prospective randomized placebo-controlled double-blinded studies are not feasible due to the complexity of pseudarthrosis patients especially because of the problem of meaningful randomization. Even for the classic operative methods ("gold standard") such studies are not available. Even in the large number of our patients with tibia non-unions, only three were identified with a roughly similar x-ray (hypertrophic non-union in the distal third, treated on the day of the accident with unreamed nails). These patients, however, were completely different in terms of age, history of the non-union, the number of previous operations, accompanying diseases, sex, etc. One of the pseudarthroses was to be evaluated as infected, the other two were without clinical relevance. Without any evidence, one of the non-unions was to be assigned to the verum group, one to the placebo group and the third to an operation group and then to compare the results. As is customary in precise scientific analysis, one chooses in such cases the highest possible existing degree of evidence which we believe to meet our extended case collection. For the approval process of non-union treatments, even the highest health authority in the United States (FDA, Food and Drug Administration) requires only that trauma occurred more than 9 months earlier and the last intervention at least 3 months before.

Quality	Duration	Number	Recovered	Not recovered
Atroph/oligotr.	48	291 (55%)	223 (77%)	67 (23%)
Hypertroph	44	177 (34%)	140 (79%)	37 (21%)
Infected	42	60 (11%)	47 (78%)	13 (22%)
Total	46	528 (100%)	411 (78%)	117 (22%)

Table 10. Success rate dependence to qualify of non-union.

Impulses	Duration	Recovered	Not recovered
< = 3,000	163	143 (88%)	20 (12%)
4,000	222	174 (78%)	48 (22%)
6,000	14	7 (50%)	7 (50%)
8,000	34	21 (62%)	13 (38%)
10,000	5	5 (100%)	0
12,000	90	61 (68%)	29 (32%)
Total	528	411 (78%)	117 (22%)

Table 11. Success rate dependence to impulses (except scaphoid).

For all these reasons we are allowed to draw conclusions about the safety and efficacy of ESWT in non-unions from our large patient group especially since other groups [28-36] reported similar results in similar treatments.

Our results (Figure 1) clearly contradicted those of Biedermann [37] who cast doubt on the efficacy of ESWT since it follows only a natural healing process.

Apart from the known side effects of shockwave therapy (local swelling, petechia, hematoma), none of the more than 1,000 patients treated by us suffered complications. ESWT is effective, uncomplicated, less time-consuming and less costly. Even though the very mechanism of shockwave therapy has not yet been fully explored, we consider ESWT to be the therapy of choice, compared to operative treatment, for non-unions and delayed healing bone fractures not requiring surgery.

Impulses	Number	Recovered	Not recovered
< 3,000	27	15 (56%)	12 (44%)
4,000	18	15 (83%)	3 (17%)
6,000	29	19 (66%)	10 (34%)
8,000	11	6 (55%)	5 (45%)
Total	85	55 (65%)	30 (35%)

Table 12. Success rate dependence to impulses (scaphoid).

Literature

1. Haupt G, Haupt A, Senge T. Die Behandlung von Knochen mit extrakorporalen Stosswellen - Entwicklung einer neuen Therapie. Chaussy C, Eisenberger F, Jocham D, Wilbert D (Hrsg), Stosswellenlithotripsie – Aspekte und Prognosen, Attempo Verlag 1993; Tübingen:120-126
2. Haupt G, Haupt A, Gerety B, Chvapil M. Enhancement of fracture healing with extracorporeal shockwaves. AUA Annual Meeting, New Orleans 1990
3. Haupt G. Stosswellen in der Orthopädie. Urologe A, 1997; Nr.3: 233-238
4. Haupt G. Use of extracorporeal shockwaves in the treatment of pseudarthrosis, tendopathy and other orthopaedic diseases. Urology 1997;158:4-11
5. Schaden W, Kuderna H. Extracorporeal shockwave therapy (ESWT) in 37 patients with non-union or delayed osseous union in disphyseal fractures. Chaussy C, Eisenberger F, Jocham D, Wilbert D (Hrsg), High energy shockwaves in medicine, Thieme Verlag 1997; Stuttgart: 121-126
6. Maier M, Milz S, Tischer T, Munzing W, Manthey N, Stabler A, Holzknecht N, Weiler C, Nerlich A, Refior HJ, Schmitz C. Influence of extracorporeal shockwave application on normal bone in an animal model in vivo. Scintigraphy, MRI and histopathology. J Bone Joint Surg Br.2002 May; 84(4): 592-9
7. Maier M, Averbeck B, Milz S, Refior HJ, Schmitz C. Substance P and prostaglandin E2 release after shockwave application to the rabbit femur. Clin. Orthop.2003 Jan; (406):237-45
8. Wang F.S, Wang C.J, Huang H.J, Chung H, Chen R.F, Yang K.D. Physical Shockwave Mediates Membrane Hyperpolarization and Ras Activation for Osteogenesis in Human Bone Marrow Stromal Cells. Biochemical and Biophysical Research Communications 2001; 287:648-655
9. Wang C.J., Hunag H.Y., Pai C.H.. Shockwave-Enhanced Neovascularization at the Tendon-Bone Junction: An Experiment in Dogs. The Journal of Foot & Ankle Surgery 2002 January/February; 1:Vol.41
10. Wang F.S., Yang K.D., Chen R.F., Wang C.J., Sheen-Chen S.M. Extracorporeal shockwave promotes growth and differentiation of bone-marrow stromal cells towards osteoprogenitors associated with induction of TGF-ß1. The Journal of Bone and Joint Surgery 2002 April; Vol 84-B, No.3
11. Wang F.S., Wang J.C., Sheen-Chen S.M., Kuo Y.R., Chen R.F., Yang K.D.. Superoxide Mediates Shockwave Induction of ERK-dependent Osteogenic Transcription Factor (CBFA1) and Mesenchymal Cell Differentiation toward Osteoprogenitors. The Journal of Biological Chemistry, 2002; Vol.277, No.13. Issue of March 29, pp 10931-10937
12. Chen Y.J., Kuo Y.R., Yang K.D., Wang C.J., Hunag H.C., Wang F.S.. Shockwave Application Enhances Pertussis Toxin Protein-Sensitive Bone Formation of Segmental Femoral Defect in Rats. Journal of Bone an Mineral Research, 2003; Vol.18, No. 12
13. Wang F.S., Yang K.D., Kuo Y.R., Wang C.J., Sheen-Chen S.M., Huang H.C., Chen Y.J.. Temporal and spatial expression of bone morphogenetic proteins in extracorporeal shockwave-promoted healing of segmental defect. Bone 32 (2003), 387-396
14. Wang C.J., Wang F.S., Yang K.D., Weng L.H., Hsu C.C., Huang C.S., Yang L.C.. Shockwave therapy induces neovascularization at the tendon-bone junction. A study in rabbits. Journal of Orthopaedic Research 21 (2003); 984 – 989
15. Hsu R.W.W., Tai C.L., Chen C.Y.C., Hsu W.H., Hsueh S.. Enhancing mechanical strength during early fracture healing via shockwave treatment: an animal study. Clinical Biomechanics 18 (2003): S33-S39

16. Chen Y.J., Kuo Y.R., Yang K.D., Wang C.J., Sheen Chen S.M., Huang H.C., Yang Y.J., Sun Y.C., Wang F.S.. Activation of extracellular signal-regulated kinase (ERK) and p38 kinase in shockwave-promoted bone formation of segmental defect in rats. Bone 34 (2004); 466-477
17. Chen Y.J., Wurtz T., Wang C.J., Kuo Y.R., Yang K.D., Huang H.C., Wang F.S.. Recruitment of mesenchymal stem cells and expression of TGF-ß1 and VEGF in the early stage of shockwave-promoted bone regeneration of segmental defect in rats. Journal of Orthopaedic Research. 2004 May; 22(3):526-534.
18. Chen Y.J., Wang C.J., Yang K.D., Kuo Y.R., Huang H.C., Huang Y.T., Sun Y.C., Wang F.S.. Extracorporeal shockwaves promote healing of collagenase-induced Achilles tendinitis and increase TGF-ß1 and IGF-I expression. Journal of Orthopaedic Research. 2004 Jul; 22(4): 854-861.
19. Wang F.S., Wang C.J., Chen Y.J., Chang P.R., Hunag Y.T., Sun Y.C., Huang H.C., Yang Y.J., Yang K.D.. Ras Modulation of Superoxide Activates ERK-dependent Angiogenic Transcription (HIF-1) and VEGF-A Expression in Shockwave-Stimulated Osteoblasts. The Journal of Biological Chemistry, 2004; 279(11): 10331-7.
20. Russo S., Amelio E., Corrado E.M., Suzuki H.. Meccanismi biomolecolari ed onde d'urto: an upgrade review. 5° Congresso Nazionale SITOD, Verona 13-15 Maggio 2004
21. Takahashi K., Wada Y., Ohtori S., Saisu T., Moriya H.. Application of shockwaves to rat skin decreases calcitonin gene-related peptide immunoreactivity in dorsal root ganglion neurons. Auton Neurosci. 2003 Sep 30; 107(2):81-4
22. Takahashi K., Saisu T., Yamazaki M., Wada Y., Mitsuhashi S., Moriya H.. Gene expression for extracellular matrix proteins during shockwave-induced osteogenesis in the long bone of rats. 4th Congress of the International Society for Musculoskeletal Shockwave Therapy, Berlin 24-26 May,2001
23. Marx S., Thiele R..Fallvorstellung der arthroskopisch kontrollierten Therapie der Osteochondrosis dissecans mittels ESWT. Arthroskopie 2003.16:266-271
24. Ludwig.J., Lauber S., Lauber J., Hotzinger H.. Shockwave treatment of femur necrosis in the adult. Z Orthop Ihre Grenzgeb.1999 Jul-Aug; 137(4): Oa2-5.GermanThiele R., Marx S., Ludwig J., Herbert Chr..Extracorporeal Shockwave Therapy for Adult Osteochondritis dissecans of the Femoral Condyle and the Talus. 7th Congress of the International Society for Musculoskeletal Shockwave Therapy, Kaohsiung April 1-4, 2004
25. Lauber S.. High energy extracorporeal shockwave therapy in femur head necrosis. Z Orthop Ihre Grenzgeb.2000 Sep-Oct; 138(5):Oa3-4.German
26. Ludwig J., Lauber S., Lauber HJ., Dreisilker U., Raedel R., Hotzinger H.. High–energy shockwave treatment of femoral head necrosis in adults. Clin. Orthop.2001 Jun;(387):119-26
27. Valchanou VD, Michailov P.. High energy shockwaves in the treatment of delayed and nonunion of fractures. Int Orthop.1991;15(3):181-4
28. Schleberger R., Senge T.. Non-invasive treatment of long-bone pseudarthrosis by shockwaves (ESWL). Arch Orthop Trauma Surg.1992;111(4):224-7
29. Beutler S., Regel G., Pape H.C. Machtens S., Weinberg A.M., Kremeike I., Jonas U., Tscherne H.. Die extrakorporale Stoßwellentherapie (ESWT) in der Behandlung von Pseudarthrosen des Röhrenknochens. Unfallchirurg 1999;102:839-847
30. Birnbaum K., Wirtz D.C., Siebert C.H., Heller K.D. Use of extracorporeal shockwave therapy (ESWT) in the treatment of non-unions. Arch Orthop Trauma Surg (2002) 122:324-330
31. Wang C.J., Chen H.S., Chen c.E., Yang K.D.. Treatment of Nonunions of Long Bone Fractures With Shockwaves. Clinical Orthopaedics and Related Research, 2001 No. 387, pp 95-101

32. Schaden W., Fischer A., Sailler A.. Extracorporeal shockwave therapy of nonunion or delayed osseous union. Clin Orthop.2001 Jun;(387):90-4
33. Rompe JD, Rosendahl T., Schollner C., Theis C.. High-energy extracorporeal shockwave treatment of nonunions. Clin Orthop 2001 Jun;(387):102-11
34. Schoellner C., Rompe JD., Decking J., Heine J.. High energy extracorporeal shockwave therapy (ESWT) in pseudarthrosis. Orthopäde.2002 Jul;31(7):658-62 German
35. Maier M., Schmitz C., Refior H.J.. Extracorporeal Shockwave Application in the Treatment of Pseudarthrosis. European Journal of Trauma, 2003.No.5:262-7
36. Biedermann R., Martin A., Handle G., Auckenthaler T., Bach C., Krismer M.. Extracorporeal shockwaves in the treatment of nonunions. J Trauma.2003 May;54(5):936-42

28

Use of ESWT in Adult Osteochondrosis Dissecans and a Case Study of the Treatment of Osteochondral Lesions

Sergej Marx, Richard Thiele

The following is a presentation of the treatment with ESWT of osteochondrosis dissecans in the early stages I, II and III according to Berndt & Harty, and a supplement in the form of a case study of one application in a single case.

The findings are based on the extension of a study to prove the efficacy of extracorporeal shockwave therapy on adult osteochondrosis dissecans.

Surgery seemed to be the only possibility to remove specific intracorporeal objects but lithotripsy, which has been used for decades in urology, shows the non-invasive option.

As a result, ESWT gained momentum in orthopedics. Apart from basic research on the mechanism of extracorporeal shockwaves, equipment and efficacy studies were developed in connection with different indications.

Osteochondrosis dissecans (OCD) describes a degenerative bone-cartilage disorder which results in separation of a cartilage-bone area from the joint surface. OCD appears as an intraarticular loose body and an intraarticular ulcer remains when this body is loosed. Osteochondrosis dissecans is rated in different stages. A large variety of scores have been published. Osteochondrosis dissecans is among the aseptic bone necrosis caused by vascular deficits. Overexertion and trauma appear to have a significant impact on the generation of this lesion. Depending on the phase, the patient suffers from pain, crepitation, clicks or a feeling of joint blocking by a loose body. Overall, the pains described by the patient are often viewed as uncharacteristic. In the initial stages, the main symptoms are load-related pains; in more advanced stages, intermittent blockage and signs of impingement are found. In general, osteochondrosis dissecans constitutes a prearthrosis and occurs exceedingly often in high performance athletes.

The theory to treat osteochondrosis dissecans with extracorporeal shockwave therapy is based on an extension of the experience gained on other bone diseases such as non-unions and delayed fracture healing, on studies of the efficacy for avascular necrosis of the femoral head, and especially on data resulting from numerous studies in basic ESWT research.

ESWT is described to induce the release of hydroxyl radicals, formation of new blood vessels, stimulation of bone growth and proliferation of cartilage cells as well. ESWT also induces the release of growth factors such as endothelial nitric oxide (eNO), vessel endothelial growth factor (VEGF) and proliferating cell nuclear antigen (PCNA) or OP 1 the osteogenic protein.

The rationale to indicate shockwaves in OCD is based on the above mentioned findings.

Extracorporeal shockwave therapy of osteochondrosis dissecans of the knee joint was performed under general anesthesia. Previous MRI should enable the physician to precisely locate the area to be treated. During therapy this will be accomplished through fluroscopy. In most cases, diagnostic arthroscopy prior to ESWT is to provide for an additional, more precise localization of the pain and for visual follow-up.

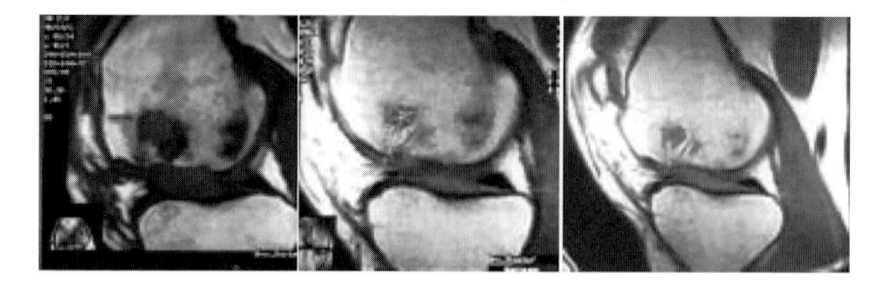

Before ESWT   3 months after ESWT   6 months after

More than 50 patients with Stage I-II osteochondrosis dissecans of the femur condyle were treated with high energetic extracorporeal shockwaves and evaluated through different scores as well as on-going MRI exams. To generate shockwaves, an Ossatron from HMT was used to apply 2500 impulses at 0.35 mJ/mm^2. Following the treatment, patients were restricted to partial weight bearing for 2 to 6 weeks. However, depending on the location of the defect, patients were allowed to walk around on crutches. If the pathological finding was ventral, the brace would be applied in 30° or 40° flexion.

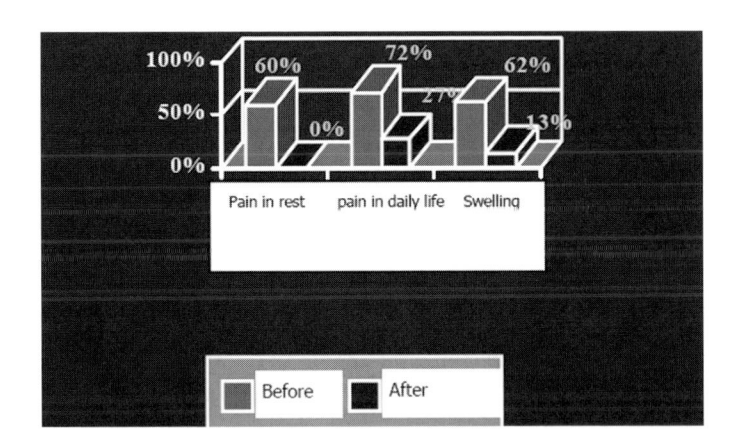

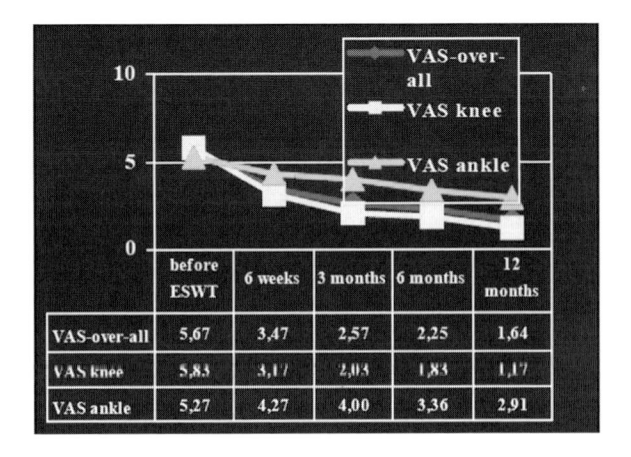

	before ESWT	6 weeks	3 months	6 months	12 months
VAS-over-all	5,67	3,47	2,57	2,25	1,64
VAS knee	5,83	3,17	2,03	1,83	1,17
VAS ankle	5,27	4,27	4,00	3,36	2,91

No undesirable side effect or complication was found in any patient. The results of the different scores showed consistently significant improvements. This represents the subjective improvement experienced by the patients. While 60% of patients suffered pain at rest and partial weight bearing prior to ESWT, only 38% complained about minor pain under strong body activity after the treatment. None of the treated patients showed any pain at rest after the treatment.

Prior to the treatment, 62% suffered from swelling on the joint while only 13% reported signs of swelling after the treatment.

More than 72% reported pain during ADL before treatment but only 27% reported minor pain in their daily activities afterward and 10% reported significant pain one year after the treatment. To classify MRI findings, patients were scored within 4 groups according to Berndt & Harty. MRI signs as described could therefore be transferred. In 40% of the cases, the MRI finding showed a complete restitution and 30% showed an improvement in the defect size and were upgraded from Grade II to Grade I.

In 30% of the cases no clear improvement was found in the course of the study. This does not necessarily coincide with the subjective finding of patients. Almost all patients (see above) reported an improvement after therapy.

The following describes one case that was observed and documented outside the study.

A 29-year-old patient had been suffering pain symptoms in his right knee joints for more than 24 months. While trauma could not be specified, a multitude of microtrauma may be assumed since he was an amateur football player. A lesion diagnosed by x-rays but not visible half a year earlier was classified as Stage III osteochondrosis dissecans in the medial femur condylus. Additionally a bone cyst and pre-arthrosis narrowed cartilage tissue in the medial knee compartment were found as well as joint effusion. Diagnostic arthroscopy revealed marked Stage III-IV cartilage damage. A histological exam showed macroscopic cartilage and bone fragments with degenerative changes and hyalines as well as fibrous cartilage. Even the bone scan exam showed similar findings.

Since the patient insisted on treatment with ESWT, shockwave therapy was performed.

The ESWT consisted of 2500 impulses applied under general anesthesia at an energy flow density of 0.35 mJ/mm². The treatment was applied with the Ossatron from HMT, an electrohydraulic shockwave generator especially designed for orthopedic use. Following the treatment, the patient was ordered to wear a Mecron-Brace in 30° flexion for 6 weeks and full weight bearing was allowed. However any sports activity by the patient was prohibited during that time.

The pain symptoms soon began to improve. Even 6 weeks after the treatment, the patient rated his pain at 2 compared to 7 on the 10-scale VAS at baseline. This was confirmed and continued to improve until complete relief from pain was achieved.

A first MRI 3 months after ESWT showed constant findings of osteochondrosis dissecans, the cartilage cyst and cartilage lesion. A second MRI 6 months after ESWT showed an improvement in the osteochondral lesion, but the bone cyst was unchanged. Due to the size of the defect a second high-energy shockwave therapy was conducted once again with 2500 impulses at an energy flux density of 0.35 mJ/mm².

A one-year check revealed a clear improvement of the osteochondral lesion to a Stage I osteochondrosis dissecans and no evidence of any cartilage damage. The arthroscopy showed the femur condylus completely covered with cartilage and showed no difference compared to surrounding hyaline cartilage of a healthy knee even with a tactile hook exam. A histological exam of the loose body removed in the second diagnostic arthroscopy showed a complete coverage with hyaline cartilage. The patient is clearly satisfied with the result and can once again engage in football without suffering from pain.

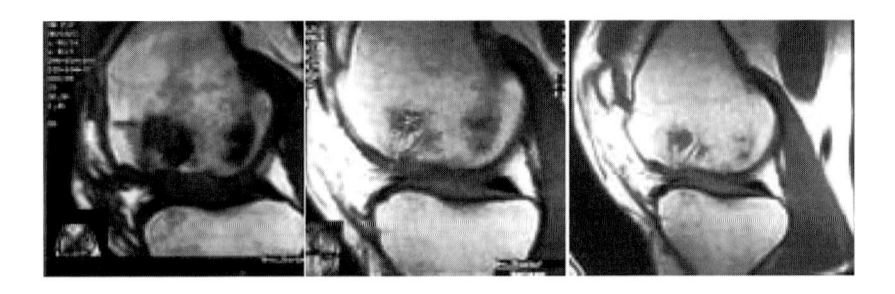

Before ESWT   3 months after ESWT   6 months after

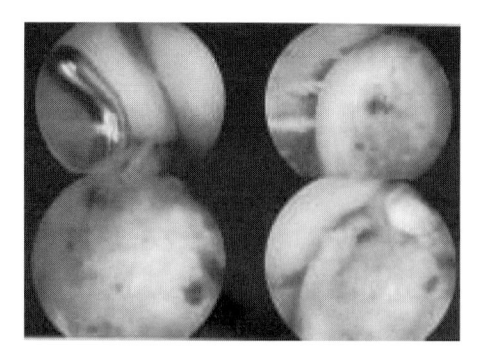

Before ESWT

The above mentioned case reports the potential effect of ESWT, but the OATS (Osteochondral Autograft Transfer System) therapy remains the gold standard for minimally invasive treatments. However, since this disease is rarely healed completely in middle age, a surgical intervention often becomes necessary. While the treatment of osteochondrosis dissecans with ESWT is still in its experimental phase, it can no longer be ignored as a method without side effects and of lesser intensity.

There is a clear tendency to the positive effect of ESWT in the treatment of osteochondral lesions such as osteochondrosis dissecans but our findings have to be confirmed by high quality studies.

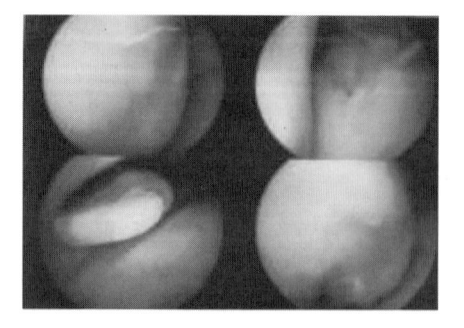

15 months after ESWT

Literature

1. Berndt AL, Harty M (1959) Transchondral fractures (osteochondrosis dissecans) of the talus. J Bone Joint Surg AM 41 A
2. Browne JE, Branch TP (2000) Surgivcal alternatives for treatment of articular cartilage lesions. J Am Acad Orthop Surg 8
3. Bruns J (1996) Osteochondrosis dissecans. Pathogenese, Diagnose und Therapie. Enke, Stuttgart
4. Buch M, Siebert W (2000) Shockwave Treatment for Heel Pain Syndrome – a Prospective Investigation. In: Coombs R, Schwaden W, Zhou S (2000) Musculoskeletal Shockwave Therapy. Greenwich Medical Media Ltd.
5. Burkart A, Imhoff AB (2000) Therapie des Knorpelschadens. Heute und Morgen. Arthroskopie 12
6. Burkart A, Schoettle P, Imhoff AB (2001) Operative Therapiemöglichkeiten des Knorpelschadens. Unfallchirurg 104
7. Delius M, Draenert K (1997) Biologische Wirkung der Stoßwellen auf Zellen, Einfluß hochenergetischer Stoßwellen auf Knochen. In: Siebert W, Buch M (Hrsg) Stoßwellenanwendungen am Knochen – Klinische und experimentelle Erfahrungen. Verlag Dr. Kovac. Hamburg
8. Gerdesmeyer L (2003) The Successful Treatment of Calcified Lesions of the Shoulder with ESWT; Influence of Different Parameters on Outcome and Clinical Results. In: Abstracts: Combined Sixth Congress Internationale Society For Musculoskeletal Shockwave Therapy
9. Gerdesmeyer L, Bachfischer K, Hauschild M (2000) Overview of Calcifying Tendonitis of the Shoulder Treated with Shockwave Treatment. In: Coombs R, Schwaden W, Zhou S (2000) Musculoskeletal Shockwave Therapy. Greenwich Medical Media Ltd.
10. Gerdesmeyer L, Hasse A, Engel A, Bachfischer K, Rechl H (2001) Der Einfluß extrakorporaler Stoßwellen auf die Osteoinduktion nach Radiatio. In: Siebert W, Buch M (Hrsg). Extrakorporale Stoßwellentherapie in der Orthopädie. Ecomed
11. Imhoff AB, Burkart (1998) Knorpelschaden – Knieinstabilität. Das instabile Knie und der Knorpelschaden des Sportlers. Steinkopff, Darmstadt
12. Jürgensen I, Bachmann G, Haas H, Schleicher I (1998) Einfluß der arthroskopischen Therapie auf den Verlauf der Osteochondrosis dissecans des Knie- und oberen Sprunggelenks. Arthroskopie 11
13. Kramer J, Stiglbauer R, Engel A, Prayer L, Imhof H (1992) MR contrast arthrography (MRA) in osteochondrosis dissecans. J Comput Assist Tomogr 16
14. Krämer K-L, Stock M, Winter M (1997) Klinikleitfaden Orthopädie, 3.Aufl. Fischer, Ulm
15. Lauber S, Ludwig J, Lauber H-J, Hötzinger H, Dreisilker U, Rädel R, Platzek P (2000) MRI after Shockwave Treatment for Osteonecrosis of the Femoral Head In: Coombs R, Schwaden W, Zhou S (2000) Musculoskeletal Shockwave Therapy. Greenwich Medical Media Ltd.
16. Lauber S, Ludwig J, Lauber J, Hötzinger J (2001) Die ESWT-Behandlung der Hüftkopfnekrose und Osteochondrosis dissecans. In: Extrakorporale Stoßwellentherapie in der Orthopädie (Siebert W, Buch M [Hrsg,]), ecomed
17. Levitt R, Alvarez R, Ogden J (2000) The FDA Studies of Musculoskeletal Shockwave Therapy for Lateral Epicondylitis and Heel Pain Syndrome. In: Coombs R, Schwaden W, Zhou S (2000) Musculoskeletal Shockwave Therapy. Greenwich Medical Media Ltd.

18. Neuland H, Kesselmann Z, Duchstein H-J, Mei W (2003) First In-Vivo Analysis of the Molecular Biological Mechanisms of Extracorporal Shockwaves and their Effects on Tendons in Close Proximity to Bony Tissue. In: Abstracts: Combined Sixth Congress Internationale Society For Musculoskeletal Shockwave Therapy
19. Ogden J, Schaden W, Thiele R (2003) Orthotripsy for Treatment of Non-Union: A Meta Analysis. In: Abstracts: Combined Sixth Congress Internationale Society For Musculoskeletal Shockwave Therapy
20. Pommeranz SJ (1997) Gamuts & pearls in MRI & Orthopedics. The Merten Company, Cincinnati
21. Rompe J-D (1997) Extrakorporale Stoßwellentherapie. Grundlagen, Indikation, Anwendung. Chapman & Hall
22. Rössig S, Schöder J, Kohn D (1998) Einfluß des Knochenreifungsalters auf die Ergebnisse der operativ behandelten Osteochondrosis dissecans des Kniegelenks. Arthroskopie 11
23. Schaden W (2000) Shockwave Treatment for Chronic Non-unions and Pseudarthrosis. In: Coombs R, Schwaden W, Zhou S (2000) Musculoskeletal Shockwave Therapy. Greenwich Medical Media Ltd.
24. Suzuki H, Amelio E, Cavalieri E, Mariotto S, Galasso O, Russo S (2003) Effect of Shockwave on the Catalytic Activity of Endothelial Nitric Oxide Synthase in Human Umbilical Vein Endothelial Cells. In: Abstracts: Combined Sixth Congress Internationale Society For Musculoskeletal Shockwave Therapy
25. Wang C-J, Wang F-S, Kuender DY, Huang C-S, Hsu C-C (2003) The Mechanism of Shockwave Therapy. Tissue Regeneration from Clinical to Basic Science Study. In: Abstracts: Combined Sixth Congress Internationale Society For Musculoskeletal Shockwave Therapy
26. Wess D (2003) Physical Principles of Shockwave Therapy. In: Abstracts: Combined Sixth Congress Internationale Society For Musculoskeletal Shockwave Therapy

Shockwave Treatment of Femoral Head Necrosis in Adults

Peter Diehl,[1] Johannes Schauwecker,[1] Hans Gollwitzer,[1] Ludger Gerdesmeyer[1]

Summary

Adults with Stages I to IV osteonecrosis of the femoral head according to the ARCO classification present an overall therapeutic challenge. Extracorporeal shockwave therapy (ESWT) has already been shown to have a promising effect on the treatment of enthesiopathies and on bone healing in pseudarthrosis. In terms of femoral head necrosis, surgical methods like intertrochanteric flexion osteotomy or drilling of the femoral head are still a matter of dispute and are without proven efficacy. One alternative approach in non-invasive treatment of femoral head necrosis in early stages is ESWT. Clinical trials have shown promising results in short-term follow-up. However, medium-term and long-term results are necessary before it is possible to determine whether this method can prevent recurrence or progression of this disease.

Introduction

Variable epidemiological data are available concerning aseptic osteonecrosis of the femoral head. In the United States approximately 10,000 to 20,000 patients develop femoral head necrosis annually[14]. Osteonecrotic lesions in adults usually have similar pathomorphologic pathways[1]. Frequently the underlying condition is a circulatory disorder accompanied by the progressive destruction of bone cells due to malnutrition and insufficient oxygen supply. However, direct damage by inflammation, radiation, or high dosage cortisone therapy also may

---

[1] Department of Orthopedic Surgery, Ismaninger Str. 22, D-81675 Muenchen

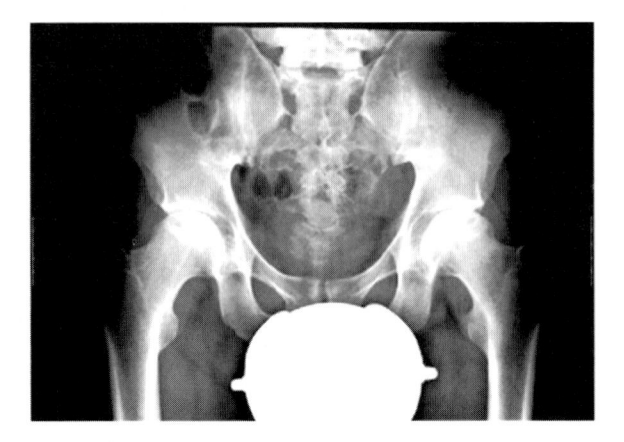

Figure 1. Radiograph with sclerotic changes of femoral head (ARCO stage III).

cause metabolic disorders that affect bone tissue adversely. The onset of the disease is heralded by micromorphologic changes that are not visible on standard radiographic studies. Nevertheless, sophisticated diagnostic technologies like magnetic resonance imaging (MRI), angiography, or bone scans may identify earlier stages of this disease.

In the joint-preserving surgical treatment of femoral head necrosis, no gold standard is proved and several treatment modalities are still a matter of dispute. The specific recent procedures are recommended primarily on the basis of the stage of the disease. In early stages, intraosseous decompression of the femur with or without transplantation of spongiosa material is recommended [8, 16] to cause a new ingrowth of blood vessels. In advanced stages, a large number of osteotomies is recommended to rotate the necrotic focus out of the biomechanical weight bearing zone[10, 28]. The results for surgical treatment of patients with femoral head necrosis with a mean follow-up of 90 months, show that total hip replacement could be delayed in only 23% of cases[17]. In addition to these findings, it has been demonstrated that surgical procedures preserved the current stage of the osteonecrosis before treatment for some time, but none led to complete recovery of the femoral head.

Until now, no therapy has been developed that addresses the cause of the disorder. In most patients, conservative therapy succeeds only in postponing implantation of a total hip replacement. The conservative methods to date consist only of symptomatic measures reducing the symptoms of the disorder without interrupting the progress itself. The promotion of new bone formation observed in patients with pseudarthrosis and related bone healing after ESWT were observed in animal models[26, 27]. The mechanism by which ESWT enhances fracture/bone healing remains to be determined. Recently other study groups have shown that ESWT has promising effects on healing and repair of chronic tendonitis[4]. The fact that ESWT enhances both bone and tendon regeneration suggests that ESWT may induce a certain signal for growth and maturation of the mesenchymal progenitors from bone marrow. It has already been demonstrated that the differentiation and maturation of bone marrow stromal cells and osteoprogenitor cells into osteoblastic lineage is involved in bone regeneration[11]. These findings are in agreement with Wang et al. who have shown ESWT to be able to promote marrow stromal cell growth and differentiation toward osteogenic lineage, presumably through TGF-ß1 induction[26]. Further investigations by Wang at al. [27] demonstrated that bone morphogenic proteins (BMP) also play an important role in signaling shockwave activated cell proliferation and bone regeneration of segmental defects. BMP are members of the TGF-ß superfamily involved in the regulation of embryonic skeletal development and in the repair of bone fracture and healing[2]. In addition, BMP also affect bone remodeling through the regulation of osteoclastic bone resorbing activity[9]. BMP have been reported as having a role in the mechanical stimulation of fracture healing and chondrocyte differentiation[29]. It has been demonstrated that ESWT of segmental defects significantly increases mRNA expression and immunoexpression in BMP-2, BMP-3, BMP-4 and BMP-7 in the callus during fracture healing[27]. In addition to these findings, it has been demonstrated that shockwaves produce a higher free radical concentration. This superoxide also plays an important role in the regulation of cell metabolism and proliferation[12]. Several physical factors such as heat, electrical field pulsatile stretch and ESWT can stimulate cell proliferation through the involvement of superoxide, thus resulting in osteoprogenitor cell growth and in osteogenesis[25]. On the other hand, the effect of high-energy shockwaves is dependent on the energy and number of impulses of the treatment. It has been reported that higher doses may cause the production of heat induced free radicals or disturbance in the homeostasis of cellular calcium, resulting in cell and tissue damage[6]. Extreme high energy shockwaves also induce aseptic necrosis and damage of osteocytes in rat bone marrow[7].

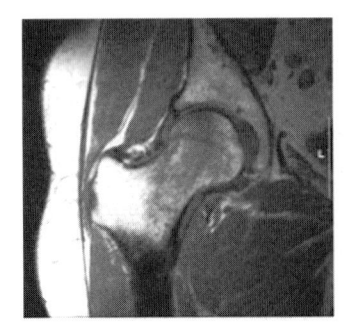

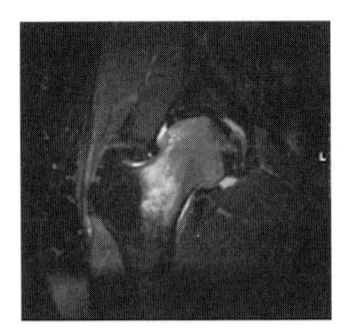

Figure 2. MRI (T1/T2) of an early stage with edema of femoral head (ARCO stage I).

The findings of this study suggest that ESWT may provide an effective noninvasive method by which to initialize bone regeneration in the treatment of femoral head necrosis.

As a result of this investigation, patients with femoral head necrosis in early stages may benefit from ESWT.

Shockwave therapy offers several important advantages over conventional surgical treatment. It is a non invasive treatment with a substantially reduced incidence of complications[20]. Moreover, hip endoprosthesis implantation could be performed in better bony conditions with higher bone mass density due to ESWT and patients would have better overall surgical conditions because no previous surgery was performed. Additionally, follow-up treatment and rehabilitation is shortened considerably for patients who have received shockwave therapy. The success of ESWT is clearly dependent on the stage of the femoral head necrosis.

A commonly used classification is based on the Association Research Circulation Osseous (ARCO) scale[22]. It is generally accepted that radiography and MRI must be used to properly classify lesions according to the ARCO scale. The ARCO system was used to classify femoral head necrosis on the basis of MRI findings (Table 1).

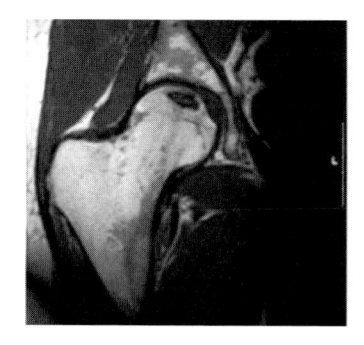

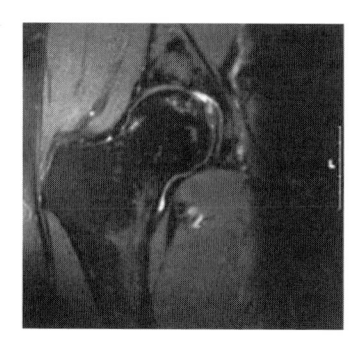

Figure 3. MRI (T1/T2) with sclerotic changes of femoral head (ARCO stage II).

To address clinical parameters like pain and function, the Harris hip score [5] is widely used, especially for follow-up. Other factors like consumption of pain killers and subjective restriction of activity are included as well as factors like type of gait, walking radius, objective restriction of activity, mobility, and ability to do every day activities.

A specific ranking system by Ficat [3] takes radiological and clinical criteria of femoral head necrosis into account.

A review of ESWT in femoral head necrosis by comparison of the medium-term results reveals widely varying success rates. Investigation by Wang et al. demonstrated 50% improvement after ESWT in patients with femoral head[24]. These findings were nearly confirmed by Ludwig et al. presenting success rates of about 65% after 1 year of follow-up[13]. Distinct therapeutic success was observed in 14 of 22 patients. This success manifested as an improvement of the pain symptoms as well as mobility and as higher scores of the Harris hip scale. The study also shows that the success rate depends on the ARCO stage. Interestingly, patients with improvement of pain are all classified as stage I and II. They showed a significantly better outcome after ESWT compared to stage III or IV. This latter group did not respond to therapy and improved only slightly in terms of pain. In addition, patient age seems to have an impact on the clinical and radiological results. This may be explained by the increasingly poor circulation and metabolism in elderly patients[13]. Better results were obtained by Russo et al., revealing complete recovery from the disorder in early stages in 85% of the patients with femoral head necrosis as confirmed by follow-up MRI[18].

Classification System	Criteria
Ficat and Arlet classification system	
Stage I	Normal
Stage II	Sclerotic or cystic lesions
Stage III	Subchondral collapse
Stage IV	Osteoarthritis with decreased joint space with articular space
University of Pennsylvania system of classification and staging [22]	
Stage 0	Normal or non diagnostic radiograph, bone scan, and MRI
Stage I	Normal radiograph; abnormal bone scan and/or MRI
A	Mild (<15% of head affected)
B	Moderate (15% to 30% of head affected)
C	Severe (>30% of head affected)
Stage II	Lucent and sclerotic changes in femoral head
A	Mild (<15% of head affected)
B	Moderate (15% to 30% of head affected)
C	Severe (>30% of head affected)
Stage III	Subchondral collapse (crescent sign) without flattening
A	Mild (<15% of articular surface)
B	Moderate (15% to 30% of articular surface)
C	Severe (>30% of articular surface)
Stage IV	Flattening of femoral head
A	Mild (<15% of surface and <2-mm depression)
B	Moderate (15% to 30% of surface or 2 to 4-mm depression)
C	Severe (>30% of surface or >4-mm depression)
Stage V	Joint narrowing and/or acetabular changes
A	Mild
B	Moderate
C	Severe
Stage VI	Advanced degenerative changes

Table 1. Radiographic classifications of osteonecrosis of the femoral head.

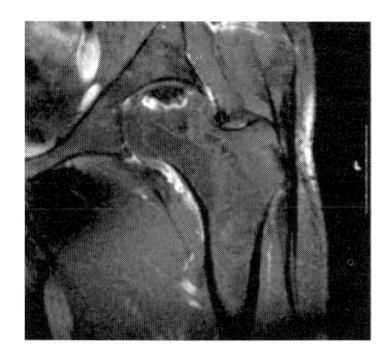

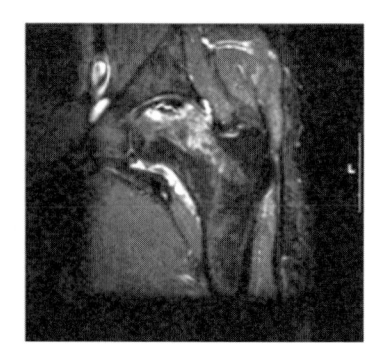

Figure 4. MRI (T1 fat sat i.v.Gd/T2 fat sat) of an advanced stage with sclerotic margin around the zone of necrosis and joint narrowing (ARCO stage V).

It seems reasonable to compare these data with operative procedures like drilling or intertrochanteric flexion osteotomy which have less effective success rates in the range of 36% to 65%[15, 19, 21]. Only the application of pedicled bone transplants revealed good results in 62 to 89% of patients[19, 23].

Interestingly in some patients, reduction of pain was noticed but the zone of necrosis on MRI was unchanged. This may be due to the known pain reducing mechanisms after ESWT[13].

Recently Wang et al. published a randomized controlled study to evaluate the effects of shockwave therapy on AVN of the femoal head[30]. Patients with stage I, II, or III osteonecrosis were randomly assigned to be treated either with shockwaves or with core decompression and nonvascularized fibular grafting. The shockwave group consisted of twenty-three patients (twenty-nine hips), and the surgical group consisted of twenty-five patients (twenty-eight hips). The patients in the two groups had similar demographic characteristics, duration and stage of disease, and duration of follow-up. The patients in the shockwave group received a single treatment with 6000 impulses of shockwaves at 28 kV to the affected hip. The evaluation parameters included clinical assessment of pain with a visual analog pain scale, Harris hip scores, and an assessment of activities of daily living and work capacity. Radiographic assessment was performed with serial plain radiographs and magnetic resonance imaging. Their publication reported that both groups showed similar values at baseline prior to ESWT. At an average of twenty-five months after treatment, the pain and Harris hip scores in the shockwave group were significantly improved compared with the pretreatment scores (p < 0.001). In this group, 79% of the hips were improved, 10% were unchanged, and 10% were worse. Of the hips treated with a nonvascularized fibular graft, 29% were improved, 36% were unchanged, and 36% were worse. In the shockwave group, imaging studies showed regression of five of the thirteen lesions that had been designated as stage I or II before treatment and no regression of a stage III lesion. Two stage II and two stage III lesions progressed. In the surgical group, four lesions regressed and fifteen (of the nineteen graded as stage I or II) progressed. The remaining nine lesions were unchanged. Finally they concluded that extracorporeal shockwave treatment appeared to be more effective than core decompression and nonvascularized fibular grafting in patients with early-stage osteonecrosis of the femoral head but long-term results are needed to determine whether the effect of this novel method of treatment for osteonecrosis of the femoral head endures[30].

These results provide evidence that the noninvasive treatment of patients with femoral head necrosis with the use of ESWT demonstrates comparable results to invasive methods at a medium-term follow-up interval.

Literature

1. Bradway, J.K. and Morrey, B.F.: "The natural history of the silent hip in bilateral atraumatic osteonecrosis" J Arthroplasty 8 (1993): 383-387
2. Ferguson, C.; Alpern, E.; Miclau, T.; Helms, J.A.: "Does adult fracture repair recapitulate embryonic skeletal formation?" Mech. Dev. 87 (1999): 57-66
3. Ficat, P.: "[Vascular pathology of femoral head necrosis (author's transl)]" Orthopade 9 (1980): 238-244
4. Gerdesmeyer, L.; Wagenpfeil, S.; Haake, M.; Maier, M.; Loew, M.; Wortler, K.; Lampe, R.; Seil, R.; Handle, G.; Gassel, S.; Rompe, J.D.: "Extracorporeal shockwave therapy for the treatment of chronic calcifying tendonitis of the rotator cuff: a randomized controlled trial" JAMA 290 (2003): 2573-2580
5. Harris, W.H.: "Traumatic arthritis of the hip after dislocation and acetabular fractures: treatment by mold arthroplasty. An end-result study using a new method of result evaluation" J Bone Joint Surg Am. 51 (1969): 737-755
6. Howard, D. and Sturtevant, B.: "In vitro study of the mechanical effects of shock-wave lithotripsy" Ultrasound Med. Biol 23 (1997): 1107-1122
7. Ikeda, K.; Tomita, K.; Takayama, K.: "Application of extracorporeal shockwave on bone: preliminary report" J Trauma 47 (1999): 946-950
8. Iorio, R.; Healy, W.L.; Abramowitz, A.J.; Pfeifer, B.A.: "Clinical outcome and survivorship analysis of core decompression for early osteonecrosis of the femoral head" J Arthroplasty 13 (1998): 34-41
9. Kawakami, Y.; Ishikawa, T.; Shimabara, M.; Tanda, N.; Enomoto-Iwamoto, M.; Iwamoto, M.; Kuwana, T.; Ueki, A.; Noji, S.; Nohno, T.: "BMP signaling during

bone pattern determination in the developing limb" Development 122 (1996): 3557-3566

10. Langlais, F. and Fourastier, J.: "Rotation osteotomies for osteonecrosis of the femoral head" Clin. Orthop. (1997): 110-123

11. Liu, P.; Oyajobi, B.O.; Russell, R.G.; Scutt, A.: "Regulation of osteogenic differentiation of human bone marrow stromal cells: interaction between transforming growth factor-beta and 1,25(OH)(2) vitamin D(3) In vitro" Calcif. Tissue Int. 65 (1999): 173-180

12. Lopez-Ongil, S.; Senchak, V.; Saura, M.; Zaragoza, C.; Ames, M.; Ballermann, B.; Rodriguez-Puyol, M.; Rodriguez-Puyol, D.; Lowenstein, C.J.: "Superoxide regulation of endothelin-converting enzyme" J Biol Chem. 275 (2000): 26423-26427

13. Ludwig, J.; Lauber, S.; Lauber, H.J.; Dreisilker, U.; Raedel, R.; Hotzinger, H.: "High-energy shockwave treatment of femoral head necrosis in adults" Clin. Orthop. (2001): 119-126

14. Mankin, H.J.: "Nontraumatic necrosis of bone (osteonecrosis)" N. Engl. J Med. 326 (1992): 1473-1479

15. Markel, D.C.; Miskovsky, C.; Sculco, T.P.; Pellicci, P.M.; Salvati, E.A.: "Core decompression for osteonecrosis of the femoral head" Clin. Orthop. (1996): 226-233

16. Mont, M.A.; Carbone, J.J.; Fairbank, A.C.: "Core decompression versus nonoperative management for osteonecrosis of the hip" Clin. Orthop. (1996): 169-178

17. Rader, C.P.; Gomille, T.; Eggert-Durst, M.; Hendrich, C.; Eulert, J.: "[Results of hip joint boring in femur head necrosis in the adult—4 to 18 years follow-up]" Z. Orthop. Ihre Grenzgeb. 135 (1997): 494-498

18. Russo, S.; Galasso, O.; Scognamiglio, D.; Corrado, E.M.: "Bone Necroses Treated with Shockwaves" 5th Congress of the International Society for Musculoskeletal Shockwave Therapy Winterthur, Switzerland (2002): 33

19. Scully, S.P.; Aaron, R.K.; Urbaniak, J.R.: "Survival analysis of hips treated with core decompression or vascularized fibular grafting because of avascular necrosis" J Bone Joint Surg Am. 80 (1998): 1270-1275

20. Sistermann, R. and Katthagen, B.D.: "[Complications, side-effects and contraindications in the use of medium and high-energy extracorporeal shockwaves in orthopedics]" Z. Orthop. Ihre Grenzgeb. 136 (1998): 175-181

21. Smith, S.W.; Fehring, T.K.; Griffin, W.L.; Beaver, W.B.: "Core decompression of the osteonecrotic femoral head" J Bone Joint Surg Am. 77 (1995): 674-680

22. Steinberg, M.E.; Hayken, G.D.; Steinberg, D.R.: "A quantitative system for staging avascular necrosis" J Bone Joint Surg Br. 77 (1995): 34-41

23. Urbaniak, J.R.; Coogan, P.G.; Gunneson, E.B.; Nunley, J.A.: "Treatment of osteonecrosis of the femoral head with free vascularized fibular grafting. A long-term follow-up study of one hundred and three hips" J Bone Joint Surg Am. 77 (1995): 681-694

24. Wang, C.-J.: "Shockwave Therapy for Patients with Avascular Necrosis of the Femoral Head" 6th Congress of the International Society for Musculoskeletal Shockwave Therapy Orlando, FL, USA (2003): 55-56

25. Wang, F.S.; Wang, C.J.; Sheen-Chen, S.M.; Kuo, Y.R.; Chen, R.F.; Yang, K.D.: "Superoxide mediates shockwave induction of ERK-dependent osteogenic transcription factor (CBFA1) and mesenchymal cell differentiation toward osteoprogenitors" J Biol Chem. 277 (2002): 10931-10937

26. Wang, F.S.; Yang, K.D.; Chen, R.F.; Wang, C.J.; Sheen-Chen, S.M.: "Extracorporeal shockwave promotes growth and differentiation of bone-marrow stromal cells towards osteoprogenitors associated with induction of TGF-beta1" J Bone Joint Surg Br. 84 (2002): 457-461
27. Wang, F.S.; Yang, K.D.; Kuo, Y.R.; Wang, C.J.; Sheen-Chen, S.M.; Huang, H.C.; Chen, Y.J.: "Temporal and spatial expression of bone morphogenetic proteins in extracorporeal shockwave-promoted healing of segmental defect" Bone 32 (2003): 387-396
28. Willert, H.G.; Buchhorn, G.; Zichner, L.: "[Results of flexion osteotomy on segmental femoral head necrosis in adults (author's transl)]" Orthopade 9 (1980): 278-289
29. Wu, Q.; Zhang, Y.; Chen, Q.: "Indian hedgehog is an essential component of mechanotransduction complex to stimulate chondrocyte proliferation" J Biol Chem. 276 (2001): 35290-35296
30. Wang CJ, Wang FS, Huang CC, Yang KD, Weng LH, Huang HY. Treatment for osteonecrosis of the femoral head: comparison of extracorporeal shockwaves with core decompression and bone-grafting. J Bone Joint Surg Am. 2005 Nov;87(11):2380-7.

ESWT – A Prospective Double Blind Study on Bilateral Plantar Fasciitis

Lowell Weil, Jr., DPM, MBA, FACFAS, Lowell Scott Weil, Sr., DPM, FACFAS, Wendy Benton-Weil, DPM, FACFAS

Introduction

Extracorporeal Shockwave Therapy (ESWT) has become a common treatment modality for chronic plantar fasciitis worldwide. All studies in the literature evaluate ESWT for unilateral plantar fasciitis with comparisons to placebo treatment on a separate control group.

The purpose of this study was to use a patient as their own control to assess the value of ESWT in chronic bilateral plantar fasciitis.

Materials & Methods

Thirty-six patients with bilateral plantar fasciitis of greater than 6 months duration that failed to respond to conservative care consisting of non-custom inserts or custom orthotics, shoe modifications, activity modifications, oral anti-inflammatory medications, corticosteroid injections, and stretching exercises were eligible to participate. Additional systemic and neurologic causes of heel pain were ruled out in all cases.

All patients were suffering from bilateral heel pain of > 6 on a VAS for both feet.

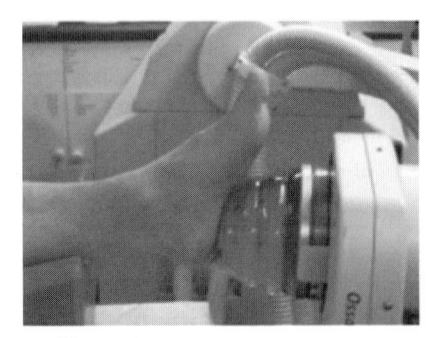

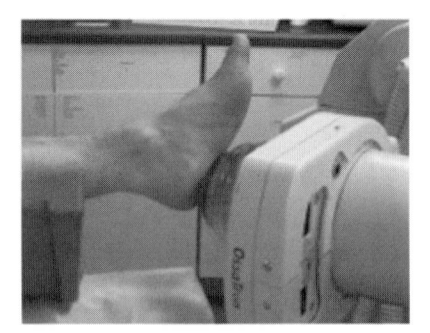

Figure 1.

Figure 2.

After obtaining consent, patients were brought to the operating room and intravenous sedation was introduced followed by an infiltrative heel block bilaterally with 8 cc of 0.5% bupivicaine plain. Both feet were blocked in the same manner.

After the patient was anesthetized and both heels numbed, a computer randomization was opened, determining which foot was to be treated and only that foot was treated. The non-treated foot was utilized as placebo.

Utilizing an Ossatron by Healthtronics, the appropriate foot was treated with 1000 pulses at 19 kV from directly inferior to the heel (Figure 1). Another 1000 pulses at 19 kV was then introduced at a 45 degree medial angle to the heel (Figure 2).

After the treatment, patients were told to continue all aspects of previous therapy. Patients were told to continue wearing the appropriate shoe gear with their custom or non-custom inserts, to continue with their stretching exercises, and to make activity modifications to their tolerance.

The patients followed-up with a blinded investigator at 1 week, 6 weeks and 12 weeks following the treatment.

End point evaluation parameters were reduction in VAS and the Roles and Mauldsey quality of life assessment.

Results

Overall the active group outperformed the sham group. The treated foot improved 70% of the time while the sham foot improved 52% of the time. Of the treated feet 67% improved by >50%, while 47% of the sham feet improved by >50%. Of the treated feet 65% attained a VAS of <3, while only 39% of the sham group achieved <3 on a VAS. In 39% of the patients, both feet improved and in 4% of the patients, neither foot improved.

Discussion

While showing that ESWT is a viable treatment alternative to chronic plantar fasciitis, this study illustrates the high incidence of the placebo effect on patients.

ESWT has been held to a higher scientific standard than surgical alternatives to studied pathologies. It is impossible to predict the placebo affect of surgical intervention for the same pathologies, but one can extrapolate a high incidence.

Gerdesmeyer studied placebo vs. placebo in a prospective analysis of patients who expected treatment vs. those who did not expect treatment and found a statistical difference in improvement in those expecting treatment.

Conclusion

This study, utilizing patients as their own control, shows that ESWT is a valuable and efficacious treatment for chronic plantar fasciitis.

Placebo success is significant but not equal to treated subjects following ESWT for plantar fasciitis.

While there are many inconclusive studies on the effectiveness of ESWT, more well-designed studies are being conducted and published showing its efficacy on many different musculoskeletal pathologies.

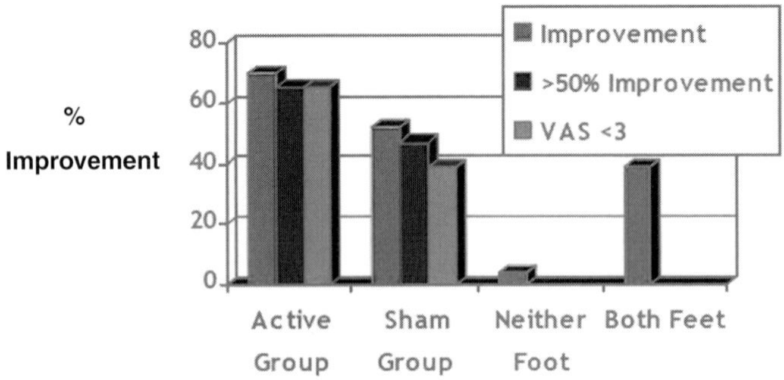
%
Improvement
80
60
40
20
0
Improvement
>50% Improvement
VAS <3
Active Group
Sham Group
Neither Foot
Both Feet

Extracorporeal Shockwave Therapy (ESWT) in Skin Lesions

W. Schaden, R. Thiele, C. Kölpl, A. Pusch

Introduction

Since 1981 extracorporeal shockwaves have been used very successfully for the disintegration of calcified deposits in urology as well as in orthopedics. Due to high efficacy and few side effects, this therapy soon became very popular around the world. Since 1990 [1] shockwaves have also been used for a variety of orthopedic indications. The therapy proved effective for tendon insertion conditions such as fasciitis plantaris (heel spur) and calcific tendonitis of the shoulder. Shockwave therapy is also widely used for lateral epicondylitis (tennis elbow) as described within previous chapters. Due to the few side effects, shockwaves have gained ground for the treatment of pseudoarthrosis (non union) and delayed union. Non-invasive and without clinically significant side effects, ESWT has also been used successfully in pilot studies for the treatment of osteochondritis dissecans (OCD) [2] as well as aseptic bone necrosis (AVN)[3, 4, 12]. In Japan, shockwaves were used successfully in animal experiments for the treatment of ischemia-induced myocardial dysfunction[5]. Even skin flap survival in rats improved as a result of shockwave treatment[6].

When treating septic pseudoarthrosis (osteomyelitis), often linked to skin lesions (fistula formation, skin defects, etc.), bone tissue would consolidate and skin defects would heal particularly fast in many cases. In addition, Gerdesmeyer [7] found an in vitro bactericidal effect of shockwave therapy. Encouraged by such findings, a pilot study on the treatment of skin lesions with ESWT was conducted.

Causes of skin lesions	Number
Posttrauma lesions	44
Postsurgical healing disorders	10
Venous ulcer	25
Arterial ulcer	15
Decubital ulcer	5
Burns	5
Total	104

Table 1. Skin pathologies.

Material and Methods

To conduct the study, an OrthoWave 180c from MTS was used. Since most often surface defects are involved, the shockwave head was modified in that the shockwave would no longer be focused but be roughly planar to the treatment area. Low energy flow densities were used to treat the skin lesions. Depending on the size of the defect, the number of impulses varied from a few 100 to several 1,000. No anesthesia was necessary due to the defocusing and low energy of the shockwaves. In principle, the treatment was performed on an outpatient basis except for those patients already admitted for other reasons. Between September 2004 and January 2005, 83 treatments were performed at the Trauma center Meidling Austria on 81 patients (2 patients were treated in 2 areas). Mean patient age was 61 years. The patient group was made up of 37 women and 44 men. At the same time, 21 patients (13 women and 8 men) were treated at Berlin's Center for Extracorporeal Shockwave Therapy. The mean age was was slightly younger (54 years). The skin pathologies are listed in Table 1.

Since no empiric data were available, treatments were carried out in weekly intervals, in part in biweekly intervals. After the first treatment, the same wound dressing was used in principle as before the shockwave therapy. Only after the second or third treatment when wound conditions had improved, adequate options were indicated.

Causes of skin lesions	Number	Healed	>50%	<50%	Dropout
Posttrauma lesions	44 (42%)	39 (89%)	1 (2%)		4 (9%)
Postoperative healing disorders	10 (10%)	10 (100%)			
Venous ulcer	25 (24%)	9 (36%)	8 (32%)	6 (24%)	2 (8%)
Arterial ulcer	15 (14%)	10 (67%)	2 (13%)	1 (7%)	2 (13%)
Decubital ulcer	5 (5%)	4 (80%)			1 (20%)
Burns	5 (5%)	5 (100%)			
Total	104 (100%)	77 (74%)	11 (10%)	7 (7%)	9 (9%)

Table 2. Results of the treatment.

Results

Table 2 lists the results by lesion cause.

In the beginning of the treatment, all of the treated skin lesions were to be considered as infected. Particularly striking was a lessening of the infection after the first treatment because of the shockwave related bactericidal effect. None of the patients received any antibiotics. None of the patients experienced any worsening of the wound conditions. Only one patient dropped out after the first therapy because she expected herself to fail. Dropouts involved for the most part very old, in part decrepit patients who, after the improvement of their wound, preferred to avoid the strenuous transportation to the hospital.

Discussion

Based on the initial encouraging results of our pilot study, a completely new potential of shockwave therapy appears to emerge. The patients enrolled in our pilot study are reported as a negative selected patient group because all cases refused to get any surgical intervention. Patients willing to get surgery were referred to the proper physicians and shockwave therapy was not offered. The promising outcome after this non invasive treatment option in chronic wound care justifies the indication of shockwave therapy in those soft tissue conditions as described above. Further studies have to be performed to determine optimum treatment parameters. Finally, subsequent prospective, randomized controlled double-blind studies may demonstrate the efficacy and safety of ESWT in treating skin lesions.

Literature

1. Haupt G, Haupt A, Gerety B, Chvapil M., Enhancement of fracture healing with extracorporeal shockwaves. AUA Annual Meeting, New Orleans 1990
2. Thiele R., Marx S., Ludwig J., Herbert Chr..Extracorporeal Shockwave Therapy for Adult Osteochondritis dissecans of the Femoral Condyle and the Talus. 7th Congress of the International Society for Musculoskeletal Shockwave Therapy, Kaohsiung April 1-4, 2004
3. Ludwig.J., Lauber S., Lauber J., Hotzinger H.. Shockwave treatment of femur necrosis in the adult. Z Orthop Ihre Grenzgeb.1999 Jul-Aug; 137(4): Oa2-5.German
4. Lauber S.. High energy extracorporeal shockwave therapy in femur head necrosis.Z Orthop Ihre Grenzgeb.2000 Sep-Oct; 138(5):Oa3-4.German
5. Takahiro N., Hiroaki S., Keiji O., Toyokazu U. et al., Extracorporeal cardiac shockwave therapy markedly ameliorates ischemia-induced myocardial dysfunction in pigs in vivo, Circulation; Vol.110: pp 3055-3061, 2004
6. Meirer R., Kamelger F.S., Huemer G. M., Wanner S., Piza-Katzer H., Extracorporeal shockwave may enhance skin flap survival in an animal model, British Journal of Plastic Surgery, V. 58; pp 53-57, 2005
7. Gerdesmeyer L., von Eiff C., Horn C., Henne M., Roessner M., Diehl P., Gollwitzer H., Antibacterial effects of extracorporeal shockwaves, Ultrasound in Med. & Biol. Vol. 31, pp 115-119, 2005
8. Wang CJ, Wang FS, Huang CC, Yang KD, Weng LH, Huang HY. Treatment for osteonecrosis of the femoral head: comparison of extracorporeal shockwaves with core decompression and bone-grafting. J Bone Joint Surg Am. 2005 Nov;87(11):2380-7.

Figures

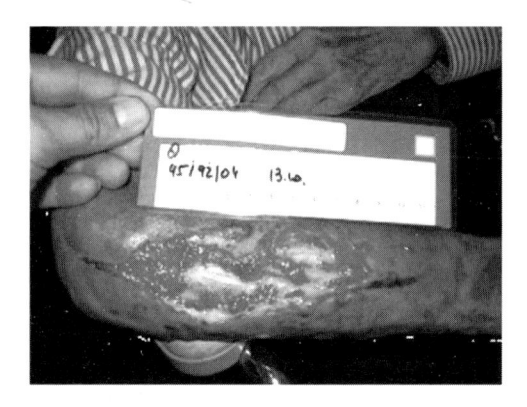

Figure 1. The forearm of a 94 year old female patient after a para-venously applied infusion and two septic revisions. An abating infection with penicillin-resistant staphylococcus aureus was diagnosed (positive smear test). Because of a chronic COPD the patient is being treated with cortisone. The patient also suffers from chronic lymphatic leukemia. The first shockwave treatment was applied on 10/13/2004 as an outpatient procedure without anesthetics.

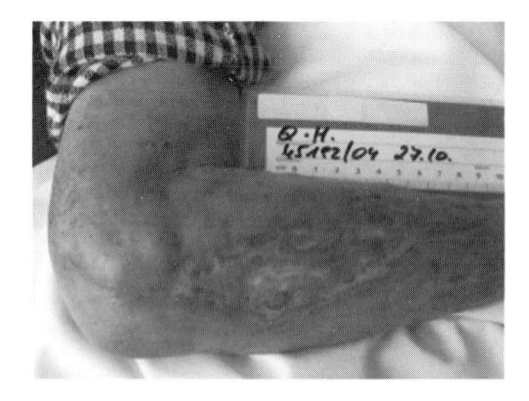

Figure 2. The same patient 2 weeks after the first shockwave treatment. A preexisting therapy with antibiotics was discontinued and the second shockwave treatment (again without anesthetics) was applied.

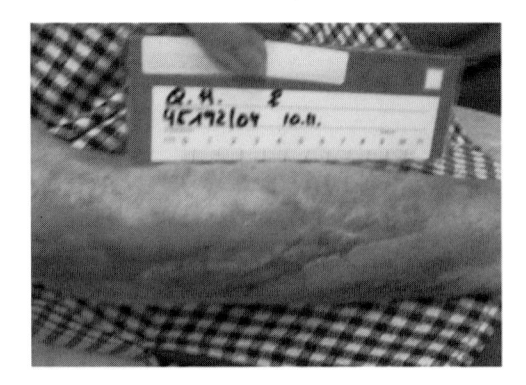

Figure 3. The lesion of the same patient after the third shockwave treatment on 11/10/2004.

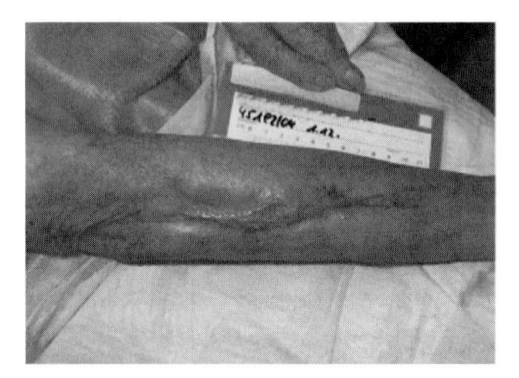

Figure 4. The healing status 6 weeks after starting the therapy with a total of 4 shockwave treatments. In total, the 4 treatments lasted just about 12 minutes.

32

Radial Shockwaves and Autologous Growth Factors-Combined Therapy for Bone Delayed Unions

Carlos Leal, MD, Michelle Cortes, MD

Tissues in the musculoskeletal system have a wide variety of healing properties, that give our specialty a particular need of understanding each organ in fields as different but yet important as molecular biology or biomechanics. Muscle and ligament tend to heal completely most of the time, while nerve and cartilage seem to heal only as functionally sufficient scar tissues. Most medullary lesions result in irreversible paralysis and cartilage loss in joint replacements. Bone is somehow in the middle of these two scenarios, having a good rate of healing in most of the cases, but with many biological and biomechanical variables that can change the final outcome in terms of healing and functional recovery. Nature has designed a nearly perfect system of bone healing, that involves bleeding, cell migration, differentiation and activation, and finally the delicate process of bone remodeling, matrix maturation and biomechanical stabilization[1-3]. If one of these steps is disturbed, bone healing is in jeopardy. It is well known that poorly vascularized bone heals slowly and has more chances of delayed unions. High energy trauma, open fractures, infection or unstable fixations may also result in difficult healing environments[4-6].

The best opportunity an orthopaedic surgeon has to treat a difficult fracture is his first approach and intervention. Science and technology have provided the tools to give biomechanical stability in most of the cases, and the knowledge of cellular and molecular biology has also changed the vision of our interventions in the past two decades. However, even the best possible treatments sometimes fail, and the biological consequences of our interventions can result in non-healing.

This is a real problem that opened research lines for many groups in the world, trying to prevent and treat delayed unions and pseudoarthrosis[7].

Successful bone healing in delayed unions and nonunions is a challenge for the orthopaedic surgeon. There are many treatment options ranging from simple immobilizations to open fixation and grafting. Treatment is based in the biological and biomechanical "re-stabilization" of the fracture. It requires a particular approach in every case, analyzing the causes of the nonunion, the type of fracture, the anatomical and biomechanical considerations of the lesion, and the best treatment option available for each situation[6].

Surgical interventions in delayed fracture healing and nonunions involve large operations that significantly increase pre and postoperative risk factors, and also represent a longer, more difficult recovery period and rehabilitation process. Bone grafts are commonly used as osteoconductors in fracture defects[8,9]. The use of non biological osteoconductive elements such as hydroxyapatite has also served the purpose of defect filling[10]. However, the osteoinductive properties of grafts are fully dependent on the host's capability to create a proper healing environment allowing bone graft substitute incorporation[9]. The vascularity, the amount of undifferentiated cells and the third messengers that activate the healing processes are probably as or more important than the physical filling of a tissue gap. The modulation of bone remodeling is a primary function of hormones and growth factors that could be used potentially as osteoinductors in cases where the natural process of bone healing is endangered[11,12]. Surgical procedures are necessary when the biomechanical stabilization is required. Surgery is also useful when tissue stimulation is needed to complete bone healing. It creates a new traumatic environment with bleeding, growth factor liberation, cell migration and differentiation that stimulates new bone formation. Partial decortication procedures, as the ones described by Judet [13], have been used widely in many situations. Grafting and tissue healing augmentation with Autologous Growth Factors (AGF) are currently used in surgery to provide adequate osteoinduction and osteoconduction in order to solve the clinical situation[14-18].

In cases where the biomechanical stability of a fracture has been reached, but the biological status of bone healing is delayed, many non-invasive techniques have been described in order to obtain bone callus[6]. These techniques apply biophysical enhancement elements to increase bone healing in difficult circumstances. Electrical stimulation and magnetic fields have been used successfully in some cases [19-24], but the most documented and widespread system currently used is the stimulation of endogenous growth factors by focalized high energy ultrasound single pulses, or shockwaves[25,26].

ESWT and Bone Healing

Extracorporeal Shockwave Therapy (ESWT) has been studied in both experimental [27-39] and clinical [40-49] fields, showing good and excellent results in bone healing for delayed unions and pseudoarthrosis. The use of shockwaves focalized on the fracture site increases bone formation by means of vascular stimulation, periosteal reaction and osteoblast activation, probably due to the endogenous liberation of Nitrous Oxide, growth factors and free radicals[25]. These have been proven experimentally by Wang et al. [50,51], showing significant differences in animal models. Clinical trials of Shaden, Rompe, and Wang [45-47] have shown bone healing in delayed unions and pseudoarthrosis using high energy ESWT devices in single sessions with excellent results. There are several recent clinical studies on the effect of ESWT for nonunion and delayed union. Schaden et al. [45] reported their experience with ESWT for the treatment of delayed osseous union and nonunion in 115 patients with a success rate of 75.7%. In a prospective study, Rompe et al. [47] evaluated the effect of high-energy extracorporeal shockwaves in the treatment of 43 patients with tibial or femoral nonunions. They showed 72% of bony consolidation after an average of 4 months with no adverse events besides transient local hematoma. Wang et al. [46] reported a success rate of 80% at 12 months follow-up in the treatment of 72 nonunions of long bones with ESWT. These studies, with a success rate range of 70% to 80% in the achievement of bony union, showed moreover an adequate relief of symptoms, a functional recovery and no systemic complications. Therefore, the use of ESWT in the treatment of nonunion is highly recommended.

We have used both techniques in delayed unions, having as a primary indication for surgery the biomechanical instability of the fracture, and for ESWT the biological instability of the delayed union. We have used high energy ESWT for five years and our results show a 79% rate of healing without surgery, a number that reproduces the data from our colleagues in Europe and Asia. According to literature data and the recommendations of the ISMST, the energy required for bone healing treatments using ESWT must exceed $0.3 mJ/mm^2$, and must be done in one single session of at least 2000 shockwaves. This requires a high energy ESWT electromagnetic, electrohydraulic or piezoelectric generator that can deliver this amount of energy. These high energy shockwaves are painful and the procedure must be done under sedation or anesthesia. We have used shockwaves in a protocol with 1000 impulses of progressive energy that create an anesthetic area on the field of treatment, and then we can apply the 2000 high energy shockwaves we consider necessary on therapeutic levels. We believe using lower flux densities in a larger number of impulses does not increase bone stimulation, because reaching the target areas is difficult with devices that deliver these energies. One may apply >10,000 low energy shockwaves to a bone and never be able to reach cell stimulation in the fracture site. Rompe, Wang and Schaden have shown excellent results with high energy in one session, and there are no reports of similar results with lower energy protocols.

Radial shockwaves have been ruled out for bone treatments because of the low energy they deliver and the depth of the tissues that need to be treated[52]. Radial shockwaves spread from the contact point in the skin and lose power as they go deeper. Furthermore, due to its physical properties, this type of shockwave is not able to be focused on a deeper point[25,26]. However, the vascular and cellular effects of radial shockwaves on insertional tendinosis have proven superficial and periosteal revascularization in bone, and probably the good results of this technology in soft tissues is also caused by the stimulation of endogenous growth factors[50,51]. Using radial shockwaves should also create proper environments for healing stimulation in certain areas of bones close to the application site, but probably not on the whole fracture, especially in large bones like the femur or tibia.

AGF and Bone Healing

One of the turning points in orthopaedic surgery has been the growing interest in biological enhancement and orthobiologic procedures to improve bone healing. Ever since Marshal Urist described Bone Morphogenetic Protein in 1965 [53, 54], orthopaedists have been aiming for the "holy grail" of a substance that could easily and rapidly consolidate a fracture. Research in PTH, PTHrp, OP1 and AGF is growing, and an important number of papers and presentations today deal with this particular line of research[5, 55, 56]. Many forms of bone healing enhancers are commercially available, and the experience is getting stronger in evidence worldwide. The use of stem cells and haematopoietic concentrates are also very popular in many other tissues, and slowly growing into bone healing as a therapeutic tool[6]. The traditional enhancement factor used in the treatment of nonunions has been the autogenous bone graft in spite of its limited availability and the high rate of morbidity in the donor site (10 to 30%)[5,16]. Now, bone tissue engineering based therapies are emerging and increasing the current treatment choices[11].

AGF is a preparation of autologous plasma with a very high platelet concentration. The alpha granules in these platelets contain several biologically active growth and differentiation factors known by their important effect on bone tissue regeneration and neovascularization[57,58,5]. Moreover, the local hematoma produced with AGF activation serves as an osteoconductive scaffold to the repair process[59]. The uses of native growth factors offer various advantages to recombinant ones. Even if AGF contains a higher concentration of native growth factors, their biological proportion remains unchanged as well as their possible interactions[57,16]. Because of its autologous origin, AGF is safe from transmissible diseases and is free from immunological reactions[57]. The only possible adverse event with the use of AGF is the development of antibodies against bovine thrombin[16]. Therefore, we prefer the activation of human thrombin to avoid this undesirable complication.

We obtain our AGF from the own patient's blood, prepare it in a cell saver in order to obtain the PRP (platelet rich plasma) and the puffy coat, and then concentrate platelets rich in alpha granules to at least 1,000,000 platelets/µL[57]. This concentrate of PRP/AGF is then ready to prepare in the operating room in the consistency that the surgeon requires for each particular procedure[57]. In mixtures with powder grafts or with bone chips it is used in a liquid form, and in arthroscopic procedures it is concentrated to a thick gel that can be managed easily inside the joint. In bone reconstructive surgery like total hip revisions it is also gelled with grafts so the handling of the AGF is easy and delivered into the proper site the surgeon desires. The gellification process is aided with calcium gluconate that reacts with the patient's blood and thrombin to create the gel in the form we need. This concentration varies according to the surgical needs and is a simple procedure.

Using AGF in percutaneous applications should be able to enhance the healing process in bone. However, the vascular stimulation and the local bleeding is absent in percutaneous procedures, and is probably a key factor in the stimulation of bone formation. ESWT has proven a vascular stimulation and the generation of endogenous growth factors, and could be used to create the proper environment for AGF to act as osteoinductors in percutaneous procedures.

Our experience with autologous growth factors (AGF) in surgical procedures for delayed unions and pseudoarthrosis is very encouraging. Using the osteoinductive power of AGF with bone grafts has reduced bone healing time and resulted in stable consolidations. On the other hand, our experience with ESWT in delayed unions has reproduced the data from the literature, and our protocols for each treatment are well defined and followed. However, we would like an easier scenario for certain fractures that are stable, in superficial bones and show signs of delayed union. We came up with the idea of using a combined therapy of low energy shockwaves and the percutaneous application of AGF and wanted to determine if this approach would have similar results to those obtained from open surgery or high energy ESWT. With solid scientific background, it seemed feasible to obtain good results with this protocol, reducing treatment time and costs.

ESWT & AGF Combined Therapy

For stable delayed unions in superficial bones, we have used a combined therapy of radial shockwaves followed by the injection of percutaneous AGF. If delayed unions are seen as unfertile soil, shockwaves would act as a plow and AGF as a seed. We believe the combination of these therapies can result in the stimulation of bone healing in the same way high energy ESWT or surgical procedures do. The potential advantages are a short minimally invasive procedure with low cost. Having this in mind we started a pilot trial in voluntary patients booked for surgery for delayed stable non unions in 2004. The patients selected to receive the treatment with radial shockwaves and injection of AGF were skeletally mature with nonunions or delayed unions of long bones not deeper than 1.5 inches, like tibia, ulna, fibula, distal femur and humerus. The contraindications to undergo this treatment were basically the same of high-energy shockwave treatments but since anesthesia is not required, criteria are less demanding. A patient was not treated with radial shockwaves and AGF if he met one of the following criteria: inadequate stabilization, local bone infection, pathologic fracture, tumor within the shockwave field, coagulopathy, use of anticoagulants or pregnancy.

We have treated 16 delayed unions since February 2004. They were 5 females and 11 males with an average age of 39 years (range, 17 to 61 years). One patient received treatment for two delayed unions: a supracondylar fracture of the humerus and an olecranon osteotomy from the original surgical approach. Five fractures had delayed healing (3 to 6 months from the initial injury or the last operation), and 11 fractures had an established nonunion with an evolution of more than 6 months (range, 6 to 13 months). We treated 6 tibias, 4 humeri, 5 ulnas, and 1 metatarsal. All nonunions were atrophic and did not show signs of established pseudoarthrosis or hyperthropic radiological changes, and had defects under 3 mm. (Table 1)

We have developed a protocol for the application of radial shockwaves supplemented with AGF. This single ambulatory procedure is done in an operating room under aseptic conditions and takes between 30 and 40 minutes.

Our process to prepare AGF is the standardized autologous procedure. With a double centrifugation technique, a platelet rich plasma with at least 1,000,000 platelets/μL in a 5ml volume is obtained[57]. This procedure requires a sterile management and pyrogen free disposable materials. Since the technique lasts approximately 1 hour, the patient blood sample (25 cm^3) has to be taken at least one hour before the shockwave application.

We do not use local anesthesia in these cases, and we prefer to use our progressive shockwave protocol to generate a reasonable anesthetic level to both apply therapeutic shockwaves and inject the AGF. With the patient placed on a standard operating table, the fracture site is localized with an X-Ray image intensifier.

With no anesthesia, we applied the following protocol: 4000 continuous impulses with 1 to 4 Bar, equivalent to 0.03 to 0.18 mJ/mm^2 energy flux density at a frequency of 6 to 10 Hz. In all cases we have used the Swiss Dolor Clast® radial shockwave generator produced by EMS in Switzerland. Once the fracture is localized in position and depth, a lubricating gel is applied over the skin. The shockwaves are delivered with a 15mm hand applicator in direct contact with the skin, with circular movements in order to achieve stimulation in all the fracture area. The initial pressure of wave application is 1 Bar (<0.03mJ/mm^2) at 10 Hz, and it is gradually increased. Then, at 500 impulses the pressure is raised to 2 Bar (0.06 mJ/mm^2) and at 1000 impulses to 3.5 Bar (0.16mJ/mm^2). Simultaneously, the frequency is decreased initially to 8 Hz and then to 6 Hz. After the first 2000 shockwaves that are used for analgesia, we start the treatment with 2000 continuous impulses with 3.5 to 4 Bar (0.16 to 0.18 mJ/mm^2) at 6 Hz. During the procedure the patient can experience some pain that is used to check the positioning of the device. Major vascular and neural structures and areas with metallic internal fixation are avoided.

Patient	Age	Gender	Site	Type of Fracture	Months Post Fx	Rx Healing at 12 weeks
1	30	F	Ulna	Transverse single diaphyseal – No hardware	5	Yes
2	43	M	Tibia	Segmentary & Double plate	10	No
3	42	F	Tibia	Macquet osteotomy - Allograft & screw	5	Yes
4	24	F	Tibia	Diaphyseal oblique & IM nail	13	Yes
5	26	M	Ulna	Diaphyseal segmentary & 3.5 DCP plate	5	Yes
6	24	M	Tibia	Diaphyseal transverse & IM nail	11	Yes
7	52	M	Humerus	Diaphyseal transverse & IM nail	6	Yes
8	20	M	Ulna	Transverse single diaphyseal – No hardware	4	Yes
9	61	F	Humerus	Supracondylar & double plates	12	Yes
9	61	F	Ulna	Trans-olecranon approach & K wires	12	No
10	55	M	Tibia	Distal metaphyseal & MIS plate	10	Yes
11	17	M	Humerus	Diaphyseal & no hardware	5	Yes
12	36	F	4th Metatarsal	Proximal osteotomy & no hardware	10	Yes
13	42	M	Humerus	Diaphyseal & 3.5 DCP plate	12	Yes
14	26	M	Tibia	Diaphyseal prox. third transverse & 4.5 Plate	13	Yes
15	24	M	Ulna	Transverse dyaphiseal & 3.5 LC-DCP plate	6	Yes

M = male; F = female; Fx= Fracture

Table 1. The epidemiological data of our patients. Only one did not show signs of radiological healing after 12 weeks of radiological follow up. Three of them were complications of osteotomies in previously healthy bones.

When the application of shockwaves finished, 10 ml of the previously prepared AGF is activated with calcium gluconate and injected percutaneously under fluoroscopy in different points of the fracture soft callus. In the fractures with a gap larger than 3 mm, the AGF is mixed with lyophilized cryopreserved 300 micron bone allografts.

The rehabilitation process starts from the first day after treatment. All patients were immobilized for at least two weeks, and weight bearing was allowed in tibial fractures using leg braces. Patients clinical follow-up was made weekly during the first month and monthly during the first year. The intensity of pain before and after the treatment was assessed with a visual analogue scale from 0 to 10, having 0 for no pain and 10 for worst pain. Radiologic images were taken to assess callus formation, fracture defects and the presence of bone union at 6 weeks and 3, 6, and 12 months after treatment.

Bone union after delayed fracture healing or established nonunion was assessed by clinical and radiological evaluations. Clinical assessment included pain intensity, fracture stability and range of motion. Radiologic evolution was determined by defect size, callus formation and stability. We considered an excellent result when both clinical and radiological stability has been achieved at 12 weeks after the treatment. We considered a good result when radiological stability is incomplete at 12 weeks, but the clinical and radiological evolution shows improvement during the follow-up. Bad results are patients with clinical or radiological instability or those who required surgical treatment.

Patients were evaluated blindly by a group of radiologists to determine the evolution of the healing process. The clinical follow-up was not blinded due to the nature of the procedure and the patient's knowledge of the type of treatment he received. We had excellent results in 14 cases (87.5%). This group had both clinical and radiological stability of the fracture at 12 weeks, even after periods as long as 17 months with no response to previous treatments. Most of the patients had stable delayed unions or nonunions that were on the limit for surgical revision. (Figure 1) We performed this treatment even in patients with serious conditions around the fracture, like vascular grafts and skin flaps. (Figure 2)

We had no healing in one tibia, originally an open segmentary high energy fracture treated with double plates and grafts. One of the fractures healed and the other one did not. We treated the nonunion, but the patient showed no signs of bone callus after six months. A revision surgery was performed and the stabilization was done with an IM nail. The other bone that did not heal was an olecranon osteotomy that had a 3 mm gap. Even though the elbow was immobilized, the K wires broke, a sign interpreted as fracture instability. The patient required surgical revision and grafting. (Figure 3)

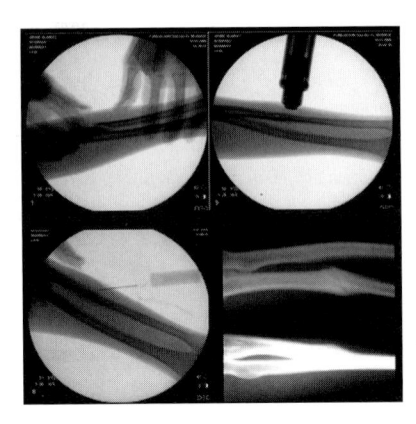

Figure 1. Patient # 8, 20 year old male, sports related accident with single diaphyseal mid-third ulnar fracture. Initially treated with closed reduction and immobilization. Four months after injury there is pain in prono-supination and X-Rays show no signs of healing (Upper Left). An open procedure is proposed with open reduction and internal fixation with a 3.5 DCP plate. Instead, we performed our protocol with rESWT (Upper Right) and AGF (Lower Left). Twelve weeks after the procedure there is a stable callus and the patient is pain free (Lower right).

Our preliminary results were so encouraging that we have stopped the treatments of delayed unions with high energy ESWT on these particular indications: stable delayed unions or nonunions in superficial bones. However, we must be sure if the effect of one of our treatments is enough by itself, or if the combination of rESWT and AGF is the one that is giving us these promising results. We have already started an experimental study in an animal model of nonunions in dogs, to determine the differences between groups treated only with rESWT, only with AGF, a third group treated with a combined therapy, and a control group. This study will tell us the role of each therapeutic variable in order to go further in its use.

The development of effective and safe methods to enhance the complex process of bone healing is one of the most important research questions in present orthopaedics. Biophysical stimulation of bone by means of extracorporeal shockwaves induces regenerating responses in bone tissue[25]. The use of recombinant or autologous growth factors in bone is also well documented and widely used today.

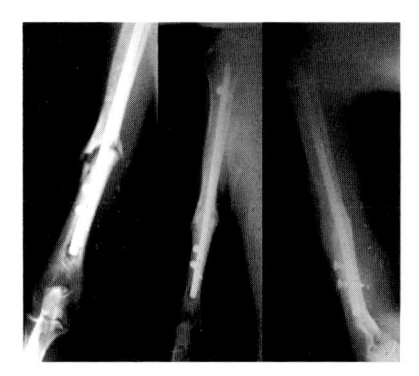

Figure 2. Patient # 7, 52 year old male, motor vehicle accident with massive skin loss that required grafting. Open GIIIC fracture with loss of humeral artery that required Dacron graft. Six months after stabilization with an IM nail shows no signs of healing and the patient has permanent pain (Left). Infection is ruled out by labs and bone scans. rESWT&AGF is performed. Six weeks after treatment there is no pain and X Rays show signs of healing (Center). Twelve weeks after treatment there is a stable mature callus and the patient is painless (Right).

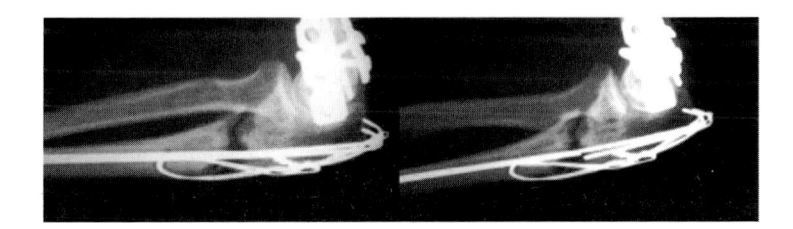

Figure 3. Patient # 9, 61 year old female, motor vehicle accident. The initial diagnosis was an inter-supracondylar fracture treated with double plates. The surgical approach required an olecranon osteotomy that did not heal. The Supracondylar fracture did not heal as well. rESWT&AGF was done in both Supracondylar and olecranon nonunions (Left). The humerus healed properly after 12 weeks post treatment, but the olecranon did not show any signs of bone callus. There is probably a mechanical instability left because the K wires were broken in the 12 week X Ray control (Right).

We propose the use of a combined therapy of low energy radial shockwaves and autologous platelet derived growth factors in the treatment of biomechanically stable delayed unions and nonunions in superficial bones, as another minimally invasive tool that represents lower costs and in our experience is giving similar results as of those obtained with open grafting procedures or high energy ESWT. Further research is absolutely necessary, not only in the animal model we are currently working on, but also in multicentric clinical trials. Not everything new is always good, but one must remember that everything good was new once.

Literature

1. Einhorn TA. The Cell and Molecular Biology of Fracture Healing. Clin Orthop Rel Res 1998 Oct;355(Suppl):S7-S21
2. Miclau T, Helms JA. Molecular aspects of fracture healing. Curr Opin Orthop 2000 Oct;11(5):367-371
3. Bostrom MP, Yang X, Koutras I. Biologics in bone healing. Curr Opin Orthop 2000 Oct;11(5):403-412
4. Einhorn TA. Clinically Applied Models of Bone Regeneration in Tissue Engineering Research. Clin Orthop Rel Res 1999 Oct;367(Suppl):S59-S67
5. Lieberman JR, Daluiski A, Einhorn TA. The role of Growth Factors in the repair of bone: biology and clinical applications. J Bone Joint Surg Am 2002;84:1032-1044
6. Rodriguez-Merchan EC, Forriol F. Nonunion: General Principles and Experimental Data. Clin Orthop Rel Res 2004 Feb;419:4-12
7. Rodriguez-Merchan EC. Editorial comment. Clin Orthop Rel Res 2004 Feb;419:1
8. Perry CR. Bone Repair Techniques, Bone Graft, and Bone Graft Substitutes. Clin Orthop Rel Res 1999 March;360:71-86
9. Bauer TW, Muschler GF. Bone Graft Materials: An Overview of the Basic Science. Clin Orthop Rel Res 2000 Feb;371:10-27
10. LeGeros RZ. Properties of Osteoconductive Biomaterials: Calcium Phosphates. Clin Orthop Rel Res 2002 Feb;395:81-98
11. Boden S. Bioactive factors for bone tissue engineering. Clin Orthop Rel Res 1999;367(Suppl):S84-S94
12. Beasley LS, Einhorn TA. The role of growth factors in fracture healing. In: Canalis E. Skeletal Growth Factors. Philadelphia: Lippincott Williams & Wilkins. 2000:311-322
13. Judet R, Judet J. [Osteo-periosteal decortication. Principle, technic, indications and results]. Memoires de l'Académie de Chirurgie 1965 May; 91(15):463-70
14. Anitua E. Plasma rich in growth factors: preliminary results of use in the preparation of future sites for implants. Int J Oral Maxillofac Implants. 1999 Jul-Aug;14(4):529-535
15. Hom DB, Thatcher G, Tibesar R. Growth factor therapy to improve soft tissue healing. Facial Plast Surg 2002 Feb;18(1):41-52
16. Sanchez AR, Sheridan PJ, Kupp LI. Is platelet-rich plasma the perfect enhancement factor? A current review. Int J Oral Maxillofac Implants 2003 Jan-Feb;18(1):93-103

17. Tozum TF, Demiralp B. Platelet rich plasma: a promising innovation in dentistry. J Canadian Dental Association 2003 Nov;69(10):664
18. Thorn JJ, Sorensen H, Weis-Fogh U, Andersen M. Autologous fibrin glue with growth factors in reconstructive maxillofacial surgery. Int J Oral Maxillofac Surg 2004 Jan;33(1):95-100
19. Day L. Electrical stimulation in the treatment of ununited fractures. Clin Orthop Rel Res 1981 Nov-Dec;161:54-57
20. Jorgensen TE. Asymmetrical slow-pulsating direct current. Clin Orthop Rel Res 1981 Nov-Dec;161:67-70
21. Sharrard WJ. A double blind trial of pulsed electromagnetic fields for delayed union of tibial fractures. J Bone Joint Surg Br 1990 May;72B(3):347-355
22. Scott G, King JB. A prospective, double-blind trial of electrical capacitive coupling in the treatment of non-union of long-bones. J Bone Joint Surg Am 1994 Jun;76A(6):820-826
23. Rogozinski A, Rogozinski C. Efficacy of implanted bone growth stimulation in instrumented lumbosacral spinal fusion. Spine 1996 Nov;21(21):2479-2483
24. Aaron RC, Ciombor DM, Simon BJ. Treatment of Nonunions With Electric and Electromagnetic Fields. Clin OrthopRel Res 2004;419:21–29
25. Ogden JA, Alvarez R, Levitt R, Marlow M. Shockwave Therapy (Orthotripsy(R)) in Musculoskeletal Disorders. Clin Orthop Rel Res 2001 June;387:22-40
26. Thiel M. Application of Shockwaves in Medicine. Clin Orthop Rel Res 2001 June;387:18-21
27. Yeaman LD, Jerome CP, McCollough D. Effects of shockwave therapy on the structure and growth of the immature rat epiphysis. J Urol 1989; 141:670-674
28. Van Arsdalen KN, Kurzweil S, Smith J, Levin RM. Effect of lithotripsy on immature rabbit bone and kidney development. J Urol 1991;146:213-216
29. Rompe JD, Kirkpatrick CJ, Kullmer K, Schwitalle M, Krischek O. Dosed-related effects of shockwaves on rabbit tendo achillis. A sonographic and histological study. J Bone Joint Surg Br 1998 may; 80-B(3):546-552
30. Ikeda K, Tomita K, Takayama K. Application of extracorporeal shockwave on bone. J Trauma 1999; 47(5):946-950
31. Wang FS, Wang CJ, Huang HJ, Chung H, Chen RF, Yang KD. Physical shockwave mediates membrane hyperpolarization and Ras activation for osteogenesis in human bone marrow stromal cells. Biochem Biophys Res Com 2001 Sep;287(3):648-55
32. Wang FS,Yang KD,Chen RF,Wang CJ,Sheen-Chen SM. Extracorporeal shockwave promotes growth and differentiation of bone-marrow stromal cells towards osteoprogenitors associated with induction of TGF-beta1. J Bone Joint Surg Br 2002 Apr;84(3):457-61
33. Wang FS, Yang KD, Kuo YR, Wang CJ, Sheen-Chen SM, Huang HC, Chen YJ. Temporal and spatial expression of bone morphogenetic proteins in extracorporeal shockwave-promoted healing of segmental defect. Bone 2003 Apr;32(4):387-96
34. Maier M, Averbeck B, Milz S, Refior HJ, Schmitz C. Substance P and Prostaglandin E2 Release After Shockwave Application to the Rabbit Femur. Clin Orthop Rel Res 2003;406:237-245
35. Martini L, Giavaresi G, Fini M, Torricelli P, Pretto M, Schaden W, Giardino R. Effect of Extracorporeal Shockwave Therapy on Osteoblastlike Cells. Clin Orthop Rel Res 2003;413:269–280
36. Chen YJ, Kuo YR, Yang KD, Wang CJ, Sheen Chen SM, Huang HC, Yang YJ, Yi-Chih S, Wang FS. Activation of extracellular signal-regulated kinase (ERK) and p38

kinase in shockwave-promoted bone formation of segmental defect in rats. Bone 2004 Mar;34(3):466-77

37. Chen YJ, Wang CJ, Yang KD, Kuo YR, Huang HC, Huang YT, Sun YC, Wang FS. Extracorporeal shockwaves promote healing of collagenase-induced Achilles tendinitis and increase TGF-beta1 and IGF-I expression. J Orthop Res 2004 Jul;22(4):854-61

38. Chen YJ, Wurtz T, Wang CJ, Kuo YR, Yang KD, Huang HC, Wang FS. Recruitment of mesenchymal stem cells and expression of TGF-beta 1 and VEGF in the early stage of shockwave-promoted bone regeneration of segmental defect in rats. J Orthop Res 2004 May;22(3):526-34

39. Wang CJ, Yang KD, Wang FS, Hsu CC, Chen HH. Shockwave treatment shows dose-dependent enhancement of bone mass and bone strength after fracture of the femur. Bone 2004 Jan;34(1):225-30

40. Haupt G, Haupt A, Ekkernkamp A, Gerety B, Chvapil M. Influence of shockwaves in fracture healing. Urology 1992;39:529-532

41. Haupt G. Use of extracorporeal shockwaves in the treatment of pseudoarthrosis, tendinopathy and other orthopedic diseases. J Urol 1997;158:4-11

42. Vogel J, Hopf C, Eysel P, Rompe JD. Application of extracorporeal shockwaves in the treatment of pseudarthrosis of the lower extremity. Preliminary results. Arch Orthop Trauma Surg 1997;116(8):480-3

43. Vogel J, Rompe JD, Hopf C, Heine J, Burger R. [High-energy extracorporeal shock-wave therapy (ESWT) in the treatment of pseudarthrosis]. Zeitschrift fur Orthopadie und Ihre Grenzgebiete 1997 Mar-Apr;135(2):145-9

44. Beutler S, Regel G, Pape HC, Machtens S, Weinberg AM, Kremeike I, Jonas U, Tscherne H. [Extracorporeal shockwave therapy for delayed union of long bone fractures - preliminary results of a prospective cohort study]. Unfallchirurg. 1999 Nov;102(11):839-47

45. Schaden W, Fischer A, Sailler A. Extracorporeal Shockwave Therapy of Nonunion or Delayed Osseous Union. Clin Orthop Rel Res 2001 June;387:90-94

46. Wang CJ, Chen HS, Chen CE, Yang KD. Treatment of Nonunions of Long Bone Fractures With Shockwaves. Clin Orthop Rel Res 2001 June;387:95-101

47. Rompe JD, Rosendahl T, Schollner C, Theis C. High-Energy Extracorporeal Shockwave Treatment of Nonunions. Clin Orthop Rel Res 2001 June;387:102-111

48. Birnbaum K, Wirtz DC, Siebert CH, Heller KD. Use of extracorporeal shockwave therapy (ESWT) in the treatment of non-unions. A review of the literature. Arch Orthop Trauma Surg 2002 Jul;122(6):324-30

49. Schoellner C, Rompe JD, Decking J, Heine J. [High energy extracorporeal shockwave therapy (ESWT) in pseudarthrosis]. Orthopade 2002 Jul;31(7):658-62

50. Wang CJ, Huang HY, Pai CH. Shockwave-enhanced neovascularization at the tendon-bone junction: an experiment in dogs. J Foot Ankle Surg 2002 Jan-Feb;41(1):16-22

51. Wang CJ, Wang FS, Yang KD, Weng LH, Hsu CC, Huang CS, Yang LC. Shockwave therapy induces neovascularization at the tendon-bone junction. A study in rabbits. J Orthop Res 2003 Nov;21(6):984-9

52. Ogden JA, Tóth-Kischkat A, Schultheiss R. Principles of Shockwave Therapy. Clin Orthop Rel Res 2001;387:8-17

53. Urist MR. Bone: Formation by autoinduction. Science 1965;150:893-899

54. Gibble JW, Ness PM. Fibrin glue: the perfect operative sealant? Transfusion 1990 Oct;30(8):741-7

55. Geesink RGT, Hoefnagels NHM, Bulstra SK. Osteogenic activity of OP-1 bone morphogenetic protein (BMP-7) in a human fibular defect J Bone Joint Surg Br 1999;81B:710-8
56. Friedlaender GE, Perry CR, Cole JD, Cook SD, Cierny G, Muschler GF, Zych GA, Calhoun JH, LaForte AJ, Yin S. Comparing rhOP-1 with Fresh Bone Autograft of Tibial Nonunions : A Prospective, Randomized Clinical Trial. J Bone Joint Surg Am 2001; 83(Suppl 1):151-158
57. Marx RE. Platelet-Rich Plasma (PRP): What Is PRP and What Is Not PRP? Implant Dentistry 2001 Dec;10(4):225-228
58. Glowacki J. Angiogenesis in fracture repair. Clin Orthop Rel Res 1998 Oct;355(Suppl):S82-S89
59. Watson JT. Autologous growth factors combined with demineralized bone matrix used as an alternative to autograft for the treatment of recalcitrant nonunited fractures of long bones: a report of six cases. Depuy Orthopaedics, Inc. 2002

33

Results of Three Prospective Studies in Patients with Neck Pain, Shoulder and Arm Pain, Lumbago and Ischial Bursitis

W. Bauermeister

Introduction

Trigger points correspond to a neuromuscular disorder referred to as Myofascial Trigger Point Syndrome (MTS). They are characterized by regional pain, sensory disorders and functional disorders of the musculoskeletal system which, in the initial phase, occur only when subjected to extraordinary stress. Later, in the chronification phase, pain is caused by performing activities of daily living, stress and even changing weather conditions. The final phase is marked by permanent pain, minimal stress threshold, increasing social isolation and reactive depression syndrome. This evolution coincides with an ever-expanding dysfunction of the motoric end plates of the muscle fibers. What is suspected is an excessive release of acetylcholine and a contraction of the sarcomere[1]. An accumulation of these contracted sarcomere is known as the trigger point complex (Figure 1) and brings about a shortening of the entire muscle. A pathological end plate noise (EPN) is identified electrophysiologically in the EMG and a histological exam of muscle biopsy shows the contraction of the sarcomere as well (Figure 2)[2,3]. Based on the hypothesis of energy crisis, accompanying vasoconstriction releases sensitizing substances which affect the nociceptors and bring about a lowering of the pain. The development of a local pathological pain transfer system may bring about the muscular trigger point[4].

Depending on their clinical effect, active and latent trigger points can be distinguished. Active triggers shorten the muscle and cause transfer phenomena such as pain in another part of the body. This is know as referred pain. Like active

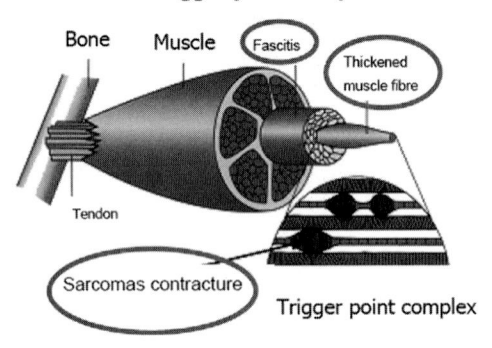

Figure 1. Trigger point complex.

triggers, latent triggers also cause muscle structures to shorten but they do not bring about any referred phenomena causing patients to suffer. In muscles that are accessible for palpation, both types of trigger can be identified as a sharply painful knot in a hardened muscle. In case of active triggers, pressure applied to this knot causes significant pain. Applying pressure on a latent trigger causes no pain in general, or pain not known by the patient or pain not previously existing.

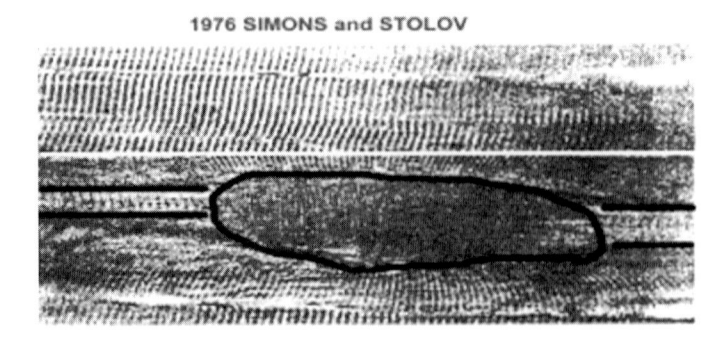

Figure 2. Trigger point histology. Longitudinal cross-section of a canine M. The outlined area encompasses some 100 sarcomere forming a knot. The sarcomere on both sides of the knot appear to be longer as compensation.

The trigger point complex is locted in the end plate zone and is referred to as central trigger points.

Inclusion criteria

Patients with chronic, therapy-resistant pain caused by active triggers.

Exclusion criteria

Patients with fibromyalgia, tumors, disc protrusion with neurologic deficits, peripheral nerve lesions or other significant diseases.

Drop-out criteria

Patients were required to get 6 treatments in total. Patients who refused the full treatment cycle were excluded for efficacy analysis.

Patient selection

For each group 20 patients were selected randomly.

Evaluation criteria for response to treatment

The evaluation criterion "Pain" was measured by the patients on the 100 mm Visual Analog Scale VAS. VAS PRE at baseline was documented before the first treatment, VAS POST (re-exam) at the end of the treatment. VAS FU was determined in a telephone follow-up.

Trigger point diagnosis

A first step consisted of measuring the range of motion (ROM) of the joint. A limitation in mobility or a right/left variation appears to indicate MTS. As a result of muscle shortening, there is restriction in the range of motion in muscles (the antagonists) extended during the exam. Included in the study were the rotation, lateral flexion, flexion and extension of the neck spinal column; inner and outer rotation and abduction of the shoulder; rotation and lateral flexion of the lumbar spine; and internal and external rotation of the hip. Muscle groups responsible for limitations in range of motion (ROM) were examined for trigger-specific characteristics: taut muscle fiber bundle (Taut Band TB), sharply painful knot within the TB, trigger of patient-specific pain patterns (Referred Pain RP) by pressure stimulation with the TRIGGOsan key on the Trigger Points. TBs or Trigger Points could not be detected in deeper or very large muscles. In these muscles, diagnosis was limited to triggering RP by applying pressure with the TRIGGOsan key[5].

Treatment

The muscles identified through trigger point diagnosis were treated with radial extracorporeal shockwaves using the Swiss DolorClast®. The number of impulses per treatment depended on the effect of the treatment as well as on increased mobility and decrease in pain. Treatment intensity was just below the pain tolerance threshold and no local anesthesia was required.

Results

A summary of the results is shown in Table 1.

Cervical spine and shoulder

VAS PRE (Chart 1) and VAS POST (Chart 2) were compared to evaluate the effect of the treatment. The comparison revealed a subjective improvement of about 56.6%. A follow-up (Chart 3) was conducted in 15 patients of this group. The subjective improvement was 43.7% in a mean follow up period of 135 days. The mean treatment number was 6.8 within a period of 71 days.

Shoulder

A comparison of VAS PRE (Chart 4) and VAS POST (Chart 5) in 20 patients showed a subjective improvement of about 68%. A follow-up (Chart 6) conducted in 8 patients of this group showed an improvement of about 74.5% on the VAS. The treatment number was 4.45 within a treatment period of 39 days.

		Cervical n=20	Shoulder n=20	Lumbar n=20
		Mean value	Mean value	Mean value
1	VAS PRE	8.40	7.1	7.0
2	VAS POST	3.65	2.27	2.65
4	VAS FU	4.73 n=15	1.81 n=8	2.81 n=16
3	VAS PRE/VAS POST Change in %	56.6	68.0	62.1
5	VAS POST/VAS FU Change in %	43.7	74.5	50.8
6	Days FU	135	187	112
8	Total Impulses	30,400	13,162	27,250
7	Number of Treatments	6.80	4.45	6.1
9	Impulses/Treatment	4470	2957	4467
11	Treatment Period (Days)	71	39	64
10	Duration of Pain (Months)	103	30	76
12	Age (Years)	51.55	55.45	54.2

Table 1. Results of treatment.

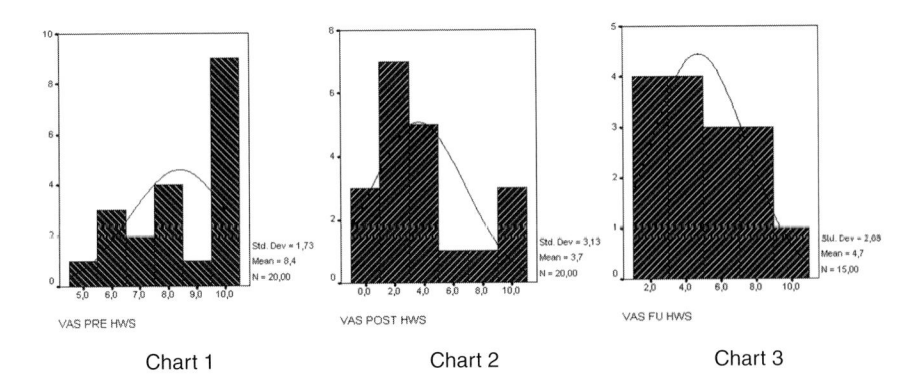

Chart 1

Chart 2

Chart 3

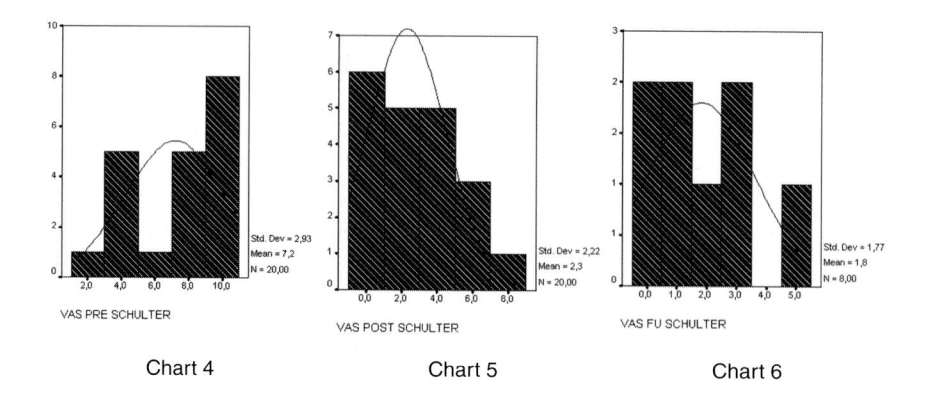

Chart 4 — VAS PRE SCHULTER (Std. Dev = 2,93; Mean = 7,2; N = 20,00)

Chart 5 — VAS POST SCHULTER (Std. Dev = 2,22; Mean = 2,3; N = 20,00)

Chart 6 — VAS FU SCHULTER (Std. Dev = 1,77; Mean = 1,8; N = 8,00)

Low back pain

A comparison of VAS PRE (Chart 7) versus VAS POST (Chart 8) in 20 patients showed an improvement of about 62%. A follow-up (Chart 9) in 16 patients of this group showed a subjective improvement of 59.8% on the VAS. The treatment number was 6.1 within a period of 64 days.

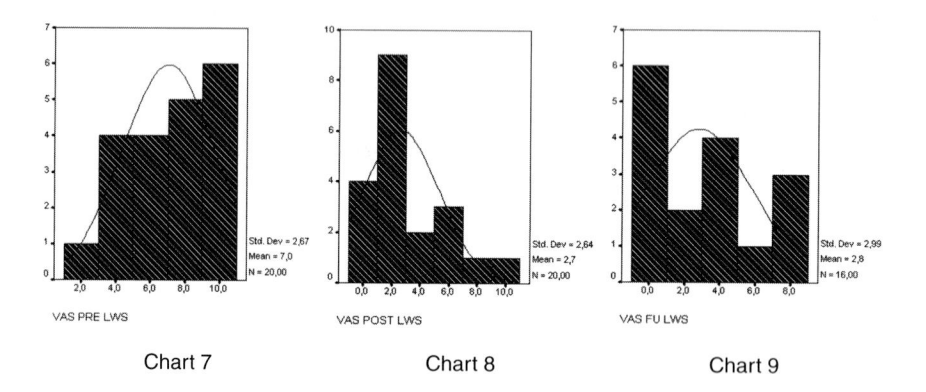

Chart 7 — VAS PRE LWS (Std. Dev = 2,67; Mean = 7,0; N = 20,00)

Chart 8 — VAS POST LWS (Std. Dev = 2,64; Mean = 2,7; N = 20,00)

Chart 9 — VAS FU LWS (Std. Dev = 2,99; Mean = 2,8; N = 16,00)

Discussion

The results indicate that the application of radial extracorporeal shockwaves may affect the symptoms of myofascial trigger point syndrome even over a longer period of time. The results for the cervical spine/shoulder area appear poorer and this observation coincides with our experience in practice. Treatment results may be improved by increasing the number of impulses per treatment and by refining diagnosis of MTS in muscles with difficult access. A combined use of ballistic shockwaves and mechanical pressure could further improve the treatment's success. Finally, the treatment parameters (number of shockwaves, energy flux densitiy, interval, etc.) have to be specified by prospective controlled studies, but rESWT could be indicated in patients suffereing from trigger point related musculoskeletal disorders as shown in our preliminary study.

Conclusion

These studies could be the basis for further evidence-based research to bring scientific evidence of the efficacy of the application of radial shockwaves for the treatment of myofascial trigger point syndrome.

Literature

1. Simons, D.G., & Stolov, W.C., (1976) Microscopic features and transient contraction of palpable bands in canine muscle. Am J Phys Med 55: 65-88
2. Simons D., Travell J., Simons L., Myofascial Pain and Dysfunction, Second Edition, 1999 Lippincott Williams&Wilkins
3. Travell J., and Simons D., Handbuch der Muskel- Triggerpunkte Untere Extremität, 1. Auflage 2000 Urban & Fischer Verlag München Jena
4. Mense S, Simons DG, Russell IJ 2001 Muscle Pain: Understanding its Nature,
5. Diagnosis, and Treatment. Lippincott, Williams &Wilkins, Philadelphia. (Endplate hypothesis,pp.240 –259)
6. Bauermeister W., (1999) Trigger – Osteopraktik, Physikalische Therapie in Theorie und Praxis, 20/8, 487-490

ATRAD - Association for Radial Pain Therapy
Felix Egloff

ATRAD is an international association dealing with musculoskeletal issues related to radial Shockwave Therapy (rESWT).

The association was founded by Swiss physicians in 2003. It acts as a negotiating partner and protects the interests of members where official bodies, insurance companies, organizations, public authorities and industry are concerned. It also offers all users an identification platform for the high-level exchange of scientific knowledge and ideas. It runs working seminars and sends out newsletters to support these objectives and to improve opportunities for contact between users.

Across the field of Shockwave Therapy as a whole, ATRAD aims to gain general recognition for this modern form of treatment and to achieve positive collaboration. On the basis of various studies and in-depth evaluations, we have decided to use the Swiss DolorClast® radial methods exclusively.

ATRAD, the medical association for pain therapy, promotes research and application of radial Extracorporeal Shockwave Therapy (rESWT) using the Swiss DolorClast® method and national and international dissemination of knowledge from science and practice in the interests of improving patient care.

The high satisfaction rate of our patients suffering from musculoskeletal disorders confirms our excellent results. We have become established in professional sports medicine, scientifically proven in many studies and economical with respect to time and money.

ATRAD purpose

In the light of the core competencies of our association and our legally specified goals we are working to

- disseminate knowledge from science and practice
- conduct research and application
- provide training with working conferences and exchange of experience
- assist scientific studies of new indications
- provide continuous education of our members
- represent the interests of our members to outside organizations and do publicity work
- encourage targeted development of improved patient orientation

ATRAD combines the providers of the radial Extracorporeal Shockwave Therapy with the new and very successful Swiss DolorClast® method.

ATRAD mission

Our patients are of course at the center of our mission. We want to provide a highly effective method, a short rehabilitation time, minimal time out of work and a high positive impact on their personal life. This is also important for the economy as a whole. Our patients also pay insurance premiums. We are aware of the cost developments in the international health system.

We know that treatments for orthopaedic problems will increase. This is for demographic reasons and also as a result of the renewed interest in sport and fitness. Our conclusion is that cost increases will be unavoidable unless we concentrate on improved and more economical treatment methods. This makes our mission an unmistakable message to legislators, associations and insurance companies because radial Extracorporeal Shockwave Therapy saves money and time.

We treat clearly defined diagnoses with unified parameters. The Swiss Dolor-Clast® method is superior to the traditional and in some cases antiquated treatments, more successful in healing and alleviating symptoms and far more economical.

Our own and international studies clearly confirm that radial Shockwave Therapy complies with usual regulations regarding

- practicality
- efficacy
- economy

The radial shockwaves as applied are superior to other treatment options. We are working towards having this method added to the catalogue of services covered by the compulsory basic insurance. This is being done for the welfare of the patient.

ATRAD's first rESWT Multicenter study (2002)

A multicentric study on radial Shockwave Therapy using the Swiss DolorClast® conducted on behalf of ATRAD has been submitted to health authorities in Switzerland.

To ensure the desirable confidence level, the study was restricted to three reference diagnoses

- Rotator cuff tendopathy (Shoulder pain)
- Epicondylopathy (Tennis elbow)
- Plantar fasciitis (Heel pain)

A total of 249 patients were treated with the Swiss DolorClast® method during 919 shockwave therapy sessions with the following results:

After completion of treatment —
    good to very good in more than 80% of cases

Ten weeks after treatment —
    good to very good in more than 80% of cases

Treatment result:

- Shoulder pain: 84.77% good to very good

- Tennis elbow: 82.45% good to very good
- Heel pain: 85.06% good to very good

This study result is superior to all traditional methods.

And the costs?

To compare the treatment costs, the costs of three options were calculated in U.S. dollars:

- case costs of an insurance company charging basic insurance coverage
- case costs of Extracorporeal Shockwave treatment with large devices on the Internet at the time of the study
- case costs with our method using innovative, practice-oriented small devices

All costs in U.S. dollars

	Traditional	**Large device**	**Swiss DolorClast®**
Shoulder Pain	$2,090.90	$2,851.07	$298.37
Tennis elbow	$1,492.01	$3,414.66	$397.82
Heel pain	$1,030.94	$3,414.66	$298.37

ATRAD general secretary
Felix Egloff
Brühlfeldweg 8
CH-Otelfingen / Switzerland
www.atrad.ch

ISMST - International Society for Musculoskeletal Shockwave Therapy An international platform for communication and knowledge transfer

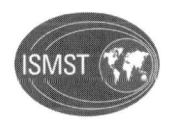

Vinzenz Auersperg
Richard Thiele

Since the end of the 1980's, musculoskeletal shockwave therapy has been researched in the field of orthopaedic trauma and administered to patients suffering from various sorts of ailments. So it was simply a matter of time before working groups and practitioners' meetings became registered associations and societies. By 1994, national organizations like the German Association for Musculoskeletal Shockwave Therapy (DGST), the Swiss Association for Orthopaedic Shockwave Therapy (SGST) and working groups within the German and Austrian Associations for Orthopaedic Traumatology (AK 10 of the DGOOC and AK-ESWT of the ÖGO) had been established. Other organizations such as the National Association for ESWT in Italy (SITOD) likewise followed suit. This new technology spread with such explosive force and demonstrated such immense success that an international coordination and communication platform for these organizations soon proved necessary. To this end, the European Society for Shockwave Therapy (ESMST) was founded on June 14, 1997, during the German Orthopaedic Association (DGOT, today the DGOOC) Congress in Vienna, for the purpose of bringing together European researchers and practitioners. Representatives of the management and advisory boards were drawn from all the then existing national organizations.

Immense interest in the technology and the first of many promising publicized results gave impetus for the association to convene on a regular basis. A decision was made for an annual conference to be held each year in a different country. To ESMST's delight, the personal efforts of its members from the various states helped make these meetings a reality and a success. The list of locations (Table 1) where the association has since met reflects this worldwide resonance. With ESWT expanding beyond the European border and Japan, Taiwan and the US on the threshold of becoming active members, the association was renamed the International Society for Musculoskeletal Shockwave Therapy (ISMST) in London, 1999.

From the inception, the expressive aim was to gather in one place, if possible, all those who are interested in shockwave therapy, in order that the transfer of knowledge not be restricted to national societies and associations or practitioners' groups that specialized in individual devices. With additional applications of this highly successful therapy, the range of healthcare professionals and scientists has broadened from trauma surgeons and orthopaedists to include those in veterinary medicine, cardiology, sports medicine, dermatology and plastic surgery. The ISMST today has grown to 492 full members, with an additional 81 awaiting membership, from 55 countries (see list).

Well attended from the start, the conferences are marked by lively discourses on the developments of shockwave therapy. While the initial focus of the conferences was on case reports and small serial presentations, the last years have been marked by the rise in scientific standard, exciting clinical trials and spectacular works in fundamental research. This has imbued the conferences with vital impetus and, in turn, greatly influenced research in ESWT clinically as well as using animal models. The talks and debates within the congresses and outside the conference halls have powerfully driven developments.

From the beginning, the ISMST has sought contact with the industrial sector in order to set itself up as an information clearinghouse and intermediary between research and business. In particular, the continual presence of a platform for manufacturers of devices provides the opportunity for discussion and collaborative development of new technology. The agreement to standardize technical specifications regarding shockwave strengths, frequencies and forms allows for the scientific comparability of studies of various sorts. As all clinical studies must employ unified rules of biometrics, works on shockwave therapy have likewise been standardized by the use of a uniform set of physical parameters.

The ISMST has been able to initiate excellent contact with all the national associations, some of which were organized within the ISMST, thereby facilitating the transfer of knowledge and scientific information as well as the presentation of local activities. The establishment of the ISMST in Vienna during the 1997 German Orthopaedic Congress is the apparent basis for the organization's closeness and intense collaboration with the German-speaking associations. One of the results of this is the cohosting of the 8th International Congress of the ISMST and 5th Joint Meeting of the German-Speaking Societies in Vienna. The collaborative effort with the DIGEST is especially to be highlighted, for example a DIGEST prize worth €3,000 was awarded to the best work done in the field. (Jan Dirk Rompe, Andrea Meurer, Bernhard Nafe, Alexander Hofmann, Ludger Gerdesmeyer: Repetitive low-energy shockwave application without local anesthesia is more efficient than repetitive low-energy shockwave application with local anaesthesia in the treatment of chronic plantar fasciitis).

The good rapport with our partner associations around the world is also affirmed by the activities of the ISMST members and executive members in national organizations. Several national conferences have benefited from the organization's assistance and scientific support (the SITOD Congress in Italy, workshops in Saudi-Arabia, the ONLAT Congress in Columbia, the SBTOC Congress and Training in Brazil, American Association of Equine Practitioners in the USA, Argentinean Orthopedic Congress, SFOCAL Congress in France, ASA in Canada). The ISMST has designed an educational training program to teach and keep physicians around the world regularly up-to-date on the new technology and treatments. (Though financed by the industrial sector, the content matter is completely independent.) These training programs have so far taken place in Naples, Dallas, Monterey, Louisville, Shanghai, New York and Lisbon.

As a result of the development of ESWT in fields like cardiology and dermatology, contact with other disciplines has grown to include not only those that are interested in the musculoskeletal system, but also healthcare professionals who use ESWT to treat circulatory ailments or to stimulate poorly healing wounds.

The exchange of information regarding the congress is also to be found online at www.ismst.com and the conference's website www.shockwavetherapy.org, along with certification and training guidelines and a regularly updated list of literature. The ISMST Newsletter, published since 2005 (available in paper version or to be downloaded from the website), offers the latest developments in ESWT and fundamental, scientific works and studies.

The association is working towards an established position in information management and knowledge transfer in cardiology and wound healing. We very much hope that every participant at the conferences as well as other events will find this platform, through the association's multidisciplinary approach to be especially stimulating and informative.

Member nations (as of December 12, 2005)

Algeria, Argentina, Australia, Austria, Belarus, Belgium, Brazil, Denmark, Cameroon, Canada, Chile, China, Columbia, Costa Rica, Czech Republic, Denmark, Egypt, France, Germany, Ghana, Greece, India, Israel, Iran, Italy, Japan,

Event:	Year	Place	President	Congress organizer
Founding meeting	1997	Vienna, Austria	Heinz Kuderna	Wolfgang Schaden
1st ESMST Congress	1998	Izmir, Turkey	Heinz Kuderna	
2nd ESMST Congress	1999	London, GB	Heinz Kuderna	Richard Coombs
3rd ISMST Congress	2000	Naples, Italy	Enzio Corrado	
4th ISMST Congress	2001	Berlin, Germany	Richard Thiele	Richard Thiele
5th ISMST Congress	2002	Winterthur, CH	John Ogden	Beat Dubs
6th ISMST Congress	2003	Orlando, USA	Beat Dubs	John Ogden
7th ISMST Congress	2004	Kaohsiung, ROC	Ching-Jen Wang	Ching-Jen Wang
8th ISMST Congress	2005	Vienna, Austria	Vinzenz Auersperg	Vinzenz Auersperg
9th ISMST Congress	2006	Rio d. J., Brazil	Ana Claudia Souza	Ana Claudia Souza
10th ISMST Congress	2007	Montreal, CN	Robert Gordon	Robert Gordon

Table 1. ISMST congresses and presidents.

Screen shot of the ISMST website homepage www.ismst.com

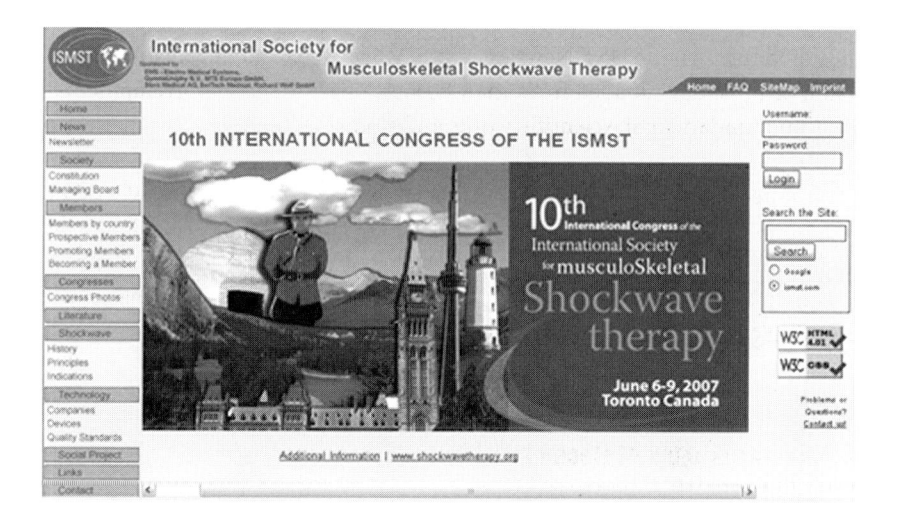

Jordan, South Korea, Luxembourg, Malaysia, Mexico, Nepal, Netherlands, New Zealand, Pakistan, Portugal, Puerto Rico, Republic of Macedonia, Republic of Slovakia, Saudi Arabia, Singapore, Slovakia, Slovenia, Spain, Switzerland, Taiwan, Thailand, Turkey, Ukraine, UAE, Venezuela, United Kingdom, USA, Venezuela

Conclusion

Shockwave treatment (ESWT) is a compelling non-surgical treatment for an expanding variety of musculoskeletal conditions. More than two decades after the first clinical shockwave treatment, many new indications have been discovered and a large number of excellent studies and basic research have been performed. The most famous shockwave researchers have written their chapters within this book on the newest technologies, treatment options and working mechanisms. Physicians as well as specialized researchers will find answers and solutions in terms of basic knowledge, biochemical pathways, standard and future indications, treatment parameters and clinical outcomes.

Index

Page numbers followed by *f* denote figures; those followed by *t* denote tables.

A

Absorption, effect of bone thickness on, 105-106*f*
Application frequency of ESWT, 2, 272
Acoustic
  - Bending, 23
  - Conductivity, 22
  - Impedance, 22-23
  - Velocity, 21
Autologous growth factors (AGF), 334-342
Analgesic
  - Effects of ESWT, 140, 218
  - Use to relieve pain of ESWT treatment, 240
Anesthesia, use of local, 25, 86, 119, 173, 196, 206, 229, 250, 269, 278*t*-279, 285, 337
Angiogenesis, 115-117
  - Angiogenic growth indicators, 37-52
Antibacterial effects, 92-95, 94*t*, 325
Antibiotic prophylaxis, 92, 95
ATRAD, 355-358
Auersperg score, 277

B

Ballistic shockwave generation, 15*f*
Biofeedback, use with ESWT, 119, 121, 249
Biological dose threshold, 25
Blue Cross Blue Shield
  - Medical Technology Assessment, 6
  - CPT/HCPCS codes, 6-7
Bone delayed unions, 331-342
  - Results from ESWT/AGF treatment, 339-342
  - Treatment options, 332
    - Treatment with ESWT, 333-342
    - AGF, 334-342
    - Combination ESWT/AGF protocol, 337-339
Bone morphological protein (BMP-2), 37, 42-43, 45-46*f*, 47, 50*t*, 52*f*, 334

C

C-fibers
  - Muscle, 71
  - Polymodal nociceptor, 71
Capsaicin, 32-33
Cavitation, 14, 24-25, 94, 112, 116, 242
Chaussy, 11, 129, 139
Chivers, 18
Cholecystokinin, 75-76
Constant-Murley Score (CMS), 230-238
Contraindications, 87*t*, 270*t*
  - reconsidering bone infection as contraindication, 91
Coupling mediums, use with ESWT, 14-16, 119, 121-127, 229

INDEX-365

D

Defocusing, 21
Dorsal horn, as sensory integration system 73

E

Endocannabinoids, 75-76
Endothelial nitric oxide synthase (eNOS), 37, 39, 40-43 (40-41*f*), 45-46*f*, 47-48, 50*t*, 51-52*f*, 66
Energy
 - Conversion of acoustic, 24, 94
 - Comparisons of low, medium, high levels, 5, 25, 43*f*, 44*f*, 64, 189-190, 200, 218-223, 226-243
 - Energy flux density, 242
Electrical sensors for measurement, 18-19
Electromagnetic currents, 15-16, 16*f*, 17*f*
Epicondylitis humeri radialis/lateral epicondylitis/tennis elbow, 2, 3, 4, 11, 38, 83, 86, 120*t*, 121, 131*t*, 141, 156-157, 205-215, 259-265, 267-273
 - Causes, 259
 - Diagnosis, 260
 - Prevalence, 205
 - Results of ESWT treatment, 206-215, 261-265
 - Symptoms, 205, 259
 - Treatment methods with ESWT, 206, 260-261
Equipment, orthopedics
 - Comparisons, 150
 - Dornier Epos Fluoro, 228, 255
 - Dornier Epos Ultra Lithotripter, 256
 - EMS, 119, 129-130
   - Dolormeter, 168*f*, 255, 262
 - Swiss DolorClast®, 119-137, 150*f*, 153-158, 166, 181-183, 194-195, 205, 219, 249, 268, 350, 355-357
   - Accessories, 134
   - Applicator, 181, 269
   - Components, 132-133
   - Control unit, 135
   - Energy range, 130
 - General recommendations, 119
 - Handling, 135-137
   - Handpiece, 131*f*
   - Indications for use, 131*t*
   - Mechanism of action, 130-131*f*
   - Propagation, 132*f*
 - Swiss LithoClast®, 129-130
 - Evolution of, 85-86
 - History, 85-86
 - OrthoWave, 326
 - Osetostar, 214
 - Ossatron, 214, 254, 265, 292, 305, 322
 - MFL 5000, 215
 - MPL 9000, 215
 - Requests to industrial partners, 129
 - Siemens Lithostar Overhead Module, 214
 - Sonocur®, 219
Extracorporeal shockwave therapy,
 - Application on nerves, 28
 - Cost efficacy, 243, 358
 - Duration of effects, 241
 - Effects on biological tissues, 11, 27-28, 37-52, 52*f*, 190
 - Effects on bone, 55-67, 99-108, 148, 331-342
 - For treatment of: (*also see separate detailed listings for some conditions*)
 - Achillodynia, 120*t*, 126, 161-174
 - Arterial vessel disease, 125
 - Arthrosis

INDEX

- AC joint, 123
- Ankle joint, 125
- Coxarthrosis, 127
- Elbow, 121
- Femoropatellar cartilage, 124
- Glenohumeral joint, 123
    - Aseptic bone necrosis, 5
    - Brain tumors, 1
    - Biological tissues, 1
    - Bone degeneration diseases, 66
    - Bone fractures, 11, 38, 64, 125-127, 289-299
    - Bursitis
        - Pes anserinus, 124
        - Prepatellar, 124
- Subacromial, 123
- Subachilleal, 126
    - Calcalneal stress fracture, 122
    - Calcaneo navicular, 122
    - Calcific tendinitis, 15, 83-84, 141, 144-146, 154-155, 177-190
        - Of the shoulder, 225-243
    - Calcified shoulder, 11, 38, 84, 217-223
    - Chronic venous insufficiency, 125
    - Chronic wound healing, 5, 64
    - Compartment syndrome, 125
    - Dupuytren's contracture, 131t
    - Enthesiopthies, 147
        - Chronic Achilles tendinitis, 5, 38, 131t
- Epicondylitis humeri radialis/lateral epicondylitis/tennis elbow, 2, 3, 4, 11, 38, 83, 86, 120t, 121, 131t, 141, 156-157, 205-215, 259-265, 267-273
        - Iliotibial band, 120t, 127, 131t
- Patella tendon syndrome, 5, 267-273
- Plantar fasciitis/heel spur, 3, 4, 11, 38, 83-85, 120t, 122, 126, 31t, 141, 146-147, 155-156, 193-201, 247-256, 275-279, 321-324
- Rotator cuff, 120t, 123, 131t
- Epihyseolysis capitis femoris, 127
    - Femoral head necrosis, 99-108, 311-318
    - Gallbladder stones, 2, 11
    - Hernias
        - Femoralis, 127
        - Inguinalis, 127
- Muscle, 125
    - Hip dysplasia, 127
    - Ischemic cardiomyopathy, 111-117
- Kidney stones/nephrolithiasis, 1, 11, 23, 83, 139-140
- Morton's interdigital neuroma, 281-286
- Myofascial trigger point syndrome (MTS), 347-353
- Os trigonum, 126
- Osgood-Schlatter, 124
- Osteochondrosis, 121
- Osteochondritis dessicans, 125-126, 303-308
- Osteomyelitis, 125
- Pain therapy, 2, 16, 69-81
    - Pancreatic duct stones, 2, 11
    - Patella tendiopathy/patella tip syndrome, 120t, 124, 131t, 161-174, 267-273
    - Plica syndrome, 124
    - Pronator teres syndrome, 121
    - Pseudoarthrosis, 2, 11, 15, 66, 83-84, 85, 141, 143-144
    - Meniscal tears, 124
    - Morbus Paner/vascular bone necrosis, 121
    - Morbus Sinding-Larsson, 124
    - Musculoskeletal system, 2, 140

- Myocardial dysfunction, 325
- Myogeloses, 131*t*
- Radiculopathy, 125-126
- Rheumatoid arthritis, 126
- Salivary duct stones, 2, 11
- Skin lesions, 325-328
- Soft tissue disorders, 66
- Supinator slit syndrome, 121
- Tarsal tunnel syndrome, 122, 125
- Tendinitis calcarea of the shoulder, 2
- Tibial edge syndrome/tibialis anterior syndrome, 120*t*, 125, 161-174
- In sports medicine 87-88, 161-174, 267-273
- Mechanism of action, 5, 140, 267, 270
- Microorganism growth, effect on, 91-93
- Molecular effects 27-33

F

Federal Office of Public Health and Insurance, 141
Femoral head necrosis, 99-108, 311-318
- Causes, 311-312
- Diagnosis, 312
- Ficat and Arlet classification system, 316*t*
- Prevalence in U.S., 311
- Rationale for treatment with ESWT, 313-314
- Results of ESWT treatment, 317-318
- Treatment of, 312-313
Focused hand piece, use of, 154-158
Free radicals, 25, 313

G

GABA, 75
Galanin, 75-76
German Orthopedic and Traumatology Society, 3
Glycin, 75-76

H

Hip replacement, 99-100
Hydrophones, 18*f*, 101-102*f*, 106-107, 229-230
Hyperstimulation analgesia, 27-28

I

Impulse width, 13
Inflammatory process, 71
Infections, 91-93
Insurance
- Coverage of ESWT, 3, 6, 141
- Federal Physician and Insurance Commission, 3
International Society for Musculoskeletal Shockwave Therapy (ISMST), 359-364
- Member nations, 362-363
International standards of ESWT, 12
Ischemic cardiomyopathy, treatment of, 111-117

J

Jet streams, 24-25, 94

K

Karpmann, 2

L

Lamina/laminae, 73
Lewin, 18
Lorentz effect, 16

M

Measuring techniques, 18-19, 106-107
Mechanical generation of shockwaves, 15
Melzack's concept of hyperstimulation analgesia, 27-28
Microorganism growth, effect on, 91-95
Morton's digital neuroma, 281-286
- Clinical presentation, 281-282
- Definition, 281
- Diagnosis, 282-284
- First identified, 281
- Etiology, 281
- Treatment, 284-285
    - ESWT as treatment, 285-286

N

Negative peak pressure, 13
Neovascularization, 37-51, 52f, 248
Neuromodulators, 73
Neurotransmitters, 73, 75
Nociceptors
- A-delta, 71-73
- C-fibers, 71-72, 76
- C-multimodal, 71

O

Ohm's laws, 22
Orthopedics, 201
- Number of applications of ESWT, 2
- Number of orthopedic treatments per year, 140
- Clinical objectives, 12
- Equipment features, 140
Osteochondrosis Dissecans, Adult, 303-308
- Causes, 303
- Description, 303
- Rationale for treatment with ESWT, 304
- Results of treatment, 307-308
- Side effects from ESWT treatment, 306
- Stages, 303
- Symptoms, 303-304
Osteogenesis, 55, 60, 61-63f, 64-67, 84, 140

P

Pain, 69-81
- Acute vs. chronic, 79-81
- Mechanisms, 70f, 70-71
- Modulation, 74-77
    - descending control systems, 77
- Neuropathic, 69-70
- Nociceptive, 69-70
- Perception, 77-79
- Receptor systems, 72, 79f
- Somatic, 69
- Transmission, 72-74
- Visceral, 69
Peptides, opioid, 75
Periaqueductal gray (PAG)/rostral ventromedial medulla (RVM) system, 77
Physical parameters of ESWT, 12
Piezoelectric principle, 16-17, 17f, 189-190
Piezocrystals, 101
Plantar Fasciitis, 3, 4, 11, 38, 83-85, 120t, 122, 126, 31t, 141, 146-147, 155-156, 193-201, 247-256, 275-279
- Bilateral, 321-324
- Definition, 275
- Diagnosis, 275
- Treatment, 275
    - with ESWT, 276-279
Positive peak pressure, 13, 23

Pressure amplitude, 104-105f
Proliferating cell nuclear antigen (PCNA), 37, 39, 40-43 (40-41f), 45-46f, 47-48, 50t, 51-52f, 66
Properties of ESWT, 12, 13f
Prostaglandins 28, 71
  -Prostaglandin E2, 27, 29-33
  Protocols
  - Calcific tendonitis, 144-146
  - Enthesiopathies, 147
  - Heel spur 146-147
  - Murnau, 142, 148
  - Pseudoarthrosis, 143

R

Radial extracorporeal shockwave therapy (rESWT), 4, 55-57, 64, 86, 88, 130, 167-168f, 355-358
  - Comparison with focused ESW, 153, 201
  - Costs, comparison, 358
  - Devices, 150
  - First multicenter study, 357-358
  - For treatment of
  - Achillodynia, 161-174
  - Calcific tendinitis of the rotator cuff, 177-190
  - Epicondylitis humeri radialis, 259-265
  - Lateral epicondylitis, 205-215
  - Patella tip syndrome (jumper's knee), 161-174
  - Plantar Fasciitis, 193-201, 247-256
  - Tendinopathies, 267-273
  - Tibialis anterior syndrome, 161-174
  - Side effects, 201
  - Use in veterinary environment, 267
Radial shockwave, 15, 64

Regional myocardial blood flow (RMBF), effects on, 111,115
Research on ESWT
  - Biological response in bone 37-43
  - Femoral head necrosis, 99-108
  - First studies, 1
  - Molecular effects 27-33
  - Shockwave Work Group studies, 3-4
  - Tendon-bone interface, 43-51
  - Effects on bone, 55-67, 99-108
  - Effects on heart, 111-117
  - Effects on soft tissue pain, 214
Riber, Frank, 1
Rise time, 13
Roles and Maudsley Score, 250-252, 256-265, 277, 322

S

Shear stress, 112, 117
Shockwaves
  - Definition of, 12
  - Frequency effects, 24-25
  - Frequency spectrum, 14, 119
  - Generation techniques, 14-17
  - Time span, 14
  - Treatment parameters, 119, 120t
Shockwave Therapy Consensus Group, 12
Shockwave Work Group, 3
Side effects, 12, 28, 65, 86t, 86-87, 119, 197t, 201, 208t, 222, 240, 242, 263, 299, 325
Skin lesions, 325-328
  - Number of impulses used in ESTW, 326
  - Results of ESTW treatment, 327
Steepening, 21
Substance P, 27-33, 30f, 71, 140, 190

T

Tendinopathies, 267-

- Indications and contraindications, 270-271
- Mechanism of action, 267
- Results with ESWT, 271-273
- Treatment protocol with ESWT, 268-269

Therapy patterns, 2

Traumatology, 289-299
- Biological effects of ESWT treatment, 291
- ESWT mechanism of action in treating, 290-291
- Number of impulses used, 290, 299t
- Results of ESWT treatment, 293-297
- Side effects from ESWT treatment, 299

U

U.S. Federal Drug Administration (FDA)
- Approval of ESWT for plantar fasciitis, 4
- Approved equipment, 6
- Approval process for non-union treatments, 298

V

Valchanov, 2, 11, 84, 139

Vascular endothelial growth factor (VEGF), 113, 115

Vessel endothelial growth factor (VEGF), 37, 39, 40-43 (40-41f), 45-46f, 47-48, 50t, 51-52f, 66

Visual analog scale (VAS), 209-211f, 250-252, 254-256, 259-265, 276-277, 286, 321-322, 349-352t

Von Willebrand factor, 42, 47

W

Wall thickening fraction (WTF), effects on, 114f

Water bath, 21-22, 101